Flower Essence Repertory

by Patricia Kaminski & Richard Katz

1994 Edition

A Comprehensive Guide to North American
and English Flower Essences for Emotional
and Spiritual Well-Being

published by

The Flower Essence Society

a division of the non-profit educational and research organization

Earth-Spirit, Inc.

P.O. Box 459, Nevada City, CA 95959 USA

Telephone: 800-548-0075 916-265-9163 Fax: 916-265-6467

Translated editions of the *Flower Essence Repertory* are available in a number of languages. Please contact the publisher for further details.

Earlier editions printed in 1986, 1987, and 1992.
This revised and expanded edition first printed in 1994.

ISBN 0-9631306-1-7

Front cover photograph of California Poppy and back cover photographs
   of Indian Paintbrush and spring foothills flowers: Wayne Green
Other photographs: Richard Katz
Line art: Catalina O'Brien
Technical editor: Jan Evers

 Printed on recycled paper.

Printed in USA.

Acknowledgments

To Dr. Edward Bach for his original indications regarding the 39 English remedies which are included in this Repertory; and for the further insights of many practitioners, especially the written insights of Julian and Martine Barnard (*The Healing Herbs of Edward Bach*), Mechthild Scheffer (*Bach Flower Therapy*), and Phillip M. Chancellor (*Handbook of the Bach Flower Remedies*).

To Matthew Wood, a long-time colleague and member of the Flower Essence Society for his insights into the properties of seven major flower remedies contained in this Repertory (*Seven Herbs, Plants as Teachers*).

To the countless practitioners throughout the world whose names would be too numerous to list here, but who have generously supported the research efforts of the Flower Essence Society. Through their many case reports, letters, conversations, phone interviews, and anecdotal comments, we are continuously able to deepen and refine our understanding of the flowers and their therapeutic benefits.

Finally, our gratitude is given to the flowers themselves, for they are the precious soul expressions of She who is called *Natura* or *Gaia*. We acknowledge the many hierarchies of Creation who guard and guide the goodness of the Earth, and especially the *Christos*, that Sun-Spirit who has united His inmost essence with the being the Earth. May the human heart and mind ever seek to be aware of the soul-spiritual identity of Natura, and may Her healing essence always renew and inspire us.

Saint John's Wort

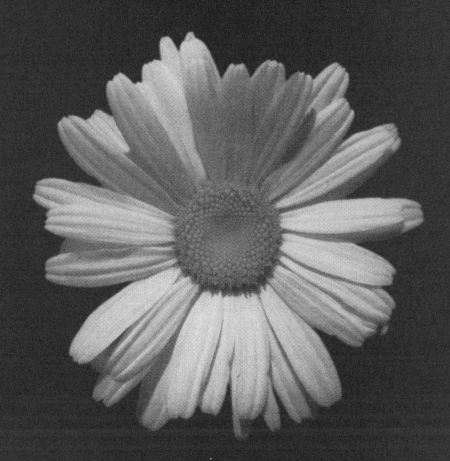

Shasta Daisy *Chrysanthemum maximum*

. . . When you no longer know how to go further, let the plants tell you, the plants that you let spring up, grow, blossom, and fruit within you. Learn the language of the flowers.

All earth-dwellers are able to understand the language of the flowers, for their teacher is the Sun-Spirit who speaks to every human heart. The plants point the way from grave to resurrection through whatever clefts and abysses, over whatever pastures and to whatever heights the path may lead: elderberry, wild rose, chrysanthemum, aster — they are the stairsteps of transformation, of purification, and of healings from the wrongs and woes of the world.

Albert Steffen, *Journeys Here and Yonder*

Table of Contents

Part I
Overview of Flower Essence Theory and Practice

Chapter 1: What is Flower Essence Therapy?

Chapter 2: Can We Verify the Properties of Flower Essences?

Chapter 3: How Are Flower Essences Selected?

Chapter 4: How Are Flower Essences Used?

Part II
Soul Issues: Categories and Themes

Part III
Flower Essence Qualities and Portraits

Foreword

The *Flower Essence Repertory* is a selection guide for professional and home use of flower essences. It is written with the understanding that a full appreciation of this health modality requires thoughtful study as well as openness of heart; and with the recognition that what is written here is only one step in an on-going process of research and discovery of this many-faceted subject.

This *Repertory* is published by the Flower Essence Society (FES), a world-wide organization of professional health practitioners and interested laypersons who are devoted to the development of flower essence therapy. Although this work is written by Patricia Kaminski and Richard Katz, co-directors of FES, it reflects the research and insights of many flower essence practitioners throughout the world who have contributed their case studies and other clinical data over the past sixteen years.

The indications presented in the *Repertory* are not meant to take the place of professional, medical, or psychotherapeutic care when appropriate. Rather, use of the flower essences described here is intended to complement and enhance well-balanced health programs in clinical practice, as well as in home care.

The *Repertory* is composed of three major sections. **Part I** gives an overview of flower essence theory and practice. Each of the subjects discussed is worthy of further elaboration, and it is our intention to develop these themes in future publications. Our aim in this writing is to provide both beginners and experienced practitioners with a philosophical, cultural, and practical context for flower essence therapy. **Part II** contains comprehensive listings of essence indications arranged by categories. **Part III** consists of in-depth profiles of each essence, summary statements of their positive qualities and patterns of imbalance, and cross-references to the categories in Part II.

The *Flower Essence Repertory* is intended to be freely accessible to those who wish to work with it in a variety of ways. Although reference is made throughout the *Repertory* to various philosophical and metaphysical concepts, it is not a pre-condition that one believe in any particular cultural or spiritual teaching in order to benefit from flower essences. What is most important is that each person consider the merits of this therapeutic modality, and apply those beliefs or concepts which are living *within* his or her own heart and mind. Regardless of one's philosophical outlook, the *Repertory* can always be used in a very basic and direct way, by simply becoming sensitive to the feeling life of the human soul, and learning the qualities of the flowers which reflect the soul's condition. We sincerely hope that the *Repertory* will be a tool for true soul healing, and for your own further exploration and discovery.

In spite of our assiduous efforts over the past sixteen years to expand and deepen our research, we are acutely aware of its pioneering nature. We welcome the active participation of our readers in developing knowledge of flower essence therapy through contributions to the Flower Essence Society research program. We also welcome your comments on how the *Repertory* can be improved in future editions. *(Please fill out and return the reporting form located inside the back cover.)* Most of all, we pray that the flowers may always be a source of inspiration and healing. If this *Repertory* helps in even some small way toward that goal, our efforts will not have been in vain.

Patricia Kaminski and Richard Katz
Nevada City, California
May, 1994

Part I

Overview of Flower Essence Theory and Practice

Introduction:
What are Flower Essences?

Flower essences are subtle liquid extracts, generally taken in oral form, which are used to address profound issues of emotional well-being, soul development, and mind-body health. While the use of flowers for healing has many ancient antecedents, the precise application of flower essences for specific emotions and attitudes was first developed by an English physician, Dr. Edward Bach, in the 1930's. Today, flower essences are gaining world-wide professional recognition for their significant contribution to holistic health and wellness programs.

Flower essences are generally prepared from a sun infusion of either wildflowers or pristine garden blossoms in a bowl of water, which is further diluted and potentized, and preserved with brandy. Quality preparation requires careful attention to the purity of the environment, the vibrancy and potency of the blossoms, celestial and meteorological conditions, and sensitive study of the physical and energetic properties of the plant through its cycles of growth.

Although flower essences resemble other health remedies which come in dropper bottles, they do not work because of the chemical composition of the liquid, but because of the *life forces* derived from the plant and contained within the water-based matrix. Like homeopathic remedies, flower essences are *vibrational* in nature. They are highly dilute from a physical point of view, but have subtle power as *potentized substances*, embodying the specific energetic patterns of each flower. Their impact does not derive from any direct bio-chemical interaction within the physiology of the body. Rather, flower essences work through the various human energy fields, which in turn influence mental, emotional, and physical well-being.

The action of flower essences can be compared to the effects we experience from hearing a particularly moving piece of music, or seeing an inspirational work of art. The light or sound waves which reach our senses may evoke profound feelings in our soul, which indirectly affect our breathing, pulse rate, and other physical states. These patterns do not impact us by direct physical or chemical intervention in our bodies. Rather, it is the contour and arrangement of the light or sound which awakens an experience within our own soul similar to that which arose within the soul of the creator of the musical or art form. This is the phenomenon of *resonance,* as when a guitar string sounds when a matching note is sung. In a similar way, the specific structure and shape of the life forces conveyed by each flower essence resonate with, and awaken, particular qualities within the human soul.

Another model which may be useful in understanding the vibrational resonance of flower essences comes from *holography*. A holographic photograph consists of light-wave interference patterns, any portion of which contains information from the whole and can be used to re-create the original three-dimensional image. Thus, we can describe the water containing the blossoms as receiving a kind of holographic imprint of the essential qualities of the plant. Each drop of water contains the whole configuration of the plant's archetype. As we dilute the flower essence, we attenuate the physical substance of the infusion so that it is no longer biochemically significant. However, the full etheric "message" of the plant essence remains in the few highly dilute drops we take into our bodies.

Working with flower essences requires a stretch in our thinking beyond the materialistic assumption that "more is better." Flower essences, like other vibrational remedies, illustrate the principle that "small is beautiful." They are part of an emerging field of non-invasive, life-enhancing subtle therapies, which promise to make a major contribution to health care in coming years.

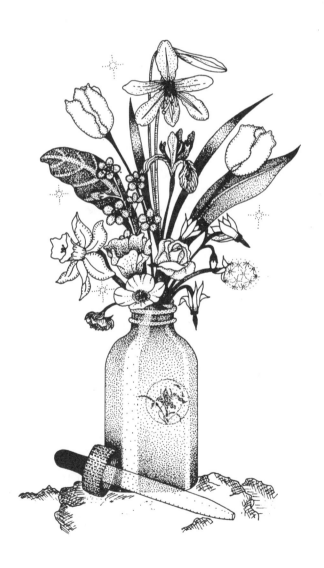

Chapter 1: What is Flower Essence Therapy?

Flower essence therapy involves the application of flower essences in the context of an overall program of health enhancement, either in professional practice or home care. Although the word "therapy" is typically used to mean the treatment and cure of disease, the Greek root *therapeia* had a wider, soul-spiritual meaning of "service," related to the word *therapeuein*, meaning "to take care of." It is in this sense of service and care that we speak of flower essence therapy; it is a way to nurture and sustain health with the beneficent forces of Nature, in the context of wise and loving human attention.

To understand the therapeutic uses of flower essences, it is important to ask some basic questions about the nature of health and illness. What is the goal of health care? What causes illness? What is the relationship between mind and body? What are our assumptions about human nature? Our answers to these general questions will determine whether we have the understanding and insight to use flower essences in their full capacity as catalysts for mind-body wellness.

The Nature of Health

The freedom to experience life

Health is the ability to fully participate in the rhythms of life, feeling the glory of the dawning day, celebrating the yearly cycle of the seasons, and sensing Nature's pulse of life quickening within us. True health is more than just "getting by." It means plunging into life, fully engaging body and soul in all that we do — in work, family and social life, creative expression, and inner contemplation.

There is no one fixed model of what it means to be a healthy person. To be healthy is to be completely ourselves — not the identity defined by social conditioning, nor the persona adopted to meet the expectations of others. Rather, it is the Self which uniquely expresses all that we can be. This will be different for each person, and thus presupposes the development of self-knowledge and understanding.

Health is the acceptance of life, with all its imperfections and contradictions. It is an expansiveness of being which grows strong by embracing all experiences, rather than trying to banish limitation, pain, or suffering. In fact, suffering has the potential to lead to a deeper appreciation of life, and an awakening to our own greater potential. Sickness can be viewed not as a scourge to be eradicated, but rather as a teacher, showing us sources of imbalance in our lives, or aspects of our being we have ignored. The challenges which we face can evoke inner virtues, and motivate us to make needed changes. At its deepest level, illness can be an *initiatory experience*, felt not merely as a loss, but also as an opportunity for a new beginning.

Health presumes an inner freedom. Responsibility is the process which leads to true freedom, the *ability to respond*. When we are simply passive recipients of illness or medical treatment, merely reacting or feeling acted upon, we become objects to be manipulated, rather than active participants in our health care. True health requires active self-awareness, in which each of us takes responsibility for life's challenges and lessons.

Medical Paradigms of Healing

Health is commonly defined in our culture as the absence of symptoms, or the elimination or control of disease. Because this definition lacks a positive image of wellness, our medical system is preoccupied with treating sickness, rather than creating health. Understanding the limits of this symptomatic approach to health is essential for anyone who uses flower essences. Without this awareness, it is easy to approach the flower essences merely as remedies to fix emotional symptoms, rather than as catalysts for awareness and transformation.

Mechanistic model of the human being

The symptomatic approach to health is based on a paradigm of medical practice which has a mechanistic view of the human being. Its philosophic roots lie deep in the seventeenth century world-view, exemplified by René Descartes, who postulated the duality of mind and body, and by Isaac Newton, whose theories led to a mechanical, clock-like model of the universe. As this scientific paradigm developed in the following centuries, the Industrial Revolution filled our world with increasingly elaborate machines, and the human body came to be viewed as the most remarkably complex machine of all. This mechanistic model regards healing as a matter of fixing broken machinery, similar to tuning-up an engine or replacing a defective part.

As computers have proliferated in recent decades, the mechanistic paradigm has been further extended as a cybernetic model of life. Human beings, and living beings in general, are now considered to be like super computers, made of biological genetic "chips." Through genetic engineering, modern medical technology is now attempting to redesign the very structure of living organisms.

While mechanical reductionism interprets life as being composed of physical "building blocks" such as cells, molecules, atoms, and sub-atomic particles — cybernetics reduces all intelligence to digital information, the succession of binary on/off bits which form the basis of the modern computer. The "artificial intelligence" of a computer is a powerful *instrument*, but is it the same thing as *life*? Consider a printed half-tone picture of a rose. The series of dots and white spaces on the printed page may resemble the image of a rose, but we know that a *living rose* is infinitely more complex and full of far deeper meaning and significance.

Contemporary medicine has admittedly developed an extraordinary knowledge of the workings of the various systems and structures of the physical body. This has led to a sophisticated technology to repair the body from the ravages of disease and injury through surgery, and to alter the physiological functions of the body through chemical medicine.

While this complex medical technology provides some remarkable benefits, it is also exorbitantly expensive. Moreover, there are also other, less tangible costs. Few doctors today visit their patients in their homes, or take sufficient time in their interviews to get a full picture of the patient's life, including home environment, family dynamics, and work experience. The rise of the specialist, who is an expert in one part of the human "machine," means that less attention is paid to the whole person than was the case in the day of the family doctor.

Furthermore, when we are treated simply as machines to be manipulated or computers to be programmed, our tremendous innate healing capacities are ignored, making us increasingly dependent on costly medical intervention. The contemporary health care crisis is more than a financial or political problem; it is a cultural symptom of our disconnection from the deep sources from which true health springs.

The germ theory

The underlying assumption of conventional medicine is that healing results from *fighting illness*, rather than from *fostering health*. In fact, it is striking how much of its language is borrowed from images of warfare. We try to "conquer disease" and "fight infection" with "magic bullets," and wage a "war on cancer."

The portrayal of medicine as a military campaign derives its impetus from the germ theory of disease, culminating in the nineteenth century with the work of Louis Pasteur, the founder of microbiology. He established not only the scientific but also the philosophical basis for modern disease-fighting techniques such as immunization and antibiotics. From the point of view of the germ theory, disease is caused by invading outside agents, such as bacteria or viruses, against which we must combat. Modern medicine has amassed a powerful arsenal of weapons which has won many battles against infectious diseases that once ravaged humankind.

The mechanistic/cybernetic models of the human being and the germ theory of disease contain some truths, and have lead to improvements in human health. However, the inability of contemporary medicine to significantly reduce many chronic diseases such as cancer, arthritis, or cardiovascular illness points to a need for a larger view of health and healing.

Resistance to disease

It was a contemporary of Pasteur, another French medical scientist named Claude Bernard, who was took issue with the idea that invading microorganisms are the reason for disease. Bernard stressed the importance of one's "inner environment" and the degree to which it was receptive to disease, rather than the "germ," which was merely the mechanism by which disease occurred. He spoke of the "soil" out of which human well-being could grow. He knew, as would any gardener, that without healthy soil we cannot grow robust, disease-resistant plants, no matter how much we battle against the invading pests.

Bernard's insights heralded the concept of *resistance* to disease, which recognizes that pathogenic microorganisms are widespread among the general population, but only certain people at particular times actually succumb to the diseases these germs "cause." Such an understanding is the basis of truly preventative health care, one which emphasizes diet, exercise, stress management, emotional well-being, and environmental factors as important components of a vibrant, disease-resistant way of life. Although such health-promoting lifestyle factors were articulated as long ago as the fifth century, B.C., by the Greek physician Hippocrates, they are again receiving increasing recognition as ways in which the individual can take responsibility and make an impact on his or her state of health.

It is true that not all illness is preventable, and many disease-causing factors may well be beyond individual control. Yet, we can influence how we *respond* to the challenges that life presents us. The modern understanding of the *immune system*, its role in disease prevention and recovery, and its close connection with our emotions and daily habits, teaches us that the way in which we live — our physical, emotional, and mental habits — has a profound influence on our ability to resist disease, and to create greater health and well-being.

It is in this context of overall health enhancement that we can understand the remarkable contribution of flower essences. They are not *substitutes* for the wonder drugs or high-tech miracles of modern medicine. Rather, their purpose is to establish the ground out of which good health grows, to enrich the deep soil of our lives, so that the life-affirming habits and attitudes which nourish our well-being can take root and flourish.

The Mind-Body Relationship

Psychosomatic medicine, stress and personality

Although mainstream medicine has been increasingly influenced in past century by the mechanistic and military models of healing, a strong counter-movement which recognizes the role of the mind and emotions has also made significant advances.

Homeopathic medicine, developed by the German physician Samuel Hahnemann over two hundred years ago, became a major force in medical practice in the nineteenth century. It emphasizes treating the person, rather than the disease, and homeopathic practitioners consider mental and emotional factors along with physical symptoms. Even though it is largely dismissed by conventional medicine as "unscientific," aspects of homeopathic philosophy have penetrated mainstream medicine. For example, in the late nineteenth century the famous Canadian doctor Sir William Osler described the importance of his patients' emotions and attitudes in illness and recovery. Osler has been quoted as saying, "It is better to know the patient that has the disease than the disease the patient has."

The rise of psychiatry and the clinical use of hypnotism brought a recognition of the extraordinary influence of unconscious mental processes on the functioning of the body. This understanding was reinforced by the experience of World War I, in which many soldiers returned from the front lines suffering from "shell shock" due to the extreme stress of combat. It was at this same time that Dr. Edward Bach developed his insights into the role of emotions and attitudes in disease, leading to his flower essence system in the 1930's.

The decade of the thirties unleashed the tremendous societal traumas of the Great Depression and the beginnings of World War II. With such challenges facing the human psyche, it is not surprising that this decade also brought further investigation of mind-body relationships. The concept of "psychosomatic medicine" was developed by the psychiatrist Dr. Franz Alexander and others at this time. A number of diseases — such as warts and other skin ailments, asthma, stomach ulcers, and colitis — were recognized as having emotional rather than physical causes, although their effects were definitely quite physical. It was also in the thirties that Dr. Hans Seyle began his pioneering work on *stress*, a concept which has now made its way into popular culture. Seyle showed that the "fight-or-flight" reactions of the sympathetic nervous system, which are appropriate to situations of immediate physical danger and emergency, can become debilitating when repeatedly triggered by habitual emotional attitudes or chronic stress reactions.

In the post-World War II era, mind-body research began to identify specific personality traits which correlate with a susceptibility to certain diseases. (Such an understanding has ancient roots; already in the second century the noted Greek physician Galen suggested the melancholic person was more susceptible to cancer.) One of the most famous modern studies to associate personality and disease was conducted in the 1950's by Drs. Meyer Friedman and Raymond Rosenman. They coined the term *Type A behavior* for the impatient, hostile attitude that seemed connected with a greater risk of heart disease, compared to the more easy-going *Type B*.

Dr. Dean Ornish, who is receiving increasing recognition for his program of reversing heart disease through diet, life-style, and psychological change, has conducted some of the most significant contemporary research on heart conditions. He has found that behind the compulsive drive of many heart-disease patients is the effort to create a false self which can win approval and love from others, to fill the "empty void" felt deep within the heart. For such people Ornish prescribes "emotional open heart surgery" to help let down defenses. His research shows that enriching one's feeling life, along with related lifestyle changes, contributes to a far better rate of long-term cure than conventional heart surgery.

Recent research by psychologist Lydia Temoshok suggests what she calls a *Type C personality*, characterized by unexpressed anger, hopelessness, and depression, which seems to correlate with greater susceptibility to cancer. In a landmark ten-year controlled study, Stanford University psychiatrist Dr. David Spiegel found that women with breast cancer who received group psychotherapy lived twice as long as women with the same condition and physical treatment, but who received no psychotherapy.

Additional research at Stanford with arthritis patients in a self-help program showed the importance of developing a sense of self-responsibility and mastery, described by psychologist Albert Bandura as "self-efficacy." Patients in the program who overcame feelings of helplessness and overwhelm experienced reduced pain and increased mobility.

While much study still remains to be done in order to establish the precise relationship between personality traits and specific diseases, current research clearly demonstrates that emotions and attitudes are major contributing factors to our ability to resist disease and create health.

Placebo effect

Ironically, some of the most convincing arguments for the role of attitudes and beliefs in human health comes from data that is often discarded in research. When controlled studies are done, the control group receives a *placebo*, something which looks like a medication or treatment, but which is physically inert. The idea is that the treatment or medication is effective if the subjects who receive the "real" treatment have significantly better results than those with the placebo.

Nonetheless, many of the people who receive placebos do recover, often at much greater rates than would be expected from those not receiving any treatment at all. This "placebo effect" has become well recognized in research, and is explained as the effect of the belief of the patient, reinforced by the caring attention of the medical practitioner or researcher, that some helpful treatment is being received.

Researchers are generally paid to measure the physical effect of the remedy or procedure on the patients who receive the "real thing." Yet it seems equally significant to study the responses of the placebo group, who *receive no medical treatment at all, but often experience demonstrable changes based simply on the belief that they are receiving treatment.*

The placebo effect is convincing evidence that attitudes and beliefs impact the human body in ways which are as observable and real as active physical agents. Rather than discarding this part of the experimental method, we should examine it more closely. This demonstration of mind-body influence challenges us to develop therapies which *directly* address attitudes and beliefs. Flower essence therapy is one such modality.

Psychoneuroimmunology

In the 1980's medical science began taking the mind-body connection seriously, as research began to map some of the bio-chemical mechanisms involved. With the publication of Robert Ader's book *Psychoneuroimmunology* in 1981, this term entered the medical and popular vocabulary. Psychoneuroimmunology (PNI) refers to the mind's ability, acting through the nervous system, to alter the physiology of the human immune system, which is responsible for resistance to disease. Studies have shown direct connections of the nervous system with the thymus gland, which produces the T-Cells which are basic to immune function. Numerous "biochemical messengers" have been studied, including hormones which transmit emotional responses to and from glands in the body, and various neuro-peptides such as the endorphins which have pain killing and euphoric effects.

It is extremely important that we accurately comprehend the meaning of PNI and other mind-body research. *It does not explain the mind as a purely physiological phenomenon, nor does it prove that the mind can be controlled chemically.* Such an interpretation mistakes the *brain*, which is a part of the physical body, with the *mind* or *soul*, which are aspects of Self beyond the physical body. The mind acts *through* the brain and other parts of the body, and thus affects their functioning. As well, the mind's activity is impeded or enhanced by the condition of the brain and body. This is a reciprocal relationship, far more complex and dynamic than the simplistic assertion that the mind is *nothing but* biochemical mechanisms.

If PNI research is interpreted in a reductionistic way, it becomes just another elaboration of the human being as a complex machine or bio-computer. The true significance of PNI research is that we can measure the physical *effects* of our beliefs, attitudes, and feelings, which are otherwise not directly measurable. This is analogous to physicists who study invisible sub-atomic particles by looking at their trails in cloud chambers. The biochemical pathways charted by PNI research are evidence of higher soul qualities which have their origins in a realm beyond the physical body. Thus understood, this research supports a wider understanding of the human being, in which the physical body is directly affected by what we think and feel.

In summary, we can see that modern flower essence therapy is part of a larger quest within health care professions for a more holistic view of the human being, and especially the significance of feelings, attitudes, and beliefs upon our overall health and ability to resist to disease.

The Contribution of Dr. Edward Bach

It is in this historical context of mind-body medicine that we can appreciate the genius of Dr. Edward Bach, the founder of flower essence therapy, and understand why his work speaks so powerfully to our own time.

Dr. Bach was a pioneer in understanding the relationship of emotions to the health of the body and psyche. He understood that to create health, the emotional and spiritual aspects of our being must be addressed. Ill health results when we lack an awareness of our soul-spiritual identity, and when we are alienated from others or disconnected from our purpose in life. As Bach explained in his landmark treatise *Heal Thyself,* disease is a message to change, an opportunity to become aware of our shortcomings and to learn the lessons of life experience so that we may better fulfill our true destiny.

Bach received conventional medical training in London, and practiced for many years as a bacteriologist. His approach, however, was quite unconventional, in that he based his treatment more on the emotions and attitudes of his patients than on a purely physical diagnosis. He later changed his practice to homeopathic medicine, appreciating its whole-person approach to health, and the application of remedies which energized the body's own healing powers. In fact, a series of intestinal nosodes developed by Bach are still used by homeopaths today.

In 1930 Dr. Bach left his homeopathic practice in London to go into the countryside to develop a new system of natural remedies, made from wildflowers. Through his sensitive observation of Nature and of human suffering, he was able to correlate each plant remedy with specific human states of mind.

Before his death in 1936 at the age of 50, Bach developed a range of flower essences which demonstrated a remarkable insight into human nature. At a time when the world was preoccupied with physical suffering, political upheaval, economic devastation, and the rise of Nazism and Fascism, Bach perceived the inner darkness of the human soul. He recognized the significance of destructive emotions such as depression, hatred, and fear. Along with other pioneers of psychosomatic medicine, he realized the devastating toll which unbalanced emotions and attitudes have on the human body. Bach went further, however, in that he knew that true health is based on a connection of one's life and destiny with a larger purpose. Moreover, he understood that substances could be found within Nature herself, which are capable of bringing profound change to the human soul and body.

The Holistic View of the Human Being

Life energy and health

If we recognize the human being as more than a machine to be repaired when it is broken, or a complex bio-computer in need of re-programming; can we develop an expanded view of human nature, a more "holistic" perspective? The first step is to recognize the human being as a system of *energetic forces*, as well as physical structures and biochemical activity. The ancient Oriental concepts of *chi* and *prana*, or that of *vital force* in Western tradition, describe a *life energy* which animates physical matter within living beings. A deficiency or disturbance in these life energies can lead to stress in the physical body, thus lowering resistance to disease.

By looking only at the physical systems of the human being, conventional medicine ignores the influence of transphysical energy fields. It is somewhat like trying to understand the images on a television by analyzing its parts, but without recognizing the surrounding electromagnetic energy field which carries the broadcast signal. The physical structure is fundamental, but the reductionist presumption that there is *nothing but* this structure ignores the forces which animate physical forms.

The etheric body

The electromagnetic fields with which we are so familiar in our electronic age provide a useful analogy in order to comprehend the energy fields of living beings. However, it would be a mistake to try to explain *life* in terms of the *physical energies* of electricity and magnetism. Life energies, known as the *etheric formative forces,* have their own distinct qualities, characteristics, and even their own geometry. For example, physical forces radiate out to the periphery from a point of origin, while etheric forces concentrate in from the periphery to a vital center. George Adams and Olive Whicher, in their book *The Plant Between Sun and Earth*, describe how the study of *projective geometry* gives a mathematical basis for understanding the polarity of physical and etheric forces in living organisms such as plants.

These etheric life forces envelop the physical body, and can be said to constitute the *etheric body.* One striking demonstration of the existence of this body is the "phantom pain effect," when a person retains a painful sensation of an amputated limb. The physical limb is gone, but the etheric limb remains. This phenomena is also illustrated in the "phantom leaf effect, " by which a Kirlian photograph of a cut leaf apparently shows the image of the energy field of the complete, uncut leaf. Russian researchers called this auric field the "bio-plasma" of a living being, which we can consider another name for the etheric body. *(See page 62 for more information on Kirlian photography).*

The etheric body also engenders life-building habits and rhythmic patterns of behavior. A similar concept has been advanced by Rupert Sheldrake, the pioneering English biologist and author of *A New Science of Life*. Sheldrake's *theory of formative causation* describes *morphogenic* (form-producing) *fields*, which give shape and direction to living organisms, and are molded by patterns of past experience. These are the etheric formative forces, which are common to all living organisms and are responsible for the growth and unfolding of organic forms.

It is the etheric body which distinguishes the living from the non-living. Its presence makes the difference between a vital, flourishing organism, and a lifeless heap of matter. When the etheric body withdraws from the physical body, death and dissolution occur. When the etheric body is strong and vital, the physical organism is full of life.

Homeopathy and acupuncture as energy medicines

Two health modalities which are well-established in the world today — homeopathy and acupuncture — recognize and address the human etheric energy fields. What distinguishes homeopathic remedies from conventional medicaments is that they are so physically dilute that any biochemical influence is attenuated or eliminated, while their energetic forces are enhanced through a *potentization* process of rhythmic *succussion* which accompanies each stage of dilution. These remedies then impact the human energy fields through the *Law of Similars.* This principle holds that a substance which causes a particular complex of symptoms in large doses will stimulate the body to heal that same symptom complex in homeopathic dose. Thus, homeopathy acts as a catalyst to rally the vital forces of the human being to engage in the healing process.

Acupuncture is an ancient Oriental medical science in which tiny needles are inserted along the *meridians*, which are pathways of human vital energy. Used for everything from pain relief to curing chronic disease, acupuncture treatments affect physiological systems by adjusting and toning the human energy body.

Homeopathy is a widely practiced and highly respected profession in Europe, India, South America, and Australia. After a century of suppression, it is undergoing a revival in North America. Acupuncture, practiced for thousands of years in China and Japan, has become more and more widespread in the West in recent decades. Both of these health modalities can substantiate thousands of cases in which clients have experienced healing for which conventional medical science has no explanation. Giving infinitesimal doses of substances, or inserting needles in energy meridians, makes no sense if the human being is only a biochemical mechanism. The success of these etheric therapies is powerful evidence that the human being is more than a machine, and that human energy fields are real.

The system of human energy fields

Recognizing the existence of the etheric body as a field of life energy is the first step to gaining an understanding of human *subtle anatomy*, the structure and functioning of "higher bodies" or energy fields which extend beyond the physical dimension. While there are many systems of subtle anatomy, we refer in this *Repertory* to a fundamental four-fold division of the human being which derives from various traditions of metaphysical wisdom and healing, and is summarized succinctly in the writings of the modern spiritual scientist, Dr. Rudolf Steiner.

This four-fold classification refers to 1) the physical body — the biochemical and mechanical structure of the body; 2) the etheric body — the life sheath which immediately surrounds the physical body and which is intimately connected with the vital forces of Nature; 3) the astral body — the seat of the soul, and the repository of human desires, emotions, and feelings, especially correlated with the world of the stars and other cosmic influences; and 4) the Spiritual Self or ego — the true spiritual essence or identity of each human being. These four bodies can also be regarded as comprising two fundamental polarities within the human being: that of *life* (the physical/etheric) and that of *consciousness* (the soul/spiritual). Having already reviewed the physical and etheric bodies, we now proceed to the consciousness pole of the human being.

The astral body

Consciousness is born in the *astral body*, creating an inner space wherein the outer world can be experienced. If we compare the open planar quality of a plant leaf with the enfolding interior space of an animal or human organ, we have a picture of the difference between the etheric and astral bodies. The presence of the astral body in animals is evidenced in their characteristic movements and sounds, which are outward expressions of their inner experiences. In human beings, the astral body is the home of the *soul,* and our feelings, desires, and sensitivity to others and the environment. It contains our experience of both the world around us and our interior world. The astral body is very much a place of polarities, where we are torn between like and dislike, attraction and repulsion, extroversion and introversion. While it is the etheric body which imparts vitality, it is the astral body which gives color and depth to our lives.

Although the plant is primarily an expression of etheric forces in its growth and development, we see the influence of astral qualities in the appearance of the flower, with its unique colors, forms, and fragrances. The cup-like shape of many flowers suggests an interior space, although in a more partial way than human and animal organs. We can therefore understand why flower essences are specifically made from the flowering part of the plant. When the green plant shines forth in blossom, a very extraordinary and pure form of astrality briefly touches its etheric dimension. The remedies which are made at this moment of flowering are uniquely able to address the emotional experiences of the human astral body, harmonizing them with the etheric body.

One of the ancient teachings about the astral body is that it contains seven major energy centers, or "chakras." Much literature is available about the chakra system, its relationship to the emotions, and its correlation with the endocrine gland system of the physical and etheric bodies. Flower essences clearly have a great impact on the human chakras. However, we feel that an understanding of the chakra system and its relationship to flower essences should be based upon empirical evidence, as well as metaphysical philosophy. In this *Repertory*, only a few of the major chakra relationships are mentioned for those essences in which they are particularly significant. We intend to provide a fuller discussion of the relationship of flower essences to the chakras in future seminars and publications, as our research develops.

The Spiritual Self

The crowning aspect of the human being in the four-fold system is the *spiritual ego* or *Self*, also known as the *I Am* presence or the in-dwelling individual spark of divinity. It is this inner awareness of Self, this possibility of individuation, that leads to the freedom to shape one's destiny and to develop moral forces of *conscience*, as well as *consciousness*. This *I Am*, or self-reflective presence, distinguishes human beings from the other three kingdoms of Nature — the animals, plants, and minerals.

The Spiritual Self is that divine aspect of our being which works through the matrix of body and soul, seeking incarnation into matter in order to evolve. It represents an individual identity that cannot be fully defined by demographic or hereditary factors, but which manifests in our character and personal destiny. Just as the crystalline structure of each snowflake descending from the sky to the Earth is unique, so also is the diamond-bright divinity which belongs to each human soul a sublime expression of individual spirituality.

It is also the Spiritual Self which provides a central focus to integrate the diverse elements of our being. Egotism or selfishness occurs when we identify with limiting roles, self-images, emotions, or cravings, rather than with the fullness of the Spiritual Self. Sometimes these expressions of the "lower self" are hidden from the full view of our consciousness, but nevertheless exert powerful influences as the psychological "shadow" or "double." If we can shift our identity to the Spiritual Self, we develop a *witnessing* capacity, a calm center for self-awareness and honest examination of our thoughts and deeds.

We cannot overcome selfishness through *self-denial*. An unhealthy suppression of individuality does not bring a true realization of the spiritual ego. Without a strong sense of selfhood and purpose we are subject to the random influences of shifting circumstances or to the control and direction of others; we drift through life like a rudderless ship at sea. Genuine *selflessness* is born of freedom and strength, when service and surrender to a higher purpose are the conscious choice of a strong, radiant Self.

The physical expression of the Self is the immune system. Its function is to differentiate between that which serves the totality of our being, and those unhealthy processes which selfishly serve their own purposes at the expense of the whole. It is no coincidence that at a time when true spiritual identity is disturbed or distorted in myriad ways, our culture as a whole also experiences a rapid increase in illness related to immune function. The deeper message of these physical diseases is that we need to develop an integral relationship to the Spiritual Self.

A strong but balanced sense of Self is thus vital to the health of both body and soul. By awakening our awareness of the Self as the sacred, inmost part of our being, its sun-like radiance can light our path through life.

In summary, it is through understanding the multi-dimensional nature of the human being that we can realize the full potential of flower essence therapy for facilitating health and well-being. *It is a process which engages all four levels of our being*; the Spiritual Self, our inner experiences, our life forces, and also our physical nature. We are challenged to make a conscious choice to change, to take responsibility for our health and life destiny with the full force of our spiritual Self. We must address the emotions and attitudes which constitute the astral body, developing inner balance and clarity. Furthermore, we need to nourish the etheric body, awakening vital forces which in turn can energize and strengthen the physical body. Thus understood, flower essence therapy becomes truly *holistic*, relating to each dimension of life.

Flower Essence Therapy as Soul Healing

The human soul

While flower essences can touch every aspect of human experience, they do so through the vehicle of the human soul. Just what do we mean by soul? This is a question which has preoccupied thinkers for ages, so it is not likely we can offer a definitive description here. As the American philosopher Ralph Waldo Emerson said, "The philosophy of six thousand years has not searched the chambers and magazines of the soul." Nonetheless, we do hope in this brief overview to impart a sense of what soul life is, and how flower essences enrich the soul.

In the theological discussions of philosophers, as well as in many contemporary religious and metaphysical teachings, "soul" is the immortal aspect of the human being, destined for damnation or redemption, or incarnating from lifetime to lifetime. In the words of the English poet, William Wordsworth, "The soul that rises with us, our Life's Star / Had elsewhere its setting /And cometh from afar." From this perspective, the soul is a spiritual entity.

From the point of view of modern materialistic science, what we call soul is a completely physical entity, nothing but a by-product of chemical reactions in the brain. We can trace this concept all the way back to the seventeenth century French philosopher René Descartes, who located the soul in the pineal gland.

The classical view was that the soul is neither purely spirit nor body, but rather a living *quality* of the body. The Greek philosopher Aristotle defined soul as "the initial actuality of a natural body endowed with the capacity for life." The Roman

Plotinus declared, "It is the soul that lends all things movement," echoing what Cicero said several centuries earlier, "For everything that is stirred to movement by external forces is lifeless, but whatever possesses life is moved by an inner and inherent impulse. And this impulse is the very essence and power of the soul." The medieval nun, Hildegard of Bingen, described soul as "a breath of living spirit, that with excellent sensitivity, permeates the entire body to give it life."

From these descriptions we have a feeling of soul as that which moves, or *animates*, a living body. In fact, *anima* and *animus* are the Latin words for the female and male aspects of soul. As humans we share this animating quality of soul with our fellow creatures on the Earth, the *animals*, each species of which expresses a unique soul quality in its sounds and movements.

Soul is what moves us; it is passion, desire, the striving for what is beyond our reach. Soul is also the depths of experience. It is the descent into pain, vulnerability, mortality, surrender. Like the blossom of the plant, the human soul expresses the richness of experience; it gives color, texture, and feeling. It is a chalice to receive life, an interior space in which to experience the outer world. The soul lives through contact with the heartbeat of life. We experience such soul in "soul music," or in poetry which rouses the soul.

The soul is thus strongly connected to the astral body, the home of our emotions, our likes and dislikes, our experiences. Yet it is an oversimplification to say the soul *is* the astral body, for the soul also seeks a relationship with the physical world, with Nature, and with human society.

How can it be that the soul arises from the spiritual world, yet expresses itself through the physical body? What mystery is contained in this paradox? Just where do we find the soul? The German poet Novalis said, "The seat of the soul is there where the inner world and the outer world meet. Where they overlap, it is in *every* point of the overlap." The Greek word *psyche* means both "soul" and "butterfly." This image suggests that the soul is capable of transmutation, or *metamorphosis* from earth-bound caterpillar to enclosed chrysalis and finally to unfettered heavenly wings. Soul is thus an intermediary between inner and outer; between the body (incarnation in matter) and the spirit (limitless expansion of the Self); and between life and consciousness.

This dynamic, fluid nature of soul is essential. If we confuse soul and spirit, as did many of the theologians of the past, then the soul becomes a disembodied abstraction separated from the pulse of life. If we reduce soul to a physical mechanism, as does modern materialistic science, then we deny its transcendent and mysterious attributes, conjuring a macabre vision of a colorless world populated only by machine-like creatures.

There are many descriptions and perspectives on soul. As in the well-known Indian parable of the blind men and the elephant, each perception is a glimpse of a larger totality that is beyond our view. However, with each new viewpoint, we arrive closer to the truth. Now that "soul" has escaped the obscurity of theological dissertations and crossed the frontiers of ethnic idiom to take its place in the titles of best-selling books, we have the opportunity to join with the larger culture in an exploration of the meaning of soul. We can now speak of flower essences as a soul therapy with some expectation that we will be striking a chord of recognition.

Psychology, psychotherapy, and soul healing

Psychology, in its etymological roots, is the "knowledge of the soul" (*logos* of the *psyche*). This may be hard to recognize in a culture where some psychologists exploit rats to understand human behavior, or use sexual insecurity and other emotions to sell consumer products or manipulate public opinion. These practices illustrate an approach which treats the soul as a mere mechanism which can be predictably programmed. To the extent that people act mechanically and unthinkingly, such behaviorialist methods become self-fulfilling assumptions.

Some schools of psychology and psychiatry have increasingly turned to psychopharmacology, involving the use of tranquilizers, anti-depressants, or psychotropic drugs to address the soul's struggles. While it is true that chemical manipulation of the brain can dramatically alter behavior and experience, the soul is more than brain chemistry.

Despite various attempts to reduce psychology to mechanistic programming, psychotherapy ("soul care") is ultimately concerned with enhancing self-awareness and the quality of the life of the soul. In the early development of psychotherapy, it was Sigmund Freud's psychoanalysis which recognized that the psyche has hidden or unconscious dimensions, which nonetheless exert powerful influences on our thoughts, feelings, and actions. However, psychology and psychotherapy did not really come into their own until the societal traumas of the first half of the twentieth century — two World Wars, the Depression, the Holocaust — which gave a strong impetus to shine the light of understanding into the dark recesses of the human psyche. As the generation born after World War II has matured, psychotherapy has become an integral part of our cultural life.

The soul therapy of Carl Jung

The Swiss psychiatrist Dr. Carl Jung especially developed the soul dimension of psychotherapy. Jung was originally a disciple of Freud, but took issue with his narrow emphasis on sexuality as the cause of neurosis, and as the primary basis for the soul-spiritual aspirations of humanity. Jung recognized that within the depths of the individual's experience — contacted through dreams, meditation, deep therapy, and in the mythological images of traditional cultures — are certain transpersonal *archetypes*. These recurring themes are expressed with many variations according to individual circumstances. However, they emanate from a common source, which Jung named the *collective unconscious*, or what might also be called the *ground of being* or *universal mind*, first articulated by the Greek philosopher Plato. Jung contended that conscious inner work could help one arrive at an understanding of how these archetypes play a role in the unfolding of individual destiny. He taught that by a process of *individuation*, the human soul can harmonize its various aspects and find its unique expression in life. Particularly important is the encounter with the *shadow*, the unrecognized emotions and attitudes which often run counter to our conscious intentions. Once these disowned elements of the psyche are acknowledged, they can gradually be reclaimed and integrated with the conscious Self. Jung called this process the *Union of Opposites*, borrowing an image from the tradition of alchemy.

In fact, one of Jung's major contributions was to revive a modern interest in alchemy as a language of the soul. Jung disputed the conventional view that alchemy was an attempt to magically convert base metals into gold. Instead, he viewed alchemy as a series of symbolic processes for inner work and the transmutation of the soul. Jung found correlations between transformative images which arose spontaneously in the dreams of his patients, and the archetypal forms used in alchemy. This lead Jung to conclude that alchemical processes involving the substances of Nature were basically projections of the human psyche, a kind of waking dream full of symbols of the inner life, but without any independent reality.

Unfortunately, Jung was only half correct in his assessment of alchemy. His insights led to new wisdom about the life of the human soul, but without a direct connection with the soul of Nature. The natural world is filled with living archetypes just as real as those that dwell within the human psyche. As we will discuss below, alchemical wisdom is not simply a projection of an interior world onto a blank screen; it works with the *correspondences* between the human soul and the soul of Nature. It is this very understanding which is the foundation of flower essence therapy.

Recent developments in psychotherapy

In the post-World War II period, one the most significant pioneers of psychology was Abraham Maslow, the founder of *humanistic psychology*. Maslow took issue with the misplaced emphasis within psychiatry and behavioral psychology on helping a dysfunctional individual to become "well-adjusted" in his or her work and family roles. Maslow posited a *hierarchy of needs*, which includes the basic capacity to function in the world and achieve the necessities of life. However, beyond these physical survival needs is the striving for *self-actualization*, or the full development of the *human potential* to find deeper meaning and fulfillment in life. This recognition became the basis for humanistic psychology and for what is called the *human potential movement*, which spawned a great variety of therapies designed to help the soul to find fulfillment in life.

Transpersonal psychology is a further development, in which there is a recognition of a transcendent or spiritual dimension to life which gives a wider context to our individual soul development. One of the pioneers of this work was Roberto Assagioli, the developer of *psychosynthesis*. Through this process a core sense of the Spiritual Self is developed as a center around which to constellate the various sub-selves, or subpersonalities.

As we approach the end of the twentieth century, voices are arising which question whether psychotherapy as it is practiced may be thwarting rather than enhancing the life of the soul. Archetypal psychologist James Hillman has criticized the narcissism of those whose approach to self-development leads to introversion and withdrawal from social and political involvement. He urges us to see the connection between individual neurosis and societal ills, and to become engaged in the issues of our time. Theodore Roszak has pointed out that much contemporary soul anguish has its origins in society's disconnection from the Earth. Feeling that the self-actualization of the human potential movement is inadequate, he calls for a new *ecopsychology*, in which our own healing is inseparable from healing the Earth. Robert Sardello urges us to bring meaning and beauty to our lives not only as an inner reality, but as an active and dynamic experience in the social and natural world. Thomas Moore writes of the need for "care of the soul" as a daily activity, rather than only an experience for the therapist's office. He suggests we let go of our obsession with fixing psychological problems, and instead attend to the wisdom of our soul's unique experience.

In their sometimes polemic, but always trenchant questioning of contemporary psychotherapy, these voices challenge us to develop a new psychological paradigm. The psyche should not be regarded as an isolated object for inner reflection, but a fully engaged participant on Earth and within human culture. The individual human soul is a member of the world soul (*anima mundi*). It is intimately related to *Gaia*, the living being of the Earth, and to all the beings within her. So envisioned, psychotherapy becomes genuine soul healing, true to Novalis' definition of "where the inner world and the outer world meet."

Flower essences and the world soul

Flower essence therapy embodies this expanded vision of soul care. Its fundamental tenet is that our personal wellness and sense of wholeness depend very much on the greater well-being of the world in which we live. However, this is not merely an abstract concept or a theoretical ideal. The inmost process — the very heart of meaning within flower essence therapy — is that a *dialogue or relationship is engendered between the human soul and the soul of Nature.*

Ultimately, we can view flower essence therapy as an extraordinary form of communion, one in which we receive not simply physical nourishment from the substances of the Earth, but where we allow ourselves to consciously absorb soul qualities from the Earth's living being. Such therapy affords us the opportunity not merely to be "healed" in a personal sense, but to actually experience and learn from Nature, to unite microcosmic and macrocosmic awareness.

Understood from this perspective, we can appreciate the deeper significance of the two *polychrest* (multi-use) remedies in the Bach system. Wild Oat and Holly epitomize the blending of inner and outer in flower essence therapy. Dr. Bach intended them to be widely used, to help orient the soul in the most basic way along its healing journey. Wild Oat addresses our capacity to find meaning in the world, to develop the inner commitment and focus which can strengthen and direct the soul to find its vocation or calling to serve others and to contribute to world culture. On the other hand, Holly addresses the inmost feelings of the soul which separate us from others, such as hostility, jealousy, and envy. In fact, the very name of this remarkable plant means wholeness or holiness; Holly leads the soul toward a feeling of unity, inclusiveness, and trust in relationships with others.

As we consider each of the essences listed in the *Repertory*, we see that they always address the exquisite balance of the soul: to find inner strength and meaning, but also to build compassionate sensitivity for others; to widen the consciousness, but also to focus it for practical and grounded activity; to be aware of higher and more subtle worlds, but also to be in the physical world and in the physical body. While still a pioneering effort, flower essence therapy has the potential to make a real and significant contribution to our understanding of soul healing. It promotes a truly dynamic relationship between inner and outer, personal and social, the human world and the natural world, and personal awareness and transcendent consciousness.

The divided alchemical tradition

The process of relating the individual soul to the world soul and the soul of Nature has ancient roots in the tradition of alchemy. Although considered by contemporary culture to be merely a primitive precursor of modern chemistry, and believed by Jung to be strictly psychic or symbolic; alchemy is in fact a profound system of philosophical and scientific activity which recognizes the interconnectedness of Humanity, Nature, and the Cosmos. The great Egyptian teacher Thoth (known as Hermes Trismegistus to the Greeks) was reputed to be the founder of the alchemical tradition, and is known as the originator of the axiom, "As Above, So Below."

Alchemical wisdom held that the order of the universe is expressed in the world of Nature, as well as in the human being, who can be considered a microcosm of the larger cosmos. One of the clearest representatives of this teaching was the medieval Swiss alchemist Paracelsus. He depicted Nature as a book written in cosmic script, whose forms and processes pointed to the working of higher laws. His *Doctrine of Signatures* described how the correspondences between forms of plants and humans indicated the specific healing action of plant remedies. This was based on the understanding that physical structures and processes of plants express the same universal principals which are manifest in the forms and processes of the human being. Paracelsus related celestial influences from the planets and stars to plants and metals, an understanding we can also find in the compendiums of such great herbalists as Hildegard of Bingen, Gerard, and Culpeper.

According to Paracelsus, the work of the alchemist was to take the substances of Nature and make them more refined and subtle, thus enhancing their transformative powers for the human being. He wrote, "The *quinta essentia* is that which is extracted from a substance — from all plants and from everything that has life . . . the inherency of a thing, its nature, power, virtue, and curative efficacy." Thus, for Paracelsus, a healing remedy was the refined *quintessence* of a natural substance.

The esoteric school of Rosicrucianism was an important part of the alchemical tradition, devoted to the perception of the natural world as a rich library of spiritual archetypes and transformative processes. Their spiritual practices were not designed to leave the physical body, nor to abandon the larger body of Nature or the needs of the human community in which they lived. On the contrary, each achievement along the Rosicrucian path demanded greater mastery of the physical and social worlds, and an increasingly deeper consciousness of the spiritual laws shaping these worlds. Active during the late Middle Ages and at the beginning of the Renaissance, the Rosicrucian alchemists lived in a practical way in the world, making substantive contributions in the healing, academic, and scientific professions of their time.

As we know, science forsook its metaphysical roots, and developed a mechanistic paradigm in which *matter* no longer has any connection to *being*, or to the etheric forces of Nature. *Alchemy* has become *chemistry* which, along with reductionistic biology, forms the basis for contemporary materialistic medical science. Alchemical teachings were dismissed as merely primitive superstition or charlatanism. Certainly many errors and distortions have crept into alchemical teachings through the ages, but profound wisdom permeates these teachings, for which a materialistic age has no comprehension.

Thus the tradition of alchemy, based on the relationship between the outer world of Nature's substances and the inner world of the human soul, has become divided in our time. On the one side we have a soul-devoid study of a mechanical world, and on the other side we have a disembodied system of symbols which exist only in the interior world of the psyche. Contemporary psychology reflects this alchemical split. Psychiatrists who follow the medical model work with substances and physical processes, but do not attend to the inner life of the human soul. Psychologists in the Jungian tradition are masters of the inner soul life but (with a few notable exceptions such as Dr. Edward Whitmont) generally lack a relationship to the soul of Nature, and do not work with a precise knowledge of the actual substances of Nature.

Flower essence therapy as a new alchemy of the soul

Because flower essence therapy addresses the relationship between the human soul and the soul of Nature, it reunites the two polarities of the alchemical tradition. It is a harbinger of a *new alchemy of the soul*, one which incorporates ancient wisdom with a modern awareness of the human psyche and of Nature.

The essence derived from the blossoming plant creates an alchemical *quinta essentia*, facilitating a soul dialogue between the archetypes of Nature and the archetypes within the human soul. This is not based on romantic sentimental projection, or nostalgia for a mythic golden age. Rather, it is a very precise understanding that the thoughts, feelings, and experiences of the human psyche are reflections of the same cosmic laws inherent in the growth patterns, shapes, colors, fragrances, and vital energies of Nature which are expressed in the flowering plant. This is the meaning of the alchemical teaching, "As Above, So Below." The soul life we find as we journey inward corresponds to the *anima mundi* of Nature herself.

The Unique Role of Flower Essence Therapy in Health Care

Flower essences are not drugs

Because flower essences are something we take into our bodies, it is easy to confuse the essences with drugs which are used to treat physical and emotional illness. Flower essences are not drugs. First of all, because of their vibrational nature, flower essences have no direct impact upon the body's biochemistry, as do pharmaceutical and psychoactive drugs. Tranquilizers, anti-depressants, pain-killers, mood-brighteners, and "mind-expanding" drugs affect emotional states, but they do this by changing brain chemistry, thus altering the biological vehicle through which the human soul expresses itself.

Such biochemical manipulation may be important in cases of severe illness, such as extreme suicidal tendencies. Yet, apart from the danger of side effects, we must ask profound questions about the use of mood-altering drugs to control or eliminate such typical human emotions as depression, fear, anxiety, and shyness. What is the effect on the soul of chemically-induced personality makeovers? Is something lost when the soul no longer needs to grapple with the pain of childhood abuse, or anger at the injustices of the world? Can the soul learn life's lessons if it no longer has the freedom to experience pain and transformation? Would society have fared better if its great poets had treated their introversion with mood enhancers, or if its social critics had cured their alienation with anti-depressants?

Flower essences, by contrast, leave the soul in freedom. They *encourage* rather than *compel* change, working by vibrational resonance rather than bio-chemical intervention. Their effect is evocative, much like the impact of a conversation with a wise and caring friend. The essences stimulate an inner dialogue with hidden aspects of the Self, awakening profound psychological archetypes, and giving us access to their message. As a result of such "speaking" to our soul, deep emotional and mental changes take place, which may then produce physiological alterations as well. But these changes are not imposed from without; they occur from within ourselves, through our own experience and effort.

Flower essences are *catalysts* which stimulate and energize the inner transformative process, while leaving us free to develop our own innate capacities. They are used best within a context of inner development, through self-observation, dialogue, and counseling. For this reason, they are not used to treat particular diseases. Rather, flower essences help us to learn the lessons of any ailment, to meet the challenges presented to our souls by emotional and physical pain and suffering, and thus to transform our lives. Such a health-enhancing metamorphosis may naturally eliminate many painful physical symptoms, but the ultimate goal remains the evolution of the soul. Unlike pain-killing or symptom-suppressing drugs, which can create long-term dependence when used to control chronic conditions, flower essences stimulate lasting changes in consciousness, which continue to be a part of our lives after we stop taking the essences.

Flower essences are not conventional herbal remedies

Flower essences have much in common with herbal remedies. They share a heritage of using pure ingredients directly from Nature, and a philosophy of working with, rather than suppressing, the healing process. In fact, after Dr. Bach left his homeopathic practice and discovered flower essences, he referred to himself as an herbalist, and characterized the essences as herbal remedies.

However, flower essences are a very specialized form of herbal preparation, which should be distinguished from conventional herbal remedies. Herbal products are made from many parts of the plant, including the root, stem, leaves, fruit, seed, as well as the blossom; they are made by a variety of methods, including infusion, decoction, and tincture.

Flower essences differ in their preparation method in that they are generally made by infusion, and only with the fresh blossoms of the plant within a very specific environmental matrix. In describing flower essence preparation, Dr. Bach commented, "Let it be noted in this that the four elements are involved: the earth to nurture the plant; the air from which it feeds; the sun or fire to enable it to impart its power; and water . . . to be enriched with its beneficent magnetic healing." We would also add that there is the fifth alchemical element, the *quintessential* element, which is the sensitive consciousness of the flower essence preparer. Thus, flower essences are more than simple herbal extracts; they are alchemical *quintessences* which carry the living archetypes of the whole plant, captured at its highest moment of unfolding into blossom.

Herbal remedies are generally selected on the basis of physical symptoms, and are used for their naturally occurring physical constituents. Flower essences, by contrast, are vibrational in nature, and are selected for their impact on soul qualities. Still, within the herbal and shamanic traditions of many cultures there is the knowledge that plants have deeper meanings, and are associated with spiritual forces and processes. This legacy of a more subtle herbalism can be viewed as one of the sources for understanding flower essence qualities.

Herbal properties of plants bear a relationship to their uses as flower essences, but are not identical. Often the flower essence's impact on the soul is like a "higher octave" of the physical effects of the plant, although this must be considered in the context of a complete study of the plant, as discussed starting on page 43. For example, Dill is used as a culinary herb to stimulate digestion and counteract flatulence caused by eating too much or too quickly. As a flower essence, Dill addresses "psychic indigestion," when the soul is overwhelmed by too many or too rapid sense impressions; it works to refine and clarify our experience of the sense world. Many modern herbalists use flower essences along with traditional herbal medicaments. However, they report that the essences address issues of the psyche far more directly and precisely than do conventional herbal remedies.

Flower essences differ from fragrances and essential oils

Flower essences should not be confused with fragrances, nor with pure essential oils used for aromatherapy, although the term "flower essences" is sometimes mistakenly applied to these oils. Flower essences have no particular smell, except for the brandy which is used as a natural preservative. This is because the *physical* substance of the blossom contained in the essence is highly attenuated, so that its *vibrational* qualities can be accentuated.

Fragrances are generally synthetic preparations prepared for their scent, and used in perfumery. Pure essential oils are highly concentrated natural distillations of the aromatic oils of plant substances, and are thus a specialized type of herbal remedy. Essential oils can have strong impacts on both body and soul, but their pathway is through the senses and physical body, rather than the vibrational fields of the flower essences. Aromatherapy and flower essences work well in tandem, but they should not be confused. They are complementary therapies — body to soul, and soul to body.

How flower essences and homeopathic remedies compare

Flower essences also differ from homeopathic remedies, although these modalities have much in common historically, philosophically, and in practice. Both types of remedies are vibrational in nature, and thus physically dilute. They each act as catalysts for the person's own healing process, rather than suppressing or controlling symptoms. Both modalities address the person rather than the disease, and endeavor to match the remedy to the unique individual situation. Dr. Bach practiced as a homeopathic physician before developing his flower essences, and today homeopaths are among those who most readily recognize the efficacy of flower essence therapy.

Yet there are significant differences between flower essences and homeopathic remedies. Bach clearly described his development of flower essences as a break with homeopathy, for he contended that the essences do not follow the *Law of Similars,* which is the very definition of homeopathic medicine.

According to this principle of similars, homeopathic remedies are developed by *provings*, in which large doses of a substance are given to a group of healthy individuals, and the symptoms they develop become the indications for the condition the remedy addresses. If Bach had used this homeopathic method, he would have given a test group of people large doses of Holly, and found that they became envious, jealous, or hateful, or found that Clematis in large doses produced a dreamy, unfocused state in his test group.

It is a historical fact that Bach never used provings in developing his flower remedies, nor have homeopathic provings been used to test other flower essences. Instead, Bach found that Holly flower essence brought a sense of connection and love to the soul troubled by jealousy, envy, or hatred, and that Clematis essence enhanced the quality of presence for dreamy, disembodied persons.

If flower essences do not follow the *Law of Similars* of homeopathy, can we say instead that they are an expression of the *Law of Contraries*, which is the basis of symptom-suppressing allopathic medicine? Bach apparently believed that flower remedies work by contraries within the soul, saying that they "flood our natures with the particular virtue we need, and wash out from us the fault that is causing the harm." However, our own research over the past sixteen years indicates that this is an over-simplification. Rather than working by similars or contraries, the transformative action of flower essences is an expression of the integration of polarities within our psyche, as understood in alchemy and by Jungian psychology.

For example, Mimulus flower essence addresses the fears of everyday life; it does not create fear when given in large doses to an otherwise healthy person without these fears, as would be expected if it followed the homeopathic *Law of Similars.* Nor does Mimulus essence obliterate fear, as would a tranquilizer drug operating by the *Law of Contraries.* A person taking Mimulus flower essence may become more *acutely conscious* of an existing state of fear, perhaps previously hidden from awareness. At the same time, Mimulus encourages the person to face these fears, rousing the requisite soul strength to meet such challenges. Therefore, we can say that the Mimulus works with the *polarity* of fear and courage, enabling the soul to reach a higher level of integration. Rather than *eliminating* fear, Mimulus helps us to have the *courage to face fear.* Understood in this way, flower essence therapy applies the alchemical law of the *Union of Opposites,* by which polar opposites are integrated into a higher synthesis.

Flower essences and homeopathic remedies are also prepared differently. While homeopathic remedies have been made from nearly any substance, and from any part of the plant, flower essences are made exclusively from the blossom. For this reason, flower essences should be also distinguished from various vibrational remedies made from other parts of plants, or from animal or mineral substances, such as sea essences and gem elixirs. It is specifically the flower that is used for flower essences, because it is in the process of blossoming that the soul qualities of Nature come into the form and substance of the plant. Thus, the flower essence becomes a vehicle of communication between the soul of Nature and the human soul.

Even when homeopathic remedies are made from flowers, they are prepared differently than flower essences. The homeopathic mother substance is a tincture or alcohol extraction of the mascerated plant, which is then diluted and potentized, often many times, to produce a remedy. Flower essences begin with an infusion in water of the whole blossom of the plant, in which the preparer works very consciously with the surrounding meteorological and environmental conditions. For this reason, flower essences are made in the "laboratory of Nature," in the natural wildflower habitat or in a garden where the flowers can flourish under ideal conditions.

Flower essences are used only in the first or second dilution, yet directly affect the mind and emotions. They impact the psyche in a gentle way which generally leaves the consciousness free to choose how to respond to their influence. Homeopathic remedies usually need to be raised to a much higher potency to affect mental and emotional states. Many practitioners believe that such potencies act upon the psyche in a more compelling manner than do flower essences. In this way, high-potency homeopathic remedies have some similarities to pharmaceutical drugs, and must be used with great caution by very skilled practitioners. Low-potency homeopathic remedies, by contrast, work more directly with the physical-etheric aspect of the human being, and are thus more similar to herbal remedies. Flower essences combine the safety of low-potency homeopathic remedies with the consciousness-stimulating ability of higher potency remedies. They accomplish this by creating a *dialogue* with the soul, rather than *dictating* to it.

Flower essences also differ from homeopathic remedies in the manner in which they are used. A homeopathic case involves an extensive cataloguing of symptoms, usually with a strong emphasis on physical conditions and habits, which give a picture of the etheric or life body of the person. The practitioner then seeks to find the best fit between the list of symptoms presented by the patient and the list of indications for the remedy.

By contrast, flower essence therapy correlates an "archetype" or "message" of a plant with a particular quality within the human soul or psyche. While physical and other symptoms provide clues regarding inner issues, choosing a flower essence is more than matching a list of symptoms and indications. Rather, the emphasis is on identifying underlying life issues and lessons, as a way of painting a "soul portrait" of the individual. This picture is then correlated with one or more flower essences whose vibrational configurations embody these qualities and processes.

It is thus clear that flower essences are *not* homeopathic remedies, although both belong to the larger category of energy or vibrational remedies. There may be confusion on this point because some brands of flower essences are labeled as homeopathic drugs for regulatory or import purposes. Such labeling is unfortunate and inaccurate, but it in no way invalidates the philosophical and practical differences between these two modalities.

Working with vibrational devices

Flower essence therapy also differs from systems of vibrational testing and practices which employ machines or devices to measure or adjust human energy fields according to various quantitative scales. These modalities are frequently employed to aid in the selection of homeopathic, nutritional, and herbal remedies, as well as to "tune" physiological systems by working with vibrational "equivalents" of remedies. To the extent such devices work with *quantitative* measurement, they can give useful information, particularly about relative strength or degree of vitality within human physiological and energetic systems, and how these are affected by various substances. However, these measurements are not a substitute for working with the *qualities* of flower essences and the soul issues they address. Flower essence therapy involves us in a series of conscious *relationships*; it entails inner dialogue and reflection about feelings and attitudes, sensitive conversation with a friend or therapist, and a receptive listening to the healing language of Nature.

Furthermore, using vibrational or electronic devices as substitutes for real flower essences creates a subtle field lacking a physical-etheric anchor. While the materialist ignores the soul of Nature by reducing substance to mere chemistry and mechanics, there are serious problems with the opposite impulse which utilizes purely vibrational mechanisms that disassociate one's soul from the physical substances of Nature.

Thus, at best, vibrational devices can serve a supplementary role in flower essence therapy. However, there is no substitute for developing a conscious relationship with the human soul and with the soul of Nature if we wish to truly partake of the gifts which the essences offer us.

Flower essences and the healing quest

In the beginning of this section, we defined health as the ability to completely experience life, to become fully ourselves. By awakening the innate capacities of our soul, flower essences enhance health on all levels: physical, emotional, and spiritual. They do this not by suppressing symptoms, nor by altering our biochemistry, but rather by acting as catalysts to strengthen our conscious healing journey.

This journey is a quest for wholeness, founded on the recognition that illness is a wake-up call from our soul, demanding self-discovery and sensitivity to others and to the world around us. Most of all, *it requires that we change our inner attitudes, beliefs, and perceptions.* It is here that flower essences can offer their unique contribution, no matter what other therapies we are using.

It is all too human to fear and resist change, particularly when we are unaware of its purpose or necessity. By rousing our awareness, even if it is sometimes painful, the essences provide an additional stimulus to help us past our denial and resistance. In the words of the German poet Goethe, "Unless you are constantly dying and becoming, you are but a shadowy guest on a darkened Earth." This is true for all of us, but illness makes this truth more urgent.

Therefore, while flower essences combine with and support many other health modalities, they have their own unique message to share with us. Like true friends, they challenge us to self-awareness and change, but ultimately leave the choice to us whether we seize the opportunity and heed the call toward soul metamorphosis.

California Wild Rose *Rosa canina*

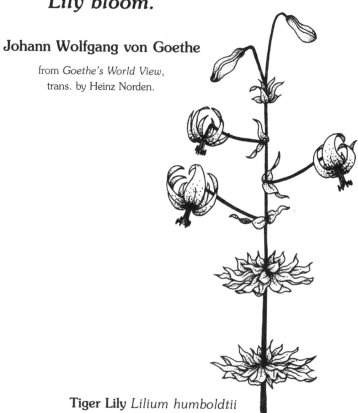

*Je älter ich werde, je mehr vertrau
ich auf das Gesetz, wonach die Rose
und die Lilie blüht.*

**The older I grow, the more I trust in
the law by which the Rose and the
Lily bloom.**

Johann Wolfgang von Goethe

from *Goethe's World View,*
trans. by Heinz Norden.

Tiger Lily *Lilium humboldtii*

Chapter 2: Can We Verify the Properties of Flower Essences?

The Need for Flower Essence Research

How do we know that flower essences have the effects attributed to them in this *Repertory*, or in other flower essence literature? In the face of recent scientific evidence, it seems indisputable that emotions and attitudes have a profound affect on health. Yet, it challenges our accepted modes of thought to say that a highly dilute infusion of flowers without any discernible biochemical mechanism can affect how we think and feel. Furthermore, even if we accept that flower essences can affect human states of mind, how can we be sure that a plant essence will have the specific effect which is claimed? These are crucial questions for anyone seeking to understand and employ flower essences in health care. It is for this reason that the Flower Essence Society is dedicated to a multi-faceted research program.

The legacy of Dr. Bach

Dr. Edward Bach's pioneering work in the 1930's is a starting point for our inquiries, but it leaves many questions unanswered. Although Bach was only able to spend about eight of his 50 years researching flower remedies, he had done considerable study of human psychological types during his years as a bacteriologist and homeopath. These insights were further developed into the particular soul typologies corresponding to his flower essences, first as a system of 12 types, then 19, and finally 38. Through Bach's sparse writings and talks, and the biography written by his assistant, Nora Weeks, we have some glimpses of how extraordinarily perceptive Bach was about the soul life of his patients. By carefully observing how his patients walked into the consulting room, he often intuited which remedies they would need.

Although he was highly critical of medical science, it is clear that Bach's professional medical training served him well in his flower essence research, for he was able to apply the scientific discipline of keen observation and systematic study to an understanding of the human soul. We may assume that Bach employed a similar approach in his Nature studies. He appears to have some connection to the alchemical tradition, and refers in his writings to the teachings of Paracelsus. We also know that Bach originally prepared his flower essences by gathering sun-potentized dew drops from the blossoms, a method favored by alchemists.

However, we have no information about Bach's perceptions of the plants used for his flower essences. Nora Weeks reports in the biography, *The Medical Discoveries of Edward Bach*, that he traveled extensively throughout the countryside in search of plants to use as herbal or flower remedies, and that he spent time observing their form, growth patterns, and habitat. But aside from her account of his extraordinary sensitivity to plant energies, Bach's actual method of plant research remains shrouded in mystery.

Bach himself bears some responsibility for this situation, as he deliberately destroyed his research notes and many of his writings. In the introduction to *The Twelve Healers and Other Remedies,* Bach wrote, "No science, no knowledge is necessary, apart from the simple methods described herein; and they who will obtain the greatest benefit from this God-sent Gift will be those who keep it pure as it is; free from science, free from theories, for everything in Nature is simple." Evidently reacting against the excesses of an overly materialistic and reductionistic science which had little place for the human soul or the soul of Nature, Bach deprived future generations of his insights into the dynamic processes which allow plant energies to enter into the metamorphosis of human consciousness. We can speculate that his attitude may also have been due to the tradition of secrecy of esoteric knowledge within the Masonic Lodge, of which Bach was a member; or perhaps Bach himself was not fully aware of how he reached his intuitive understandings of the plants.

Julian Barnard, a leading researcher, teacher, and writer about Dr. Bach's life and work, makes the following comments in his book *Patterns of Life Force:*

> . . . At a certain point Bach's research took a leap, and we find it difficult to see where and how. In 1928 he is walking on one bank of the river still working as a bacteriologist, but searching for herbal equivalents to his vaccines, and then . . . he appears on the other bank with a 'thin glass bowl' potentising certain flowers that are to hold a new healing power.

Well, we have a choice. We may decide to leave him on his side and say his was an insight and inspiration that is beyond us, or we may choose to build a bridge that will take us across to a deeper understanding of how it works and why. Those who prefer the first course of action are left with his system of healing and can rejoice in the fruits of this work. An explanation such as it is will be that he was an extraordinarily sensitive man who had wandered and was led, who found through suffering and personal affliction: a blind and painful discovery. But Bach's work, his writings and his flower remedies invite another view, and while it is more demanding, it is also more rewarding.

It is just this quest for a bridge of understanding, to learn how the archetypal language of the flowers corresponds to the language of the human soul, which led to the founding of the Flower Essence Society, and its emphasis on plant research and flower essence case studies.

The polarization of soul and science

We need flower essence research not only to satisfy our thirst for philosophical understanding. There is also a practical and moral necessity to find standards and principles for understanding flower essences, which has become more urgent in the six decades since Dr. Bach's time. Particularly in the past ten years, hundreds of new flower essences have been made available very rapidly by dozens of groups around the world. Often different people making the same essence will attribute quite different qualities to it. Claims are frequently made for essences with little or no standards of research. What criteria can we use to know which, if any, interpretations of essence properties are correct? Can we learn to distinguish between true insight, momentary subjective feelings, and psychic or sentimental projections? Can we develop a methodology for investigating the accuracy of our intuitive perceptions?

As we seek the answers to these questions, we are met with a dilemma. In our modern culture, it is science which provides the objective standards by which we test the validity of our assumptions and beliefs. Yet science appears cold, unfeeling, dehumanizing, and unrelated to what is most sacred to the soul. Furthermore, scientific research generally ignores the ecological and cultural destruction which seems to accompany its progress.

While scientific thought dominates our culture, a major counter-current has developed, reacting against the materialism of conventional science. This conflict represents a deeper fissure in our culture, one we discussed earlier in the splitting of alchemy into soul work and hard science. The division could be described variously as one between humanities and science, soul and technology, psyche and substance, or inner and outer. We meet it also in our educational system (particularly in North America), where most scientists, engineers, and technicians have little training in history, psychology, philosophy, or the arts, and so are usually blind to the human and moral consequences of scientific development. On the other hand, there are vast portions of the population who are unfamiliar with the basic concepts of science. This results not only in an ignorance of complex modern technology, but it also cripple the capacity for rigorous thinking. Without an understanding of the scientific method, it is difficult to systematically observe and inquire about the natural world, or to independently think and evaluate evidence in a quest for truth. Thus, the polarization of our inner and outer worlds has led to imbalances both in our soul life and in our understanding of Nature.

Problems with subjective knowledge

In the past our spiritual and soul life was regulated much more by cultural and religious structures. Today, we experience greater freedom, as well as increased confusion. Some gravitate to fundamentalist convictions to feel secure. Others, rejecting the need for scientific investigation and the systematic thought of the intellect, prefer to rely on feeling, vague intuition, and mystical experience as a guide for truth.

We see this latter tendency strongly within the "New Age" movement, and among many people who use flower essences, resulting in a rapid expansion of intuitive and psychic experiences. For example, many flower essence qualities have been derived from psychic impressions and channeling, inner messages and spiritual guidance, reading of subtle energies, or various vibrational testing systems such as kinesiology (muscle-testing) and radiesthesia (pendulum). Often this is without any grounding in systematic observation of the essences' actual effects on people, or careful study of the plants from which they are derived.

Relying only on personal feeling, intuition, or brief psychic experience is on the extreme *inner* side of the polarity we have described, a place of total subjectivity. It is imbalanced because we risk living in our own reality, unrelated to others or to the world in which we live. The individual soul becomes isolated from the world soul, and from the soul of Nature.

Consider, for example, the predicament if each practitioner had a totally different definition for each flower essence or homeopathic remedy. In such circumstances, we would create a veritable "Tower of Babel," in which it would be impossible for us to work together because we could not share a common language or perception of reality.

At its heart, science is a quest for truth, for a reality that can be shared collectively, because it reflects an accurate understanding of Nature rather than an egoistic projection of personal experience. It is a corrective to the confusion that can result from excessive subjectivity. Despite the limited scope in which conventional science is practiced, it is the *scientific method* which offers us a way to accurately perceive the world and define its underlying principles. Through scientific investigation we encounter the natural world and other human beings, and we link ourselves to a larger reality. Thus, despite all that is alienating about modern science, we desperately need the *spirit of science* — the search for standards of truth in the study of Nature — in our flower essence research and in related fields of inquiry.

Imbalances in scientific method

While we require the objectivity which science offers, we face very real problems with current scientific method.

Our word "science" comes from the Latin *scire,* which means "to know," but also "to discern" in the sense of separating or cutting apart. This ability of the analytic mind to divide phenomena into their component parts, as well as to separate the observer from the observed, has enabled humankind to learn much about the natural world. As Aristotle pointed out long ago, we need some *distance* in order to see anything clearly. Humankind needed to stand back from Nature in order to observe it and contemplate its meaning. Besides giving us knowledge, our intellect has granted us a powerful sense of freedom and individuality which was not possible when reality was cloaked by social or religious dogma.

Yet, this same development of detached objectivity, or *observer consciousness*, has also alienated us from Nature, from the spiritual world, and ultimately from ourselves. Complete objectivity can only be achieved by reducing the world into a collection of objects to be observed. There is a paradox here, however. If human beings are just another class of objects, then *who* is observing this world of objects? If the mind is just a biochemical product of the mechanism of the brain, then where is the consciousness that arrived at that conclusion? The German physicist Max Planck, who first developed quantum theory, put it this way: "Science cannot solve the ultimate mystery of Nature. And it is because in the last analysis we are part of the mystery we are trying to solve." Despite the perplexing questions raised by quantum physics and relativity theory early in this century, and by current new perspectives like chaos theory, mainstream science has largely ignored these fundamental epistemological issues.

Scientific study arose out of an impulse to leave the cloisters of the Middle Ages, and to venture independently in the realm of Nature to observe her and know her laws. Yet, by relying on complex instruments as a way of measuring reality, the scientific researcher of today is often separated from the direct experience of Nature phenomena through the perception of the human senses. It is ironic to see to what extent the scientist has created the laboratory as a modern cloister, an artificial environment detached from Nature and society.

Modern science has thus become increasingly divorced from the full dimensionality of the *life process*. In striving for rational objectivity, the scientific method has narrowed its field of vision to what is physically measurable and quantifiable, disregarding the *qualitative* experience of the etheric and soul dimensions of life. Because it neither perceives the wholeness of living forms nor acknowledges the living *beings* which inhabit these forms, modern science has become disconnected from Nature and from the human soul, and thus unable to comprehend the subtle forces or soulful qualities associated with flower essence therapy and other holistic paradigms.

We need to find new forms of scientific research which are appropriate to the subtle realm of the essences, yet which retain the rigor and objective truth-seeking qualities which have made scientific inquiry such an important step forward in the evolution of human culture. Thus, we are challenged on two sides. Our research into vibrational remedies needs the disciplined search for truth, which is the essence of science. Yet, our approach to science must encompass the profound multi-dimensional relationship of humanity with the world of Nature which is so lacking in contemporary scientific research. Flower essence therapy requires the development of a new, living science of Nature.

Toward a Living Science of Nature

What kind of science can comprehend the mystery of flower essences? Such a science requires the disciplined observation of systematic thinking which characterizes the scientific method, but must be broad enough to encompass the reality of the human soul and the world soul. It perceives Nature not as a collection of mechanical objects, but as *a community of beings*. It is a *holistic*, rather than a *reductionistic* science, which not only separates physical reality into its component parts, but recognizes how each part is an expression of a greater whole. This science also recognizes that while we are the observers of life, we are also active participants in life, and that the polarity of objectivity and subjectivity must find a new synthesis.

Goethean science

The scientific approach we are positing has its sources in the alchemical/Rosicrucian stream discussed earlier, before its eventual split into the psychic symbolism of contemporary psychology and the soulless substance of chemical medicine. Alchemy recognized the correspondence between the macrocosm of Nature and the microcosm of human experience. The Rosicrucian alchemists understood that the path of human spiritual development must unite itself with the world to encounter the working of spiritual laws in the forms and processes of Nature.

This path of ensouled Nature science was further developed by the German poet and natural scientist Johann Wolfgang von Goethe (1749-1832). During his lifetime, Goethe witnessed the rapid development of scientific materialism, which soon led to the Industrial Revolution. Yet he believed with the Rosicrucian alchemists that ". . . the sense-perceptible corresponds throughout with the spiritual, and is not only an evidence of it, but indeed its representative." As a poet, it was Goethe's destiny to initiate a science which recognized the soulfulness of Nature, while remaining true to the objectivity of the scientific method.

Goethe's artistic temperament allowed him to see the relationship of the part to the whole, to perceive an underlying unity within the diversity of natural phenomena. His early scientific work was devoted to geology. He became convinced that hidden in the geological strata of the mountains he studied were deep stories which Nature had to tell. As Goethe wrote in *Wilhelm Meister*, he ". . . used these figures and crevices as letters of an alphabet, had to decipher them, formed them into words and learned to read them . . ."

Goethe's full scientific genius is revealed in his studies of living Nature, particularly of plants. He was a keen observer of the myriad details of plant life, not so much with the goal of description and classification, but rather of finding the unifying principles. Commenting on the classical botanical system of Linnaeus (Carl von Linné), Goethe wrote, ". . . I therefore felt justified in concluding that Linné and his successors had proceeded like legislators, less concerned with what was, than with what should be . . . but rather intent upon solving the difficult problem of how so many inherently unfettered beings can be made to exist side by side with a degree of harmony."

Rather than just considering its parts, Goethe looked at the totality of the plant, its development in time, and its dynamic relationships with other plant forms and processes. Goethe conceived of the multitudinous expressions of plant life as variations on a universal theme, which he called the *Urpflanze* (archetypal plant). Goethe knew plants not as static forms, but as an expression of dynamic processes of continual change, existing in time as well as in space. He was able to perceive the fluidity of forms in living beings as an expression of underlying etheric patterns and cosmic laws. He referred to these forms and processes as the *gestures* of plants or animals. This is similar to Paracelsus' *Doctrine of Signatures*, an understanding that there is a correspondence between outer physical forms and the inner qualities they express.

Goethe's pioneering work provides a basis for a living understanding of the language of Nature. It is a *qualitative* science of Nature, contrasting with the strictly *quantitative* approach of the prevailing reductionistic and mechanistic view of Nature. Rather than simply measuring the chemical constituents of a plant, Goethe studied how the shape of the leaf evolved from the young to the mature plant, appeared in a new form in the flower petals, and again in the stamens and pistils. Instead of seeing the flowering and fruiting of a plant as a mere mechanism for propagation, Goethe saw it as a culmination of a dance of expansion and contraction, expressed newly in each stage of the plant's growth. Out of this understanding, he developed his well-known concept of the *metamorphosis of plants.*

In the Goethean approach to science, human consciousness actually becomes an instrument of research. Thinking itself becomes metamorphic, developing the same mobility and flexibility as the phenomena it encounters. It involves a re-creation of an inner image of what we perceive in the outer world through our senses. This capacity is an extension of the artistic imagination; but it differs from how we often understand imagination in that *it is a precise response to the actual phenomena of Nature.*

Through this process which Goethe called "exact imagination," we begin to experience not only the phenomena of Nature, but also their effect on our own being as we inwardly experience them. In this way we can perceive not only the objects and events of Nature, but also the forces and qualities which permeate them. We are thus able to comprehend the archetypes living in Nature not as intellectual abstractions, but as direct perceptions out of our living thinking.

Observation is married to thinking, allowing perception to grow into a living concept. The Goethean scientific method thus brings about a reconciliation of the dichotomy of inner and outer, of participant and observer, and of objectivity and subjectivity, in the research process.

In Goethean science, the observer becomes a conscious *participant* in the research process. It is different from conventional "observer consciousness," where the researcher pretends to be a detached, unbiased, and uninvolved spectator. In the conventional scientific method, any subjective participation in the research project is seen as an interference to be avoided. Since it is the nature of scientific observation that the observer affects what is observed (Heisenberg's Uncertainty Principle), this unacknowledged participation becomes unconscious, often leading to hidden assumptions and biases. By contrast, the Goethean scientist takes responsibility for and actively cultivates the clarity of his or her own consciousness as a scientific instrument.

However, the Goethean method is also different from the totally subjective approach, in which our inner world is naively projected on the outer world in a very self-centered way that denies the *otherness* of what is outside of us. Nor is it like a drug-induced or psychic journey which takes us out of our physical bodies into other realities, or puts us in astral contact with discarnate beings.

The Goethean method is an encounter with a very tangible natural world that has its own laws and truths. Our understanding of that world must be based on what is actually there, discovering the correspondence between the inner experience and the outer phenomena. This is a skill that takes time and patience to develop into a true scientific research technique which can discriminate between truth and error.

Spiritual science

Goethe's scientific studies became a small, underground counter-current to the mainstream of scientific thought. He was far better known for his literary work, particularly his masterpiece drama, *Faust*. About a hundred years ago, the Austrian-born philosopher and spiritual teacher Rudolf Steiner (1861-1925) edited Goethe's scientific works, bringing them to the attention of the modern world, and articulating for the first time the true significance of Goethe's scientific epistemology. Steiner recognized in Goethe a strict phenomenalism in which thinking remains true to the direct perceptions of Nature. It was not that Goethe shunned thinking, but rather that his thinking was formed by his perception. In this way he avoided the error of mainstream science which applies the mechanistic laws appropriate to inanimate objects to the metamorphic world of living beings.

Steiner was not antagonistic to modern natural science. He recognized that humanity had developed an important faculty for independent thinking in its attempt to explain the natural world. Rather than dismiss the scientific method, he wished to enlarge it, to develop a *spiritual science*, which he called *anthroposophy*, meaning the "wisdom of humanity." In his lecture series, *The Boundaries of Natural Science*, Steiner said, "We must begin by acquiring the discipline that modern science can teach us . . . and transcend it, so that we can use the same exacting approach . . . thereby extending this methodology to the investigation of entirely different realms as well . . . Nobody can attain true knowledge of the spirit who has not acquired scientific discipline, who has not learned to investigate and think in the laboratories according to modern scientific method."

Steiner's spiritual science is built on Goethean science, but has adopted a complementary approach. Whereas Goethe began with the percept and moved to the concept, Steiner started with the pure thinking and then developed perception. Goethean science is a study of Nature, but Steiner wished to bring scientific discipline to the investigation of consciousness itself.

In Steiner's book *The Philosophy of Freedom* (also known as *The Philosophy of Spiritual Activity*), he maintained that the human thinking faculty can be raised to a level where it becomes spiritual activity. As such, it is more akin to conscious meditation than to a mystical experience of merging with the divine. In its essence, this spiritual thinking activity is totally "sense-free," yet it can be directly experienced, and its truth validated. Steiner offered pure mathematics as an example of sense-free thinking, with its rigorous logical consistency and verifiability. It is through developing higher thinking, Steiner contended, that we have the possibility to win true freedom, to grow to spiritual maturity by taking responsibility for the capacity of our Spiritual Self to comprehend higher truths.

Goethean science and sense-free thinking, Steiner explained, form two sides of a polarity, matter and consciousness, both of which must be encountered and harmonized to develop true spiritual science. He likened this process to the ancient breath yoga of the Orient, which worked with the cycle of inhalation and exhalation. In this new yoga of our modern age, we "breathe in" our sense perceptions of the world, and we "breathe out" our thoughts. As Steiner described in *Boundaries of Natural Science*, "inhalation and exhalation are physical experiences: when they are harmonized, one consciously experiences the eternal. In everyday life we experience thinking and perception. By bringing mobility into the life of the soul, one experiences the pendulum, the rhythm, the continual interpenetrating vibration of perception and thinking."

By uniting perception and thinking within our soul experience, tempered with scientific discipline, spiritual science is able to avoid the problems of subjective knowledge as well as the imbalances in conventional scientific methods discussed earlier. Spiritual scientific research requires that we become free of psychic projection, emotional bias, and self-delusion in order to become clear instruments of perception and insight. Yet to obtain objectivity, we neither become a detached observer cut off from Nature and divorced from any inner experience, nor depend upon abstract technical instruments of measurement. Rather, true objectivity consists of a disciplined and systematic ability to observe and to understand what is being observed. The essence of the scientific method — objective observation and documentation of phenomena — must be integrated with the essence of the spiritual approach — reverent recognition of transpersonal and transphysical states of reality and being.

Through spiritual science, the human soul can encounter the archetypal realm of Nature and the higher realms of spirit with the same clarity and inner discipline which is practiced in the physical sciences. Just as the botanical scientist, for example, can develop the perceptive capacity to clearly distinguish the structure of a flower, so the spiritual scientist can learn to employ inner vision to "see" the forces which form the flower, and the living "idea" or archetype from higher realms which brings the plant into being.

Such a new science of Nature requires heightened capacities within the human soul for imagination (clear-seeing), inspiration (clear-hearing), and intuition (clear-feeling or sensing). All these methods of working with the phenomena of Nature need to be reinforced and amplified by a community of researchers who are working in similar ways, so that individual insights can be corroborated and refined through a collective pool of knowledge.

Goethe's and Steiner's spiritual scientific approaches have been taken up and elaborated by many contemporary researchers working in the fields of botany, animal biology, biodynamic agriculture, anthroposophical medicine, physics, chemistry, and mathematics. In our flower essence research, we face a similar challenge. Can we apply the *spirit of science* by integrating the *clarity* of scientific method with sufficient *soul sensitivity* for the inner qualities found in the plant?

Flower Essence Plant Study

Flower essence research is essentially a two-fold process: it involves study of the plants used to make essences, and study of the experiences of people using the essences. Both of these areas are vitally important, but plant study presents perhaps the greatest challenge, requiring the breaking of new ground.

Dr. Bach's development of flower remedies, and the homeopathic tradition of Hahnemann out of which Bach's work emerged, both emphasized the clinical use of the remedies, and provide few guidelines for direct study of the sources of the remedies in Nature. To some extent, our flower essence plant studies can draw upon the herbal traditions of many cultures, which are rich with useful plant information and lore. However, much herbal knowledge is fragmentary or vague, often representing incomplete remnants from past cultures. Herbology today, much like conventional medicine, frequently emphasizes physical properties and effects, without relating them to their soul qualities or subtle influences. In the alchemical teachings of Paracelsus and others we find a rudimentary approach to plant study which integrates the inner and outer worlds. However, when we look for a modern development of alchemical studies, the purely symbolic approach of Jungian psychology predominates, unrelated to the actual substances of Nature.

Therefore, our task is to forge a modern alchemy, a new science of Nature which can help us understand the plants we use for flower essences. Along this path, the nature studies of Goethe and the spiritual scientific philosophy of Steiner can be guiding lights. However, Goethe and Steiner never applied their methods to the study of the soul language of flower essences, and Bach's flower essence discoveries were never developed into a systematic plant science. Thus, while we have much to learn from those who have come before — individualities such as Paracelsus, Hahnemann, Goethe, Steiner, Jung, Bach; and traditions such as herbalism, shamanism, and folk medicine — we must ask new questions, and seek new answers. Finding our way to a spiritual science of flower essence therapy is a truly pioneering journey, on which we have taken just the first few steps.

The importance of physical observation of plants

Those who prepare flower essences (and other health remedies) for the public have a fundamental responsibility to understand the plants they use. For practitioners and those who use flower essences in home care, the research methods described below constitute important background knowledge for appreciating the complex effort required to discover and thoroughly research flower essence properties. Even for those not directly involved in plant research, it is important to understand the many research considerations that comprise flower essence field study.

In the research program of the Flower Essence Society, we begin our study of flower essence qualities with observation of the plant itself, and its relationship to its environment. In the words of Paracelsus, "if you wish to know the Book of Nature, you must walk its pages with your feet."

Before interpreting the soul qualities of plants, it is important to cultivate the discipline of actually perceiving the plant, observing its color, form, habitat, growth patterns, and seasonal cycles. All of these physical details provide a foundation on which to build more grounded insights about the subtle qualities of the plant. Once we have sensitively encountered the plant as a physical being, recording our many observations in a journal and sketch-book, we can gradually create an inner image of the plant, and begin to understand its essential nature.

This process is similar to our observant attention to the posture, facial expressions, and movements of a person, so we can understand something of his or her inner character. We must first discern in the physical forms and movements what Paracelsus called the plant's *signature* and Goethe the *gesture*, before we can know the soul qualities they represent.

To acquire such deep insights involves patient, continuous observation, and a deep love and sense of wonder for the world of plants. Just as we could not say that we really knew someone from one or two brief encounters, so it is also necessary to develop a *relationship* over time with any plant we wish to know. Furthermore, just as we need to know something of a person's connections with their family and community in order to gain a fuller picture of who they are, we should consider the plant's relationship to its habitat, other plants, the animal world, natural seasonal cycles, and environmental changes.

It is important to remember that the plant is a *time being*. We do not know a plant only by seeing it in blossom. The flower is the culmination of a process which begins with a seed, sprouts into a root and shoot, opens into leaves, grows through stages of new branches and leaves, gathers its forces into buds, and finally bursts into blossom. It continues with the fertilization and falling away of the flowers, and the ripening into fruit and seed, by which the cycle begins again.

Consequently, to make flower essences we must know more than just the flower at the moment of blossoming. Our study is of the whole plant as it extends in both time and space. This is because the flower essence is not simply an extract of the substance in the blossom; it is a distillation of the whole being of the plant. It is at the moment of flowering that the highest soul-spiritual expression of the plant surfaces; and yet only if we are willing to follow the plant in its complete journey can we truly appreciate the mystery of the blossom itself.

This deep knowledge of essence plants is important, not only so that they can be used wisely, but also because plants are living beings, who require that we represent their essence to the world with as much respect, accuracy, and truthfulness as possible. Just as we can easily misunderstand a human being by projecting our own subjective bias, or by not taking sufficient time to truly learn from and listen to his or her life biography; so also can we very easily distort our relationship with plants. If we are unfamiliar with plant observation, we may have difficulty distinguishing what is truly significant about a particular plant from what is a common property of many plants. It is easy to oversimplify the process of finding plant gestures. We must be prepared to observe and experience many plants for years before being able to truly understand the archetypal gesture and corresponding soul essence of any specific plant.

Encountering the plant: a field study of Yarrow

We first encounter a plant as a particular form, with its specific colors and aromas, in relationship to its habitat. We are interested in understanding how each part of the plant relates to the whole, and how it compares to other plants. Over time, we observe the relationship of the plant and its growth patterns to the cycles of Nature.

To give a practical dimension to our outline of plant research, we will give some general indications for studying Yarrow *(Achillea millefolium)*. This well-known wild herb is one of the most prominent and efficacious flower essences included in the *Repertory*.

We find Yarrow flourishing in sunny, open areas, and particularly exalted in alpine meadow habitats. In the early spring we see only a mat of dark green feathery leaves closely hugging the ground. Rubbing the leaves, we encounter a strong, sharp aroma. If we dig a bit, we will note the rhizomatous roots spreading underground. Later in the spring, a strong central stem emerges from the leafy matrix, until it obtains a height of 1 to 3 feet (30 cm - 1 m). Arranged alternately along the stem, which is covered with fine hairs, are more feathery leaves, up to 5 inches (13 cm) long.

In the heat and light around the time of the summer solstice the Yarrow unfolds its blossoms in a brilliant white canopy over its green foliage, seeming to glow with an almost incandescent radiance. Looking more closely, we see that the stem has branched many times to form the umbel (umbrella-like) inflorescence. The flower head is a extremely compact cluster of many flowers, each of which has five white petal-like rays, and central florets with little spots of yellow where the anthers first appear on the stamens. Remarkably, as summer ripens into autumn, the Yarrow continues to stand in full flower, only gradually drying out as the year wanes, yet still retaining its characteristic form.

Yarrow is found throughout the temperate zones of both the northern and southern hemispheres. It is a perennial herb, with a sturdy woody stem, and a strong root system which spreads vigorously from underground runners. Yarrow's traditional name "Millefoil," and its species name *millefolium* mean "thousand leaves," referring to its finely divided and highly defined leaves. Unlike many plants with broad fleshy leaves, or which have narrow or divided leaves only in the upper part of the plant, even the lower leaves of the Yarrow are feathery. The whole plant is highly aromatic, filling the air with a very pungent smell, particularly in the heat of the sun.

Besides the white Yarrow, two other Yarrows are included in the *Repertory*. Pink Yarrow is nearly identical in appearance to the common white Yarrow, except for the deep pink to rose-red flowers. Pink Yarrow is often grown as a horticultural variety, but many lighter pink Yarrows occur naturally. The Golden Yarrow is a larger, sturdier plant, which is native to Asia Minor. Its golden yellow flowers have no petal-like rays, only yellow centers very tightly clustered together. Its leaves are larger, and more fern-like than feathery.

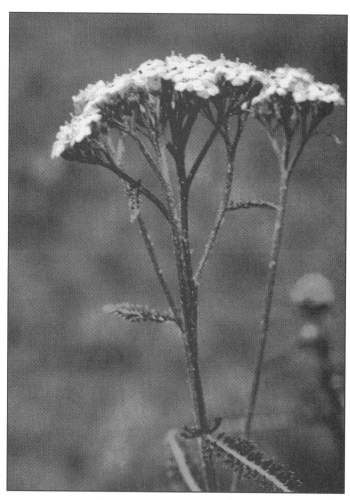

Yarrow *Achillea millefolium*

The Yarrow plant is distinguished by its feathery leaves, strong, upright stem, and its umbel canopy of radiant white composite flowers.

Elemental and alchemical forces in the plant

As we refine our plant observation, we are able to move from the physical structure to a perception of how life forces work through the plant. One of the most basic ways of seeing the plant is through the four elements of earth, water, air, and fire, a system prominent in the alchemical tradition, and which can be traced back to Aristotle. We should not confuse these four elements with the approximately 100 chemical elements of the periodic table of modern science. The four alchemical elements represent *processes* and *qualities* of Nature, not physical "building blocks." Earth is the quality of solidity and strength, water the quality of liquidity and life, air the quality of expansiveness and openness to light, and fire the principle of radiance, warmth, and transformation. In the human soul, each element expresses one of the four human *temperaments*, as they were known in classical thought. The earth-bound person is *melancholic*, the watery person *phlegmatic,* the airy person *sanguine*, and the fiery person *choleric*.

Each plant contains the working of all four elemental processes. However, we can observe that certain of the elements are more pronounced than others. In the Yarrow plant we see a strong relationship to the air in the feathery leaves and flowers, a fiery quality in the aromatic oils, a watery quality in its rapidly spreading rhizome roots, and an earthy quality in the strong structure of its woody stem. Compared to other plants, the elemental forces are exceptionally well-balanced in the Yarrow, with the water quality perhaps the least developed.

The forces working through the plant world encompass more than these four elemental qualities. Each of the chemical or nutritive constituents of a plant can be understood as a living *process*, as well as a chemical *substance*.

For example, the presence of a high percentage of potassium salt (potash) in the ash of Yarrow expresses what the alchemists call *sal*, a form-creating, earthy salt process evidenced in the strongly structured stem and roots. We know from chemical agriculture that physical potassium is used to strengthen stems and prolong the life of leaves. The extraordinary ability of Yarrow to build up a well-ordered structure, and to maintain it after having reached the stage of flowering, is testimony to formative powers of potassium. It creates a kind of "boundary" for the more cosmic, fiery forces which operate in the plant, as expressed in the aromatic oils, the feathery leaves, and brilliant light-filled inflorescence. Thus the Yarrow is able to balance the polarity of cosmic and earthly processes, thriving in the heat and light of the summer sun, while holding its earthly form strongly intact.

This understanding of the forces working through the plant has been applied in a very practical way in biodynamic agriculture, a form of organic agriculture initiated by Rudolf Steiner in 1924. Yarrow is part of the biodynamic preparations, which are applied to compost in order to enliven the soil. According to Steiner, the

Yarrow plant embodies such a remarkable balance of earthy and cosmic forces that it is able to sensitize the earth to receive quickening influences from the cosmos, and bring astral influences into the Earth in a harmonious way. This is a reflection of its effect on the human being, where Yarrow is used to strengthen weaknesses in the astral body.

Our goal in flower essence research is to become aware of these dynamic forces working through the plant, so that we can better understand how they relate to subtle properties within the human soul.

Herbal lore and medicinal uses

Besides the direct study of the plant itself, we can learn much from the accumulated human knowledge about plants, how they are used for food and medicine, and the qualities which have been attributed to them. There is a rich heritage of plant use in all traditional cultures of the earth, only a fraction of which has survived in herbal texts and reports from primitive peoples. This wisdom represents not only a long history of practical experience, but also remnants of perceptions from an earlier time in history when humankind had a clairvoyant experience of plants, through unconscious unity with the soul of Nature. Much of this oral knowledge was lost, or never recorded in written form. However, because it was a product of a pre-scientific awareness, there is much projection and inaccuracy mingled with true insight. Thus, while we can receive many clues from herbal lore of plants, it can never substitute for original and thorough spiritual scientific investigation of the essences.

Some herbal lore about the physical properties of plants has been scientifically verified; in fact, the medical pharmacopoeia earlier in this century included many herbal remedies. These medicinal properties of plants are important clues in understanding flower essences. As we described earlier, flower essence qualities often express a higher "octave" of the physical property, a parallel expression in the astral or etheric body of what the physical herb is doing in the physical body.

Yarrow is an example of an herb with an extensive history of medicinal uses and lore. One of Yarrow's folkloric names was Venus' Eyebrow, and the herb has been traditionally associated with the planet Venus, as reported by old herbalists like Culpeper. Soul qualities associated with Venus herbs include sensitivity, intuition, and compassion.

However, many plants encompass polar relationships, and this is certainly true of Yarrow. In addition to its Venusian nature, we also discern Mars-like qualities of strength and protection. Mars is associated with the "martial" arts, and Yarrow was carried into battle by soldiers as a talisman of protection. Yarrow was known by such names as "Soldier's Woundwort," "Knight's Milfoil," and "Herbe Militaris." Its botanical genus, *Achillea*, is reportedly named for the Greek warrior Achilles, who used it to heal his soldiers' wounds, but who himself was afflicted in his vulnerable heel.

Yarrow herb has the physical property of treating wounds by stanching bleeding, whether from outer injuries, internal hemorrhaging, or excessive menstrual flow. It was also believed to provide spiritual protection against one's enemies. Yarrow tea, made from the whole flowering plant except the roots, has been used traditionally for inducing sweating during colds and fevers, for indigestion and gastric inflammation, as an expectorant, and to relieve internal bleeding.

Modern chemical analysis also yields information about the properties of Yarrow, which confirm many of its traditional uses. The herb contains a bitter substance *achillein* which helps stimulate digestion, and also tannins and resins with wound-healing capacities. The essential oil is found throughout the plant, particularly in the flowers. It is blue-green and, like chamomile oil, contains *azulene*, which is a bitter, astringent principle, and *cineol*, which has antiseptic, expectorant, and stomachic attributes.

As we review the lore and herbal uses of Yarrow, we see several themes. Although it has releasing qualities in its expectorant and diaphoretic (sweat-inducing) properties, its strongest action seems to be its ability to create and hold form. This is expressed in its wound-healing and anti-hemorrhaging abilities, its astringent qualities and anti-inflammatory action. It also invigorates the fiery metabolic processes of digestion, demonstrating that its formative power is not static, but able to enter into a dynamic relationship with the mutable fire forces of life. Again we see Yarrow as an exceptionally *balanced* plant, with an outstanding capacity to integrate earthy and cosmic forces; it harmonizes the sensitivity of Venus with the strength and protection of Mars.

Botanical relationships

We can also learn much about a plant by considering its botanical classification, and its botanical relationship to other plants. The alchemical tradition teaches us to approach Nature as book written in a language whose meaning we can learn to decipher. With this background, we can then use the scientific discipline of botanical classification as an encyclopedic guide to the living forms we wish to understand.

Developed over two centuries ago by Linnaeus, our modern botanical system has established universally accepted nomenclature for the myriad species of life on Earth. Yet, there is more to the families, genera, and species of the Linnean system than a convenient method of keeping order, like the arrangement of books in a library. Botanical classification represents thousands of meticulous observations of Nature's life forms, noting which characteristics are similar, and which differentiate one plant or animal from another. Although few botanists are aware of the alchemical tradition, or even Goethe's research, the structures and forms they so carefully study are themselves expressions of the living processes working in plants, and provide clues to understanding their essential qualities. Flower essence research can thus avail itself of existing scientific systems such as botanical classification, and then infuse them with a sensitive understanding of soul messages which speak through the physical life forms and processes.

In our research, we have found that plants which are related botanically generally exhibit affinity in their flower essence qualities. The plant families, in particular, express broad archetypal properties, with members of each family representing variations on a common theme.

For example, Lily Family plants have minimally-rooted, watery bulbs. They are thus only loosely connected with the earth, holding their forces in a womb-like water of life. On the other hand, their star-shaped, typically hexagonal flowers reflect the pristine harmony of the celestial spheres. Flower essences from Lily Family plants, such as Star Tulip, Mariposa Lily, Easter Lily and Alpine Lily, generally work with the feminine, receptive aspects of the human soul, more akin to the harmony of the spiritual world, yet learning to face the challenges of earthly life.

Rose Family plants, in contrast, are strongly rooted and have flowers and fruits with five-fold geometry, representing the perfection of the human form (as in Leonardo da Vinci's

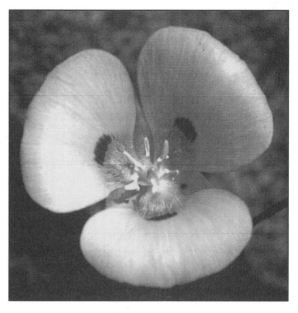

Mariposa Lily *Calochortus leichtlinii*

This delicate white and mauve wildflower is found in the mountains of western North America. Its tiny bulb grows in rocky crevices, barely attached to the earth. A member of the Lily Family, it has three cup-like petals, offset by three smaller sepals.

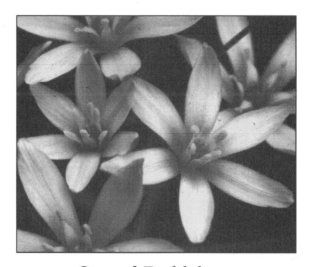

Star of Bethlehem
Ornithogalum umbellatum

Native to Europe and North Africa, the Star of Bethlehem is part of Dr. Bach's emergency combination formula. Its round bulb and perfect six-pointed star flower are typical of Lily Family plants that are related to the Onion (sometimes classified separately as the Amaryllis Family).

drawing of the star man with limbs outstretched). The Blackberry, Quince, and Rose plants, in particular, have long roots deeply anchored in the ground, thorn-covered stems, and vigorously-growing branches. These essences work with themes of incarnation, helping one to strongly take hold of life on Earth, and to bring forces of love, compassion, and commitment.

Yarrow is a member of the Compositae, or Sunflower family of Daisy-like flowers, whose essences generally deal with principles of synthesis or integration of the Self. Each composite flower is like a field of flowers in itself, containing many central disk florets, as well as petal-like ray florets. The Yarrow flower carries this principle of integration one step further, as its flower head is a tightly-organized cluster of many composite flowers, each of which is composed of ray and disk florets.

Although Sunflower family plants share a characteristic flower structure, the individual plant species exhibit a wide range of plant forms and gestures. In fact, each plant family is really a broad spectrum of

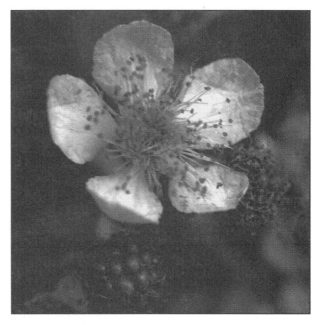

Blackberry *Rubus ursinus*

The wild blackberry has five-petaled flowers with numerous stamens, which are characteristic of Rose Family plants. Its prolific, thorny branches, dark black fruits, and tenacious roots are among the most intense expressions of this plant family.

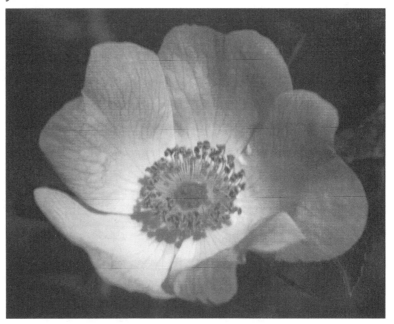

California Wild Rose *Rosa californica*

The delicate and sweetly fragrant pink blossoms of this wild rose are found on a vigorous shrub with sharp thorns and a deep, strong root system. Unlike more elaborate cultivated roses, it retains the simplicity of the five-petaled form.

qualities, or variations on a common theme. We see the Sunflower with its broad, rounded leaves and tall, radiant flower heads in contrast with the Star Thistle, with its narrow stem-hugging leaves, spiny thorns, and small clusters of tubular florets. Also within this plant family we have the contracted Tansy flowers, sometimes called "buttons" because they contain only disk florets (like the yellow centers of the daisy), contrasted with the Dandelion and Chicory, which contain only the ray florets.

The Yarrow is a particularly remarkable member of the Sunflower Family because in many ways it also resembles plants of the Umbelliferae, or Parsley family. With its umbel inflorescence, and its finely divided and aromatic leaves, penetrated by the light and air, Yarrow shares the qualities of openness and sensitivity of such Umbelliferae as Angelica, Dill, and Queen Anne's Lace. They have similar qualities of multiple branching in the finely-divided leaves and flower heads, strongly structured central stems, and aromatic qualities which penetrate into the leaves and stems. However, while these plants

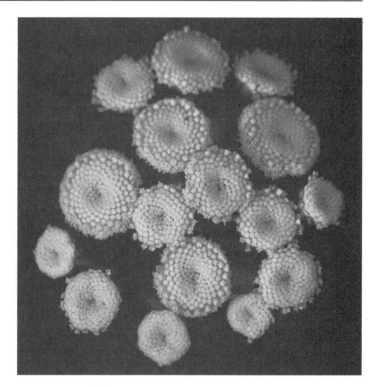

Tansy *Tanacetum vulgare*

This composite flower has only central disk florets, and thus resembles the center of a daisy, without any ray florets. The densely structured flower head gives an impression of compactness and containment.

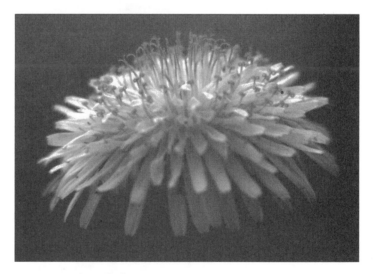

Dandelion *Taraxacum officinale*

Bursting into brilliant yellow blossoms in early spring, this composite flower has only ray florets. The stamens form the central structure; there are no disk florets. The expansive quality of the Dandelion is seen not only in the ray flowers, but also in the seed head which disperses easily into the wind.

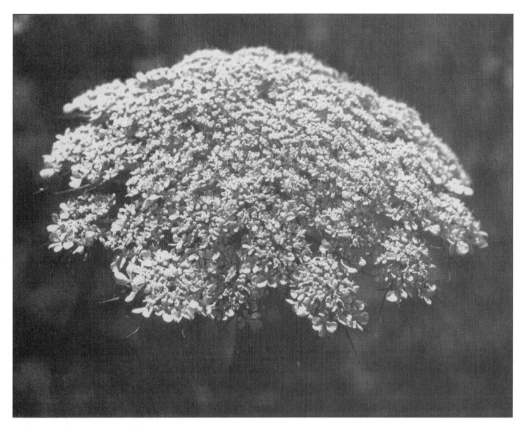

Queen Anne's Lace *Daucus carota*

This member of the Umbelliferae family has a canopy of white flowers and lacy leaves like the Yarrow. However, the individual flowers are simple and five-petaled, and thus distinguish this plant from the Yarrow's composite disk and ray florets.

have complex umbel flower heads like Yarrow, the individual flowers are quite simple, unlike the composite Yarrow flowers. Thus, we see that while botanical classification is an important guide to understanding plant gestures and signatures, we need also to consider relationships of form which cross botanical boundaries.

Within the broad themes of botanical families, plants which share the same *genus* have an even closer relationship in form. For example, the white Yarrow (*Achillea millefolium*), Pink Yarrow (*Achillea millefolium* var. *rubra*), and Golden Yarrow (*Achillea filipendulina*) are all members of the *Achillea* genus. Some other groups of essence plants in the *Repertory* which share the same genus are *Aesculus* (Chestnut Bud, Red Chestnut, White Chestnut); *Artemisia* (Mugwort, Sagebrush); *Calochortus* (Fairy Lantern, Mariposa Lily, Star Tulip, Yellow Star Tulip); *Dicentra* (Bleeding Heart, Golden Ear Drops); *Lilium* (Alpine Lily, Easter Lily, Tiger Lily); *Mimulus* (Mimulus, Pink Monkeyflower, Purple Monkeyflower, Scarlet Monkeyflower, Sticky Monkeyflower); *Penstemon* (Mountain Pride, Penstemon); and *Rosa* (California Wild Rose, Wild Rose). We invite the reader to examine the descriptions of these essences in Part III of the *Repertory*, to explore how the botanical relationships of these plants are expressed in flower essence qualities.

Within the Sunflower family, which is so large it encompasses 10% of all flowering plants, there is also an intermediate grouping of plants, known as the "tribe." For example, the genera *Cichorium* (Chicory) and *Taraxacum* (Dandelion), with their flowers of all rays, are in the *Cichorieae* tribe. The *Achillea* genus (Yarrow) belongs to the *Anthemideae* tribe, which also includes *Artemisia* (Mugwort, Sagebrush), *Anthemis* and *Matricaria* (Chamomile), *Tanacetum* (Tansy), and *Chrysanthemum* (Chrysanthemum, Shasta Daisy). We can see the relationship of Yarrow to plants within its tribe. It has finely divided leaves as Chamomile, and possesses strong aromatic oils like Mugwort and Sagebrush. The Golden Yarrow, in particular, strongly resembles the Tansy with its compact yellow, disc-only flowers and large, fern-like leaves.

Having gathered together all of these plant forms and relationships from our botanical studies, we have in effect assembled the various letters of the plant alphabet, and begun to arrange them into words. Our next step is discover the dynamic relationships among the words so we can create meaningful sentences to shape a "flower language."

Plant attunement

All of our plant observations and studies are important contributions to our understanding of the properties of a plant, but the whole is still more than the sum of its parts. As we begin to live with the plant on the many different levels which we have discussed, a higher relationship develops which builds from the sensory and mental understanding, gradually refining itself into *extra-sensory* and *meditative awareness*. In this way, we can begin to perceive the subtle energy fields of the plant, to hear its inner message or essence, and finally to experience the plant at a deep level of *being*. Such a path involves more than a brief mystical or psychic transmission; it is instead a grounded and very practical relationship with the plant, which begins in the physical dimension and only gradually becomes *meta-physical*.

Because this process of plant *attunement* is the result of a long and patient journey of discovery, it is really only possible here to give some indications, rather than a full description or "recipe." If it is to be precise, plant attunement must be built on a foundation of physical *observation*, along with the attentive contemplation and study we have already outlined. Next comes the stage of *imagination*, in which a inner image is formed of what is observed, and the image is allowed to metamorphose as it unfolds in time (e.g. the movement from seed to sprout and root, to leaf, bud, blossom, and fruit), or in its relationship to other plant forms. The next stage is one of *inspiration*, in which there is an inner listening to the qualities expressed in the previous process. Finally comes true *intuition*, which is a direct merging with the plant, in which the qualities of the plant are experienced as an inner reality.

Such plant attunement must be repeated again and again until one develops the sensitivity and clarity to understand its soul message. This exploration must become as flexible and fluid as the growth process of the plant itself. Only through such inner *metamorphic* activity can we understand the dynamic relationships of form and meaning which underlie the phenomena of life.

As an illustration of this process, let us recall the Yarrow plant, in which we observed the sensitive quality of its finely divided leaves and flowers, its strongly structured stem and roots, the aromatic oils, and the umbel of radiant white composite flowers. We recollect the strong form-building principle of the Yarrow, its sturdy stem, the well-structured flower head, and its ability to hold its form through the light and heat of summer. We can also think of Yarrow's use as a wound herb and talisman of protection, as well as the other qualities which our study has led us to consider. As we re-create the Yarrow in our imagination, we may see feathery wings floating sensitively in the air, with a strong, central axis of support, while a canopy of white light envelops us with qualities of clarity, inner strength, and openness.

Releasing the image and becoming inwardly quiet, we may hear or feel compassion and vulnerability, balanced by feelings of strength and protection. As we encounter the Yarrow inwardly, the polarities of sensitivity and strength seek integration within our soul. An image begins to emerge within our mind of the way Yarrow might work in the human soul.

These impressions from our Yarrow plant study have been developed and refined over the years, and tested against empirical results of people using Yarrow flower essence. From this research, a clear portrait of the Yarrow essence has evolved. *(A description of empirical research is presented in the following section.)*

Yarrow essence helps those who feel "vulnerable" (literally: "able to be wounded") to the influences of others and their environment. It "knits together" an overly-porous aura — the envelope of vital energy that surrounds and protects the body. Yarrow essence balances the overly sensitive Venusian qualities of the astral body with the grounded Mars-like strength and stability of physical and etheric forces. It encourages a healthy sense of Self, imparting strength, integrity, and clarity of consciousness typical of members of the Composite family.

Yarrow is particularly helpful for healers and counselors whose natural sympathy and compassion may cause them to "absorb" the tensions and problems of their clients. This essence is also widely indicated for persons suffering from many forms of psychic distress, hypersensitivity, pronounced allergic reactions, and persistent disturbances of the immune system. Yarrow facilitates the integrity and strength of a healthy ego structure, while enabling the soul to retain its innate sensitivity and receptivity. It is an extremely important essence in our time, due to the rapid pace of spiritual and psychic opening, occurring at the same time that environmental and social forces threaten to overwhelm, harden, or annihilate the sensitive capacities within the human soul.

The question often arises if the signature of a plant expresses the "problem" it addresses, or the quality which is the "solution" to the problem. This recalls our earlier discussion of similars, contraries, and the *Union of Opposites*. Remembering that flower essences embody a *polarity* of opposites, it becomes understandable that the physical plant form may express one or the other — or both — sides of the polarity. In the Yarrow we experience soul sensitivity in the plant's openness to the light and air in its finely divided leaves and volatile oils; but we also feel the strength and stability of its form, the sense of protection of its white umbel, and the integrity of the Self that characterizes the Compositae. Yarrow thus integrates within its form both sides of this polarity.

Our testing of the Pink Yarrow and Golden Yarrow essences in comparison with the Yarrow has also confirmed how variations in color and form are expressed in the flower essence qualities of these botanically-related plants. Pink Yarrow is *Achillea millefolium* var. *rubra*, a variety of the common Yarrow, *Achillea millefolium*. We recall that it is similar in form to the white Yarrow, but its characteristic deep pink-magenta flowers suggest a more emotional quality than the pure white Yarrow flowers. Pink Yarrow essence is used in situations of excessive emotional sensitivity, when we absorb the emotions of others, or allow our soul's astrality to "bleed" and merge with others.

Golden Yarrow is a different species of the *Achillea* genus, *Achillea filipendulina*. It is larger, with stronger fern-like leaves, compared to the other Yarrows. Its golden flower head is more tightly-knit, and the flowers have only the central disk florets, resembling the Tansy. Yet, unlike the Tansy plant which collapses as it flowers, Golden Yarrow has the characteristic Yarrow form-holding quality, and is less pungent.

We can now develop an image of the polarities with which Golden Yarrow works. The compact flower structure and stability of form expresses an inwardizing gesture; while the open leaf structure and the brilliant golden-yellow color of the flowers suggest an outward-radiating quality. The Golden Yarrow essence integrates the polarities of introversion and extroversion, as well as those of sensitivity and protective strength. It is often indicated for artists and performers whose creative sensitivity make them overly vulnerable in their very public roles.

There is one more Yarrow essence in the *Repertory*, Yarrow Special Formula, which is distinguished not by the plant species used, but in the preparation method. This formula was specifically devised at the request of European practitioners after the Chernobyl nuclear power plant disaster in 1986 to counteract the effects of radiation on the human etheric body. Radioactivity, which is the destruction of the physical structure of matter at an atomic level, is the very antithesis of the etheric formative forces which build up living structures. Yarrow contains potassium salts which help it maintain the integrity of its own structure. To augment this strong form-enhancing *sal* process, the Yarrow Special Formula is specially potentized from *Achillea millefolium* blossoms in a base of sea-salt water. Thus the Yarrow Special Formula strengthens and maintains the etheric formative forces which give strength and integrity to the human aura. While not a substitute for medical care, it is able to counteract the disruptive effects of radiation on human energy fields, whether from nuclear fallout, X-rays, televisions, computer monitors, electromagnetic fields, or other environmental hazards of contemporary life.

While it is not possible in this overview to present complete portraits of all the essence plants in the *Repertory*, we offer these few examples of the methods we have used in our plant studies. We do this not only to provide a small window into our field work with plants, but also with the hope that others will be inspired to join in the still embryonic work of developing a living science which can comprehend the forms and processes of Nature as a language which speaks to the human soul.

Such flower essence research requires a truly interdisciplinary investigation. It involves elements of a number of fields of study, including agriculture, astrology, astronomy, biology, botany, chemistry, ecology, geology, geomancy, herbology, mathematics (especially geometry), medicine, meteorology, nutrition, philosophy, physics, psychology, sociology, and artistic expressions such as poetry, painting, and music. In addition to these "outer" studies, self-knowledge and inner development is required for flower essence study. Only a broad collaborative effort which bridges traditional boundaries between specialized branches of knowledge can encompass the full meaning of flower essence research.

Clinical Studies of Flower Essences

Case studies

How can we be certain that our plant studies yield accurate descriptions of flower essence qualities? No matter how sincerely we may strive for clarity, setting aside pre-conceptions and biases, the fact remains that human beings are fallible. Particularly with such a pioneering discipline as researching the soul messages of flowers, the possibilities are great for error or distortion. If we are to carry the spirit of science into our work, we must develop a process of systematic verification of the insights we receive from our plant studies.

The primary means for verification of flower essence qualities is the collection of case reports from practitioners and users of flower essences who document their experiences. Although such "anecdotal evidence" may be discounted by strict science, it serves as a valuable source of information. In fact, this empirical (experience-based) approach is not only the most common form of flower essence research, it is also the sole basis by which homeopathic medicine has been verified for the last two centuries.

Just as the flower essence preparer needs to become a field scientist, making careful observation of flower essence plants, seeing how the individual parts form an expression of a whole; so also the flower essence practitioner needs to hone his or her skills as a scientific observer, starting with basic physical observations of the client such as voice intonation, body language, facial expression, and physical symptoms. A living picture of the evolving person can then be created, including the life story, aspirations and challenges, as well as thoughts and feelings. Like the plant which is observed again and again in various stages of growth, the soul also journeys through time, and its progress needs periodic review. Thus, the most successful case studies are longitudinal ones which extend over a number of months, incorporating several flower essence combinations and cycles of soul growth.

All practitioners can observe and document the effects of flower essences on their clients, gradually cultivating the discipline of scientific observation. This is a fundamental skill necessary for becoming adept in the selection of flower essences and evaluating the results of one's choices. It is essential to perceive and record the effects of the essences in order to support and guide the client's development. Often clients will forget from one visit to the next a troubling issue or painful situation which is no longer pressing. Good case notes enable the practitioner to remind the client of the progress which has been made, or to re-examine issues which are still challenging.

Skillful observation and record-keeping are also essential for the collection of empirical data which builds upon the established body of flower essence research, and reports or verifies new insights about essence qualities and effects. Any one case may seem insignificant or inconclusive, since case reports are of necessity filtered through the perceptive abilities of both the practitioner and the subject. However, with enough care and a large enough pool of data, we can gradually discern a pattern in how a particular essence works.

Empirical research is dramatically amplified when cases can be shared and cross-referenced from many sources. For this purpose, the Flower Essence Society has developed case study forms which cover the most significant aspects of flower essence therapy. These case studies are organized and entered into our computer data base, which is cross-indexed for a wide variety of therapeutic phenomena. Some of the most valuable case studies have been submitted for the FES Practitioner Certification Program, which follows the FES Practitioner Training Program. Candidates for certification are graduates of the training program who then go on to complete at least three in-depth cases and a related paper, demonstrating their record-keeping and observational skills. The cumulative weight of these cases and others submitted by numerous practitioners throughout the world, along with in-depth interviews and other surveys, form the backbone of our empirical understanding of flower essence qualities. This data can also be the basis for designing further studies which meet professional standards of scientific rigor.

Controlled clinical studies

The conventional standard for scientific verification of the efficacy of remedies involves controlled studies with placebos and double-blind procedures. As described earlier, in such studies two or more groups are tested, at least one with an inert placebo, and one or more with the substances to be tested. The procedure is "double-blind" because neither the test subjects nor those administering the tests know which group has the placebo and which has the remedy being tested.

Rigorous double-blind studies have yet to be conducted with flower essences, partly because of lack of funding and interest in the scientific community, but also because of certain procedural problems which arise. Most controlled tests administer a standard remedy or remedy combination to each person in the test group. These persons are usually selected because they suffer from the same illness or set of symptoms. However, flower essences are typically selected specifically for each individual, as a result of an interview by the practitioner. People with the same physical or emotional symptoms may need very different essences; for example, there are many essences for various kinds of depression. Thus, a particular flower essence combination may not be beneficial for most of the individuals in the test group, not because the essences themselves are ineffective, but because that combination would not contain the most appropriate and efficacious essences for each person. Thus, it remains challenging to prove the validity of flower essences for a random group, as generally required for double-blind tests.

Another dilemma involves developing testing and evaluation procedures and questionnaires which meet professional standards, yet which are also appropriate to the emotional and psycho-spiritual changes typical of flower essence use. Many psychological tests are geared to symptomatic alterations, and may not detect more subtle long-term soul growth. There is an inherent tension between the requirement of conventional scientific methodology for results which are *quantitatively* measurable, and the need for skillful evaluation of the *qualitative* experiences which characterize flower essence use. The Flower Essence Society is ready to assist any potential researchers and organizations in designing rigorous scientific studies which will successfully meet the criteria necessary for professional acceptance while remaining appropriate to the nature of flower essence phenomena.

Controlled studies can be important in communicating the value and validity of flower essences to professional and regulatory authorities, and can make a real contribution to knowledge of flower essence phenomena. However, such testing methods may be limited in their ability to truly assess and measure in-depth changes in human feeling and consciousness. Therefore, the path of spiritual scientific research for flower essence therapy can and must always depend on the trained perception skills of the practitioner who actively works with humans or other living beings in a therapeutic setting.

Research on Subtle Energy Phenomena

The challenge of studying vibrational remedies

Besides controlled studies, the other conventional method for authenticating health remedies is to study their constituents and their mode of operation in the human organism. This is a great challenge in the case of flower essences, because they are *vibrational* in nature. When one turns to a study of the actual substance of flower essences, biochemical analysis yields no meaningful results. The physical ingredients of the essences — water, alcohol, and an extremely dilute infusion of the flowers — cannot explain their beneficial effects. Their action lies in subtle forces not directly perceptible to physical senses, and thus not measurable by any physical apparatus.

Consequently, the authenticity of subtle remedies cannot be determined by typical scientific studies based on mechanistic paradigms which ignore the existence of force fields beyond the physical dimension. This limitation has both philosophical and medical implications, and very real legal and social consequences. Vibrational remedies such as flower essences and homeopathic remedies may be rejected by professional and regulatory agencies not because they lack effectiveness, but because these substances cannot be tested by methodologies which are designed for bio-chemically based medicines. Thus for flower essence therapy to gain wider acceptance, and for practitioners to have soundly based knowledge of subtle plant remedies, it is essential to develop new methods for perceiving and testing plant qualities.

We need to find methods which can bridge the gap between conventional scientific experimentation, whose materialistic premises exclude subtle energy phenomena, and purely spiritual research methods, which depend solely on the consciousness of the investigator. Such intermediary methods do not substitute for the honing of our own observational and perceptive skills in the physical world and in other dimensions. However, these research techniques are potentially important both as demonstrations to those who question the reality of flower essences, and as ways of testing and clarifying the insights derived from direct spiritual research.

Detecting subtle energies

Preliminary work has been done with several research techniques which investigate various quantifiable physical phenomena indicating the presence of subtle energy fields. Like tracking an invisible person through the snow by following his footprints, such methods are a way of perceiving the *effects* of invisible forces on sense-perceptible phenomena. These effects can then be observed, measured, and interpreted according to conventional scientific standards. Studying the physical effects of the invisible is exactly the procedure used in sub-atomic physics to study phenomena which are hidden to both the human senses and scientific instruments.

Sensitive crystallization

Sensitive crystallization is a subtle-energy testing method in which various organic substances are added to a copper chloride solution to produce distinctive crystallization patterns according to the nature of the substance. This method was pioneered by the late Dr. Ehrenfried Pfeiffer, a scientist who was a student of Rudolf Steiner, and one of the developers of biodynamic agriculture in North America. Pfeiffer was able to use the sensitive crystallization method to investigate plant saps and juices, as an indication of the vitality of the plant. He also worked with samples of human fluids such as blood, and was able to use sensitive crystallization for early detection of various diseases. This was possible because the crystallization patterns were apparently influenced not simply by the physical structure of the substance in the solution, but also by its etheric forces, the field of vital energy which indicates a state of health or disease before it manifests in the physical body.

Pfeiffer's ability to interpret the meaning of the copper chloride crystallization patterns was based on many years of exacting research, in which he examined hundreds of tests of plant extracts and human blood. He was then able to develop a language of form which could reliably indicate something about the substance being tested. Unfortunately, Pfeiffer's method does not seem sensitive enough to register vibrational remedies.

A new, more sensitive method has been developed by a researcher in Europe, which appears capable of differentiating between various homeopathic remedies and flower essences. However, compared to Pfeiffer's work, this research is still in a very preliminary stage. Not enough tests have been completed at this time to confirm whether the variations in crystallization patterns are due to the properties of the remedies themselves, or myriad other variables such as environmental influences or laboratory procedures.

If it can be established by further testing that each flower essence produces a distinct and recognizable pattern, then we may have important evidence that each flower essence carries a particular energetic pattern, a fact which cannot be demonstrated by conventional chemical analysis. Even if this is done, we will still have much more research to do before being able to use sensitive crystallization to yield any significant information about the properties of flower essences. We will need to create a sufficient quantity of data so that crystallization patterns can be correlated with flower essence qualities. Until this patient, methodical work is done, we will have no basis for interpreting the "language" of the crystallization patterns.

Kirlian photography

Another method for demonstrating life energy fields is that of Kirlian photography, named for the Russian researchers Semyon and Valentina Kirlian, who used high-voltage electrical charges to create visible photographic images of plant or human energy fields. Although etheric forces are not the same as electrical or magnetic forces, etheric energies do seem to be able to influence electromagnetic fields. Again, this is a situation of subtle energies leaving their "footprints" in the physical world.

Kirlian photography was popularized in the 1970's by Sheila Ostrander and Lynn Schroeder's book, *Psychic Discoveries Behind the Iron Curtain,* and *The Kirlian Aura,* edited by Stanley Krippner and Daniel Rubin, which featured the famous "phantom" cut leaf on the cover. Because of difficulties in obtaining verifiable and repeatable results, interest in this methodology has waned in recent years. Nonetheless, some promising preliminary results have been obtained by researchers who have taken Kirlian photographs of flower essence bottles, as well as of the finger tips of people who have taken various essences. While these experiments apparently indicate distinctive photographic patterns for each essence, we caution that much more testing will be necessary to confirm these findings, and to be able to interpret what these patterns may indicate about flower essence properties.

Just as Pfeiffer needed to repeat his experiments many times in order to establish the exact correlations between crystallization patterns and their indications, so flower essence research using techniques such as those mentioned above will require results which can be independently duplicated by different laboratories and definitively correlated with particular essences. The Flower Essence Society encourages researchers to continue to develop sensitive crystallization and Kirlian photography as tools for flower essence research.

There are also many other techniques utilizing physical measurement of the effects of subtle energies which hold promise for flower essence research. Some of these are briefly summarized below, with the hope that potential researchers will be inspired to investigate these areas.

Plant geometry and celestial patterns

Lawrence Edwards, a Scottish mathematician, has studied the geometric relationship of plant forms to the forces which shape plant growth. Early research in this area has indicated the correlation of these forces with the orbital movements of the moon and planets. Further documentation of these correspondences may help to verify the folkloric associations of plants with planetary influences, and their related properties.

Effects on plant growth

Some homeopathic remedies have been tested by measuring their effects on plant growth. This method could be applied to flower essences, with the realization that such a study would be limited to demonstrating the effects of flower essences on physical and etheric vitality. However, such tests would not address the essence's impact on the mental and emotional life of the human being.

Testing devices

Some practitioners use diagnostic devices which measure the relative disturbance of various meridians and organ systems. Other practitioners use direct methods, such as pulse diagnosis. Clinical experience shows that flower essences will balance certain disturbances. Research may be able to establish consistent patterns as verified by these diagnostic procedures. While such measures may not indicate the full dimensions of long-term soul transformation possible with flower essence therapy, they may at least confirm that some real short-term change has taken place in the energy fields of the person.

Capillary dynamolysis

The method of capillary dynamolysis, also known as chromatography, was inspired by Rudolf Steiner and developed by Lilly and Eugen Kolisko early in this century. The Kolisko method involves combining a plant extract with a metallic salt such as silver nitrate, and allowing it to rise vertically in a cylinder of filter paper. A pattern or picture is formed which is an indication of the forces at work in the extract. Plant extracts have been tested to verify the vitality of medicinal and food plants, and human fluids have been tested to detect disease states. It is possible that this technique, heretofore used with physical extracts, might be adapted to indicate some properties of potentized remedies such as flower essences.

Water drop technique

The water drop technique, developed by Theodor Schwenk, is another way of making etheric forces visible. It has been used to test the vitality of drinking water or other liquids by observing the wave patterns produced as a series of water drops impact the surface of a liquid. A similar method may be developed which can indicate the vibrational changes in water which take place as a result of it being potentized with a flower essence.

The techniques described above may need further refinement and organization in order to detect the range of effects produced by flower essences. The Flower Essence Society is highly interested in promoting and encouraging research using testing methods which detect the presence of subtle energy fields in flower essences. We have taken some initial steps to begin this research, and enthusiastically welcome the participation or added suggestions of other practitioners and researchers.

The Flower Essence Society
Research Program

It is clear that scientific investigation is still the predominant test of truth in our culture, and thus a prerequisite for the acceptance of the reality of flower essences by the general public as well as professional and governmental authorities. However, even among those who are convinced of the efficacy of flower essences through their own experience, scientific research on the essences is just as important to clarify one's knowledge of the qualities of the essences and the principles by which they work.

Although much has been done, we consider that our sixteen years of efforts in flower essence research are only a modest beginning. We urge readers to consider participating in the FES Research Program through any of a number of options, including:

1. Thorough documentation of client or home-care use of flower essences. This is the foundation of all flower essence knowledge, and we encourage every practitioner and user of flower essences to be involved in this level of research. FES will supply case study forms upon request.

2. Sharing insights and observations about various essences you have used with yourself or others. This involves keeping general notes and looking for over-all trends and patterns in your use of flower essences.

3. Developing controlled clinical studies of flower essences.

4. Studies in subtle plant properties based on the principles of spiritual science.

5. Developing research in detecting, analyzing, and interpreting the presence of subtle forces within flower essences.

To assist you in participating in the FES Research Program, we invite you to fill out and return the reporting form found inside the back cover. If your *Repertory* no longer has a form, we will gladly supply you with a new one.

Chapter 3:
How Are Flower Essences Selected?

When we first discover the essences, it is a common experience to feel overwhelmed by having so many possibilities. How can we choose the most appropriate essences for ourselves, friends, or clients? Whether in a home health care or clinical setting, the key elements are the same. We must know ourselves or those whom we are helping, and we must learn the soul language of the flower essences.

Identifying the Main Issues

Creating a dialogue

The first step in a selection process is to identify the key soul issues. This is best done through dialogue — conversation with others, or an inner examination which helps us contact our deepest feelings. In both cases, success in choosing appropriate essences is dependent on our ability to be honest and open about ourselves.

Sometimes, the soul issues with which we need to work are readily apparent. More frequently, identifying these issues takes some exploration. We may begin with a general sense of malaise, but not be able to distinguish specific problems. We may be more aware of physical distress, and need to see the inner message of our symptoms. We may experience frustration or overwhelm, but lack insight into the underlying causes.

The development of awareness in the self-reflection or counseling process can be aided by a process of questioning. Several good beginning questions to ask are: "What is my life purpose, and how is this purpose reflected in my daily work? What is my next step in life? How do I feel about my relationship with others? What lessons am I learning right now?" The questioning process itself contributes to an inner, meditative attitude, so that one can begin to see the soul life more effectively and choose priorities of development.

The importance of asking questions is illustrated by the story of Parzival's quest for the Holy Grail. He enters the castle of the ailing Fisher King, but because he neglects to ask the question, "Brother, what ails thee?" he misses the opportunity to be an agent of healing. The king has the Grail, but he cannot partake of its power until the question is asked. The ability to listen, observe, and ask questions is fundamental to every flower essence selection process.

Soul issues — past, present, and future

It is helpful to consider the development of soul issues in the light of past experiences, in relation to our present circumstances, and in terms of their influence on the future. Childhood emotional experiences or any significant episodes in past phases of life can be keys to understanding our current feelings and reactions. By bringing these often-repressed parts of our personal history into the light of consciousness, it is possible to identify the attitudes and emotional patterns which are underlying current life challenges. Such issues may involve experiences of abandonment, neglect, or abuse; they may include our response to parental or societal expectations, or deep feelings of anger, despair, or grief which the soul carries from the earliest moments of incarnation.

It is equally important to review the soul life in present time, particularly to examine the crucial areas of work and personal relationships. If we take an honest inventory of these two key areas of our life, it is likely we will discover a wealth of soul issues which deserve attention.

Besides evaluating the problems and challenges from the past and present, it is vital to consider future goals. We can ask questions such as, "How would I like my life to be in five (or ten) years? What inner potentials would I like to bring forward and develop in my life? What obstacles lie in the way of the realization of my goals?" Such questions allow us to identify those issues which can lead soul development forward toward its greater destiny.

Each person's biography chronicles a unique journey of the soul. By sensitive listening we can discern not only the particular complaints or problems of the moment, but also intuit the whole stream of life destiny, as it surges out of the past, flows through the present moment, and courses towards its future possibility.

Selecting Appropriate Essences

Learning the flower essences

Once the main soul issues have been determined, the next step is to select flower essences which best address these issues. Although the number of flower essences may seem daunting, it is possible to gradually familiarize ourselves with their qualities, beginning with those to which we are most attracted. We can read about the psychological profiles associated with the essences, and reflect on these descriptions in terms of what we know of ourselves and others.

In addition, it can be quite helpful to learn something of the plants themselves, which are the sources of the essences. Looking at a picture of the flower, growing it in a garden or finding it in the wild, can greatly deepen our relationship with the soul message of that plant. It is also very beneficial to use pictures of the essence plants to aid in the selection process. Often, the plants to which we are drawn have special significance. Apart from a knowledge of specific plants, our general willingness to experience the natural world, and especially the wonder and mystery of plant life, can open a vessel within the soul to receive the healing messages of the flowers.

The bi-polar nature of flower essences

As we become familiar with the properties of various essences, we discover that they encompass a wide range of human qualities, many of which seem contradictory. For example, there are essences such as Manzanita or California Wild Rose for coming into a closer relationship with the physical world. However, essences such as Angel's Trumpet or Chrysanthemum help release the soul from its earthly connection. Goldenrod helps us distinguish ourselves from a group identity, while Quaking Grass harmonizes individual will within a common group purpose. With such apparently paradoxical indications, how do we know in which direction to proceed?

The solution to this dilemma is that there is no pre-set answer. Each individual must strive for balance, strengthening those qualities which are weak or blocked, and moderating that which is excessive. Thus, an overly spiritualized person with too little connection with the body may need grounding essences like Manzanita or Clematis, while someone deeply enmeshed in the material world may need uplifting or sensitizing essences such as Hound's Tongue or Star Tulip. The goal is to liberate the unique potential within each person, rather than attempting to follow an external model of how we should be.

As we strive for soul equanimity, we also learn that balance is not static. It is an ever-shifting, spiral path of evolution. Each issue successfully addressed leads us to a new challenge. Thus, while at one time essences such as Centaury or Buttercup may be required to develop a strong sense of selfhood, at another time Chicory or Heather may be indicated to overcome a selfish tendency or excessive preoccupation with one's personal problems.

Soul polarities can also be found within the attributes of an individual essence. For example, Sunflower assists the person with an overbearing ego, and it also helps the self-effacing person to find a stronger ego identity. Sticky Monkeyflower helps those who are over-active sexually, as well as those who fear sexual intimacy, assisting in both cases to bring sexual integration and balance.

Furthermore, the bi-polar nature of an essence is expressed in its working with both the "problem" and the "solution" of an issue. We may choose Morning Glory to overcome addictive habits, or out of a desire to enhance our feelings of vitality. Sweet Pea may be suggested for our lack of rootedness, or we may be aware of a desire to find community. The "negative" and "positive" aspects of these issues are like two sides of a coin. When choosing essences it is helpful to switch back and forth from one perspective to the other in order to gain a fuller picture of how essence qualities can speak to us. In doing so, we are engaging the alchemical process of the *Union of Opposites* within our psyche.

Combining Flower Essences

It is possible, and often desirable, to combine several flower essences together in a personal formula. The effect of the combination of essences can be greater than any individual essence, if they balance and enhance each other.

How many essences can be used?

How many essences can be used in one combination? Indeed, it seems at times that we need all of them! However, it is important to remember that soul growth takes place gradually and progressively. It is best to focus on key issues, keeping in mind that the flowers work as catalysts which stimulate a whole process of change; when major issues shift, other minor or accompanying problems may also be transformed.

Therefore, it is best not to combine too many essences at one time, as this may confuse or unnecessarily overwhelm the psyche. Although absolute numbers cannot be given, practitioners report that the most common levels are three to six essences at one time. Experienced practitioners may be able to artfully combine and structure flower essence formulas with higher numbers of essences which work synergistically. However, for really key issues, it may be best to use only one central essence which can speak in a more archetypal way to the core part of the personality.

We can think of the repertory of flower essences as an artist's palette of colors. Combining several essences can produce some very beautiful hues. Mixing too many colors unskillfully creates a "muddy" result, without any clarity. The soul is our artist's canvas. It takes patience and practice to use the essence "colors" wisely. While guidelines can be given, there are no shortcuts to developing the *art* of flower essence combination.

Principles of flower essence combining

Flower essence formulating requires practice in order to develop skill. However, there are some basic principles which can provide a starting point. The easiest way to combine essences is to choose those in close *affinity* with a single issue, creating unity and focus in the formula. (This is particularly important when emotional chaos and confusion predominates.) For example, Wild Oat, Larch, and Blackberry might be chosen to help deal with issues of self-actualization in one's career. A mix of Golden Ear Drops, Pink Monkeyflower, and Mariposa Lily could be used to address feelings of vulnerability and abandonment from childhood.

Another more challenging principle is to work with *polarity*, choosing essences for contrasting aspects of soul work. For instance, Sunflower and Star Tulip in a formula would address the balance of the inner masculine and feminine. A combination of Yellow Star Tulip and Pink Yarrow would help someone who needs to address issues of sensitivity and compassion, while resolving inappropriate emotional merging. Polar formulas work to bring out inherent tensions in the soul, helping to resolve oppositions and bring them to higher resolution. They are usually more dynamic, and require more skill in selection and follow-up counseling.

Essences can also be added to a combination to *regulate* the speed and rhythm with which the other essences work, or to *balance and tone* their effects. For example, essences such as Black-Eyed Susan or Cayenne may be used to stimulate awareness or action for someone who is in denial or stuck. Essences such as Self-Heal or Yerba Santa can give strength and comfort for someone working with particularly challenging issues.

Another way to adjust the effects of a combination is to vary the frequency of the dosage. Taking the essences at short intervals, such as every hour, will intensify their effects, while stretching out the dosages to once or twice a day generally makes the effects more gentle and gradual.

As we become more skilled in flower essences selection, we can apply the basic principles of either affinity or polarity to include other elements which work as integrating factors in the flower essence formula. These may include color, botanical relationships, thematic structures such as past, present, and future, or basic geometric configurations. The art of successfully combining and structuring flower essence formulas is one which can be progressively developed, as we acquire insight into the qualities and dynamics of the essences.

Sometimes it is not possible to develop a single formula to address all of the major soul issues without overloading the combination. In these cases, it is best to work sequentially, starting with one combination to address a constellation of issues, and developing other formulas as needed. For those who are quite skilled in flower essence use, it is possible to use one or more formulas for different situations. For example, we might have one combination we take in the morning and during our work day to address the way we act in the world, and another for at home during evening hours to sensitize us to our feelings and relationships.

Adjusting the combination

The essence combination needs to be evaluated and adjusted as cyclical transformation occurs; quite often the original essences are still needed, with perhaps a new one added and another deleted. At other times a whole new set of essences may be indicated. However, it is best to avoid constant changes in the formula, as this creates confusion and lack of continuity in the soul's healing process. It is important to gain a living imagination of how the essences are working, and how the changes can be gradually and subtly enhanced through the artful metamorphosis of a flower essence combination.

Pre-mixed combinations

Many practitioners report using key combinations of essences for initial breakthrough or entry-level work in flower essence therapy. If such formulas are skillfully combined and structured, they have the capacity to address broad themes or emotional *miasms* which may need to be cleared before specific developmental work is undertaken.

However, we should bear in mind that flower essence therapy ultimately addresses the unique aspects of each person's situation. Generally speaking, flower essence selection must take into consideration each individual's history, goals, strengths, weaknesses, relationships, work, and life experiences, to facilitate the full transformational process.

Working with Essences on Different Levels

Type essences for life lesson and life purpose

One of the most important aims in flower essence work is to discern the major archetypal issue for one's life, and then find a single flower essence, a *type remedy*, which can address this. An analogy can be made to the *constitutional remedy* in homeopathic practice, although it is possible for someone to have more than one flower essence type remedy in the course of a lifetime.

The type remedy is used to address both our *life lesson* and *life purpose*. The life lesson is a deep soul issue which is a recurring theme in our lives. Usually it will be connected to an experience of emotional wounding in childhood, or a challenge we brought with us into this life; it will color our experience at each stage of development. If the *life lesson* is what we bring from our past, then our *life purpose* is what orients us toward the future. It is our destiny, the inner calling our soul feels to manifest its full potential in the world, and to serve others.

Life lesson and life purpose are closely intertwined, for it is often by mastering our life lesson that we are able to fulfill our life purpose. Our ability to heal or serve others generally grows out of the experience of our own wounding (the arche-type of the *wounded healer*). Thus there is often one essence which works with both life lesson and life purpose. However, in some cases it may be necessary to use a different essence for each, at least until it becomes clear how these two aspects work together.

Although it may take some time to reach the clarity of a single archetypal essence, it is nonetheless beneficial to consider the issues of life lesson and life purpose and some possible essences as type remedies. Such essences serve as "anchors" in flower essence formulas, to which we can return periodically while we address other issues. Through such an approach we set our sights on long-term soul development, rather than becoming preoccupied with transient moods and disturbances which may erupt from day to day.

Which flower essences can be type remedies? In truth, any flower essence can be a type remedy, if it is used for deep-seated, long-term patterns. The profound soul healing which is possible through the wise use of a type remedy requires a willingness to deeply examine core issues, skill in selecting the appropriate essence, and a commitment to long-term use.

Short-term use of flower essences

Although it is important to keep such archetypal use of flower essences as an ultimate goal, it is useful and often necessary to use essences for short-term and immediate situations. The descriptions of the life lessons associated with each essence, written from a more archetypal level in Part III of the *Repertory*, need to be flexibly interpreted in light of such use.

For example, as a type essence Echinacea may be chosen by someone whose sense of selfhood has been totally devastated by a lifetime of violent abuse. However, this essence could be used in much less drastic situations, such as bolstering self-esteem after becoming unemployed. As a type essence, Manzanita corrects a deep aversion of the soul to the body and to physical matter, often the result of an overly strict religious or cultural belief system. However, this essence can also be used during pregnancy, to bring more acceptance of the changes in the woman's physical body, and to embrace the new life which is incarnating through her. While Lavender as a type essence helps the high-strung, nervous personality, it might be added to a bath (along with Lavender oil) to help us relax and get ready for sleep after a particularly stressful day.

Thus, flower essences can apply to a wide spectrum of situations, from life-long challenges to day-to-day struggles. However, it would be inappropriate to use essences to "fix" every feeling or mood we experience in the course of the day or week. These surface feelings are quite changeable and ephemeral, and can distract us from the opportunity to do deeper soul work. In general, it is best to pay less attention to the fluctuating waves on the surface, and put our focus on the deeper flowing currents of the feeling life.

Special Selection Situations

Sharing the essences with others

When first discovering flower essences there is often a strong temptation, born of one's own enthusiasm, to try the essences with people we know and care about whether they want them or not. It should be remembered that, with adults, some conscious participation in the healing journey is necessary to gain real benefit from the essences. It is certainly appropriate to share our enthusiasm and experiences with others, and encourage them to discover flower essences. But we must then wait for their response, their choice to participate, or accept that they choose not to do so. It is intrusive and unethical to give flower essences to people without their knowledge. This is a violation of their free will, and can lead to emotional distress for which they are not prepared if unconscious feelings are stirred up without any understanding of what is happening. It is also ineffective to give essences to a person who has begrudgingly agreed to take them to please us, or to please a family member. Unless there is an inner openness to the flower essences, we cannot expect someone to be willing to examine painful feelings or make difficult changes.

Children

Because children have not yet developed the ego structure or self-awareness of adults, it is appropriate for parents or other care-takers to choose essences for them. Nonetheless, it is helpful to engage children as much as possible in the selection and use of the essences. Children are usually quite willing to take their "flower drops," and will often remind parents when it is time for more. Because their conceptual abilities are still undeveloped, it is not necessary to explain in detail to young children the emotional issues related to each essence. It is more appropriate to say something like "The flower drops will help you feel better," or "We're giving you some flower drops to help you relax and fall asleep at night."

In order to select essences for children, we need a variety of methods to discern the issues with which they are struggling. One very successful method is to have the child do a drawing, and then tell the story associated with the picture. A number of child therapists use Jungian sand play therapy as a way of engaging the child in an activity which expresses deeper layers of the psyche. Of course, it is helpful to talk directly with the child, as well as with parents, other family members, and teachers, in order to gain a fuller understanding of the child's situation. Yet these conversations should not substitute for the skillful observation of what the child reveals directly through art, play, body language, voice tone, and behavior.

Often the conflicts the child experiences are reflections of deeper tension and struggle in the family system. It is important to consider if there is marital conflict or a broken family, violence or substance abuse, a pattern of emotional repression and dishonesty, or a parental expectations for the child to fulfill unmet needs. The ideal situation is for the whole family to examine its issues through flower essence therapy. If the family is not open to the essences, an effort should be made at least to involve family members in counseling or discussion of conflicts which may be affecting the child.

Animals

Flower essences are used very successfully with animals, both in home care and by professional veterinarians. In these cases the selection process must be modified. The person selecting the essences must know the animal well enough to be able to identify its emotional moods and attitudes. With animals, the soul expresses itself in behaviors, so that a horse that kicks, a cat that scratches, a dog that growls, are all demonstrations of particular feelings. It is important, of course, to distinguish what is natural and instinctive in an animal, and what is excessive and out of balance. The art of selecting the essences consists of interpreting the essence qualities in terms of the animal's experience and soul states. We can be successful to the extent that we can empathize with an animal as a living being, rather than merely as an object to meet human needs. Some helpful suggestions may be found in Part II of the *Repertory*, under the category "Animals and Animal Care."

Animals, and particularly domestic pets, respond strongly to the influence of the people who care for them. Therefore, when giving essences to an animal, it is quite helpful to select essences for the human caretaker as well, if the person is willing to examine how his or her own attitudes and feelings may be impacting on the animal.

Home and Professional Use

Home, self-care, and informal use

Dr. Bach intended flower essences to be simple and safe method of home care, and in many ways this is true. The essences can become an integral part of a family home-health program, along with good nutrition and herbal home remedies. In order to skillfully select essences and other remedies for ourselves, family members, and friends, we should familiarize ourselves with general principles of health, and understand the specific properties of the home-care remedies which we use.

In flower essence therapy, it is also necessary to develop sufficient self-awareness or insight into others in order to identify key emotional issues. While it is possible to develop our ability for self-reflection and insight, generally it is difficult to see ourselves clearly, or those to whom we are quite close. We are often unaware or in denial of those issues which may be most significant for further development. Therefore, it is essential to gain the insights of another through conversation or informal counseling. Working with another person in this way provides a "mirror" which activates our own self-awareness, and helps us identify the issues which are the basis for our flower essence selection.

One possibility is to develop a co-counseling relationship with a friend or colleague, in which each can provide this mirroring function for the other. An extension of this concept is to form a flower essence study and support group in which each participant receives observations from other members of the group, and help in selecting essences. If there is not yet sufficient interest in flower essences in the local community, there may be other support groups available, which can provide perspective on soul issues and support for the changes which the essences stimulate.

Working with a practitioner

The level at which flower essences can be used depends on our skill and experience. While there are many situations in which self-care is appropriate, it is important to know when further assistance is needed from a trained health practitioner. (*The Flower Essence Society is developing a Flower Essence Practitioner Referral Network. Please contact us for details.*)

Whenever there is a serious physical or psychological disturbance, it is crucial to find professional help. The ideal situation is to find a health practitioner or counselor who is also trained in flower essence therapy. If this is not possible, it may be necessary to use the services of one health professional to monitor or treat the serious condition, and use another practitioner to help with flower essence selection.

Even without extreme problems, it can be quite beneficial to work with a practitioner to select flower essences. Those just learning about the flower essences, or who are grappling with difficult problems, can benefit by working with a practitioner whose knowledge of essence qualities, counseling, and interview skills elicit awareness of underlying soul issues. An experienced practitioner can give support and insight when flower essences evoke painful feelings or confront us with hard choices.

Selection by Vibrational Techniques

Many people employ vibrational techniques for selecting flower essences for themselves or others. These include various electronic devices, direct sensing through the hands or finger tips, radiesthesia (pendulum testing), and kinesiology (muscle-testing). Those who have developed sufficient skill with such methods may find that they have some value in flower essence selection. By contacting a deep, non-verbal level of awareness, vibrational methods may suggest issues and essences which are hidden from conscious awareness; or they may help to refine essence choices following the initial interview.

However, there are limitations in using such methods, which we have noted consistently in the practitioner case reports collected and analyzed for sixteen years. Those who rely primarily on vibrational methods such as radiesthesia or kinesiology frequently submit cases with essence combinations lacking continuity and cohesion. One flower essence formula seems unrelated to another, and the essences within each formula do not form a coherent whole.

When these cases are examined developmentally, it is difficult to discern clear metamorphic healing patterns. Instead, many chaotic symptoms or reactions to the essences may occur. Such cases generally demonstrate a lack of sensitive insight into deeper, underlying issues of the client's soul experience. Because personal knowledge or familiarity with the essences is usually absent or quite cursory, there is little understanding of how each essence is actually working in the flower essence formula, or how the client is truly progressing through the therapy.

In interviewing many practitioners who depend primarily on vibrational selection methods, we have discovered two basic assumptions. First, many people prefer a less "intellectual" approach, and so are attracted to techniques like radiesthesia and kinesiology because they appear to be more "intuitive." However, does this assumption correspond with actual experience?

In training flower essence practitioners, we have observed that the most effective intuitive flower essence selection has a solid foundation in conscious understanding of flower essence qualities and human soul issues. Over-reliance on external selection techniques can actually stymie genuine intuitive and creative capacities, which require conscious perception and deeply considered attunement using one's own powers of observation, discrimination, and judgment. Furthermore, if the selection process does not include a considered evaluation of the qualities of various essences, there is no opportunity to grow in one's wisdom and understanding of their fundamental meanings.

Secondly, some practitioners believe that vibrational selection techniques allow a more impartial process, since the conscious mind is set aside. They assume that these methods yield objective information independent of any personal bias or other limitation of the person doing the testing. This is highly ironic, for the model of the uninvolved, detached researcher is precisely the paradigm of mechanistic science that so many practitioners of "New Age" arts wish to avoid. In fact, the scientific researcher, as well as the kinesiologist and the pendulum dowser, are all very much participants in their respective testing processes.

Our own empirical evidence — through case studies and various tests — has verified that one's level of knowledge and understanding of flower essences and of the client's issues greatly impacts one's ability to choose essences, especially when using vibrational methods. We have repeated an experiment in many different groups, whereby a number of practitioners independently choose essences for the same person using various vibrational methods. Invariably, each practitioner chooses an entirely different set of essences, whether they use the same or different vibrational selection methods.

In another test, some practitioners use vibrational selection techniques within the context of interview and counseling practices, referencing descriptions of essence qualities; while other practitioners use the same vibrational techniques in a "blind" manner, without talking with the client or considering the essence indications. The results show a wiser, more perceptive and effective choice of essences when the practitioner uses vibrational selection techniques in the context of full awareness of the essences used and of the client's issues.

Our experiments indicate that vibrational selection techniques are *subjective* methods, whose accuracy very much reflects the knowledge, skill, experience, inner clarity, and empathetic attunement which the practitioner brings to the selection process. Even if it were possible to eliminate all unconscious projection or personal bias, there would still be no single definitive choice of essences for a particular person and situation. Whether or not vibrational techniques are employed, the essences chosen are always an expression of the practitioner's perception of the client's issues, familiarity with the essences, and the therapeutic goals which are established with the client. Similarly, vibrational selection techniques used for self-selection are no more accurate or objective than selection by other means, and thus are not substitutes for the insight and perspective which is to be gained by working with a practitioner, friend, or colleague.

In all therapeutic work, it is most important that we acknowledge and take *responsibility* for the choices we make. We need to ask fundamental questions: "What is the source of information used to make my selection? Can it yield reliable and consistent results? Have I tested that? If results differ with different practitioners, what does this mean? If the process is intimately related to my own state of consciousness, then *how* do I take responsibility for my own awareness and knowledge? What is my level of knowledge of the essences? How willing am I to perceive the needs of those I wish to help?"

Appropriately used, vibrational methods may *supplement* our conscious understanding of the essences and the issues they address; but they do not replace the process of attentive listening to our clients or developing our own perception and knowledge. Whatever choices are suggested by these procedures must be consciously tested in light of what we know about the flower essences and the appropriateness of the selection as the next step in soul development.

A similar caveat applies to use of electronic, radionic, and other related testing mechanisms, as well as computer selection programs. The accuracy of such devices and systems derives in large part from the abilities of the operator. In any case, they are supplementary, and not a substitute for personal dialogue with clients or for developing a conscious relationship with the healing language of the flowers.

Ultimately, flower essence therapy is a serious, soul-based *relationship* between practitioner and essence, between practitioner and client, and between client and essence. For these relationships to be effective, we must be willing to engage heart and mind, and to develop empathetic presence and sensitive attunement. It would not be appropriate to have fixed rules about which selection techniques to use, or how, when, or even whether to use them at all. Nonetheless, we urge those who use flower essences in professional practice and in home care to develop a thorough knowledge, love, and respect for the essences and for those whom they seek to help. The selection techniques used should be objectively tested and evaluated for one's ability to use them effectively, so that each practitioner can stand fully and responsibly behind his or her role in the therapeutic process.

Using the *Flower Essence Repertory*

Part II — Soul Issues: Categories and Themes

Part II of the *Flower Essence Repertory* contains over 3200 entries, grouped according to basic soul issues, situations, and age or population groups which share common themes. This section includes a broad range of topics, but it should not be viewed as an exhaustive compendium. It would hardly be possible to capture the countless subtle states of consciousness associated with flower essences, requiring a book not unlike a dictionary or encyclopedia. Instead, the *Repertory* is intended to survey general categories which can be considered in a practical yet creative manner, to assist flower essence selection.

The first step in using the *Repertory* is to identify the major soul issues through counseling and self-reflection, as described earlier. During a client interview, it can be helpful to jot down key words or phrases used by the client, and impressions of gestures and voice qualities, which give clues to important emotional issues.

The next step is to look under each appropriate listing of Part II to find the descriptions of specific soul issues and corresponding flower essences within that category. This should be done with an attitude of exploration and dialogue. "Is it a fear of things which are known (Mimulus) or unknown (Aspen)? Is it a fear of the hostility of others (Oregon Grape), or a fear that one's own powerful emotions may erupt (Scarlet Monkeyflower)?" These inquiries can be part of the questioning process used to select essences for another person, and can help elicit further conversation and insights. As the essence choice is narrowed down, such questions can help confirm the accuracy of the selection.

Note that some entries address the negative state of mind, some the transformed state which is the goal, and some include both polarities. It is important that we become familiar with the bi-polar nature of flower essences: both the state of imbalance and the positive or transformative potential. In selecting appropriate essences we may start with the positive goal, and then uncover the emotional or mental pattern which blocks this purpose. Alternatively, we may start with the client's pattern of imbalance or suffering, and then determine the positive quality which needs to be developed.   Therefore, the listings in Part II are a mixture of both positive and negative indications for the essences.

Consider each statement and evaluate whether it is appropriate.   If a description seems close, but not totally applicable to the situation, make note of it anyway. You may find another interpretation of the essence's qualities which seems more suitable.   As you survey the various categories related to the main soul issues, note any essences which appear in several listings.   These may be important ones to consider.

Study also the related categories cross-referenced in the listings you check, marked as *"See also . . ."*   You may find other appropriate essences, or new perspectives on essences you are considering.   Be aware of the various kinds of categories: emotional and mental states (Anger, Clarity), situations (Emergency, Study), conditions (Alcoholism, Eating Disorders), themes (Materialism, Personal Relationships), practices (Massage, Meditation), populations (Animals, Children), or stages of life (Adolescence, Aging).   The listing at the beginning of Part II can be of assistance in locating appropriate categories.

Part III — Qualities and Portraits of the Flower Essences

After selecting a number of essences for consideration, consult Part III of the *Repertory* for an in-depth description of their qualities.   Each entry begins with a succinct summary of the positive qualities and patterns of imbalance of each essence.   This is particularly helpful if the entry read in Part II indicated only the positive or negative side of the polarity.   Next, there is a listing of all of the categories from Part II under which that essence is listed.   These cross-references can be helpful in understanding further applications of the essence, or may suggest related issues to consider.   This can lead to a study of new categories in Part II, possibly revealing essences which can complement the selection.   In this way Parts II and III can be used reciprocally to create a more accurate selection.

Part III contains expanded portraits of each flower essence.   Please note that these descriptions are written from an archetypal level — from the point of view of the soul itself — characterizing the major life lesson and transformative journey addressed by each flower.   If we can perceive the broad strokes contained within these archetypal pictures, it is then easier to comprehend the detailed symptoms and finer distinctions which are contained in Part II.   We may not always need an essence at the archetypal level of soul healing; yet we should always be aware of its spiritual depth and potential.   Flower essences have the capacity to arouse profound soul metamorphosis, and such healing should be our ultimate goal.

When using an essence in a supportive role, or in a less intense situation, it may be necessary to creatively interpret or "tone down" the essence's description, so that it applies to that particular situation.   In any case, we should not be limited by the exact words used to describe the essences. The messages of the flowers originate in a realm beyond human language. In our descriptions we can only capture a dim reflection of the fullness of its being, something like attempting to capture in words the beauty of a great painting or a musical masterpiece. With this understanding, try to use the essence descriptions in the *Repertory* to contact the underlying archetype of the essence, and then translate it into words which speak to the particular human experience for which it is being used.

Essences included in the *Flower Essence Repertory*

The *Flower Essence Repertory* is a reflection of the FES Research Program. All of the essences listed in this *Repertory* have been selected for inclusion based on extensive reports from practitioners over the years, validating the accuracy of the essence qualities. As our knowledge of plant qualities has increased, along with our ability to verify the properties of the plants through empirical documentation, we have been able to expand the contents of the *Repertory*. This edition contains the following sets of essences:

The English flower essences

During the 1930's in England, Dr. Edward Bach developed a range of 38 flower essences and one emergency combination formula. Since Dr. Bach's death in 1936 his original indications for the English flower essences have been substantiated by six decades of use in home and professional health care. However, our knowledge of their therapeutic benefits continues to grow, and the reader will find new themes and insights on the use of these classic English remedies. Today the range of English Flower Essences formulated by Dr. Bach is available from several companies under different brand names. However, the indications for their use apply regardless of which line of English essences is used.

The FES Professional Kit of North American flower essences

These 72 essences were developed by FES since 1978 based on the dual foundation of plant study and practitioner reports. They were released in sequential groups of 24 as Kits #1, #2, and #3. After they had received convincing documentation in a variety of clinical and therapeutic settings in many countries of the world, they were consolidated into one major set, called the *Professional Kit*. While the general archetypes of these essences are known, we are continually able to refine and expand our understanding of them through direct plant research and empirical case studies. These additional insights are reflected in this edition of the *Repertory*.

Supplemental research essences

This edition contains 31 additional essences which have been added to the *Repertory* in several stages, as we collect case reports and develop definitive information about them. These essences have been selected from a larger grouping of nearly 200 research essences which are in various stages of investigation and review. Some of these research essences have remained in this preliminary status for over a decade, awaiting sufficient confirmation of their qualities by practitioners. The Flower Essence Society intentionally withholds the release of preliminary findings regarding essences until sufficient research and empirical data are collected to verify their descriptions.

The 31 supplemental essences listed in this edition of the *Repertory* have already received extensive study as live plants and empirical documentation of essence use. Nevertheless we feel it is important to alert practitioners to their newer status so they can participate in our on-going efforts to collect case studies and observations about their qualities and effects. Among these supplementary essences is the *Research Kit* of 24 essences introduced in the 1992 edition of the *Repertory*. Also listed is the unique Yarrow Special Formula, an adaptation of the Yarrow flower essence for protection against noxious environmental influences. Three promising research essences have been added to the 1994 edition of the *Repertory*: Love-Lies-Bleeding, Nicotiana, and Purple Monkeyflower. The remaining essences included are part of the Seven Herbs Kit described below.

The Seven Herbs Kit

The *Seven Herbs Kit* was developed by Matthew Wood, a long-time friend and colleague of the Society. Matthew Wood has researched and written extensively about these essences and they have been made available to a wide circle of practitioners. Four of these remedies are already included in the FES Professional Kit — Sagebrush, Iris, Star Tulip (or Cat's Ears), and Yerba Santa. Matthew Wood used the Blue Flag Iris, *Iris versicolor,* in his research, while FES uses the wild Iris of the Pacific Coast, *Iris douglasiana,* in the Professional Kit. Both Irises exhibit similar properties, and are listed together. The three remaining essences in the Seven Herbs Kit — Black Cohosh, Easter Lily, and Lady's Slipper — are included in the *Repertory* as supplemental essences. Matthew Wood has recently reported good results using Showy Lady's Slipper *(Cypripedium reginae)* instead of Yellow Lady's Slipper *(Cypripedium parviflorum)*. Therefore, both species are listed for Lady's Slipper.

Making new flower essences

There are hundreds of thousands of plant species. Which ones should we make as flower essences? On the other hand, why make new essences at all? Some believe that Dr. Bach considered his 38 remedies to be a complete system, addressing all possible states of mind.

The only genuine reason to offer new flower essences is if they can meet real human needs and can provide healing for the suffering of the human soul. This was why Bach, during his eight years of flower essence research, constantly revised and expanded his repertory of flower essences. As he noticed attitudes and emotional states which were not adequately addressed by his existing remedies, he found new plants which would provide the needed qualities. Similar to Dr. Bach's experience, new flower essences have been developed by FES in response to deep questions about the nature of human suffering. These questions may arise from the needs of a particular client, or a broader theme addressed by many practitioners. At other times, we find a plant with especially potent qualities, and as its message becomes clear through study and attunement, we come to recognize its particular gift for soul healing.

It has been sixty years since Dr. Bach's pioneering work. During this time, many portals for appreciating and understanding the life of the soul have been opened. At the same time grave conflicts and challenges beset our world and demand our utmost psychic strength, bodily health, and spiritual service. Now, as we approach the millennial threshold, humanity is wrestling with profound problems of social, sexual, and psychological pathology stemming from substance abuse and addiction, sudden psychic and spiritual openings, changing sexual roles, childhood abuse and family dysfunction, increasing psychic and physical violence, social and economic injustice, ethnic, racial, religious, and geopolitical conflicts, and the ecological destruction of the Earth. The flower essences we have developed, and which are described in this *Repertory*, are a response to these challenges of our time, helping the individual soul find its right connection to the world soul.

While we recognize that there are other significant vibrational remedies besides the ones included in this *Repertory*, we are confident, based on our research, that each of the essences included here has an important contribution to make to the alleviation of suffering and the soul evolution of humankind. The authors stand fully behind all research presented in this *Repertory*, and take responsibility for any possible errors or oversights. In the spirit of scientific inquiry, we continue to strive to clarify our research through updated editions of the *Repertory*. Because research is a process, rather than a static body of information, we urge practitioners and others to join in this effort, so that flower essence therapy may become a truly professional and respected health-care modality.

Chapter 4: How Are Flower Essences Used?

Flower essences are most commonly taken orally from a dropper bottle directly under the tongue, or in a bit of water. In addition to oral use, flower essences are also quite effective when absorbed through the skin in baths or topical applications. The dosage preparation methods described below are guidelines for flower essence use, based on several decades of experience. Keep in mind, however, that there are many creative and effective ways to use flower essences.

There are several levels of dilution in the preparation of flower essences. The *mother essence* is derived from fresh blossoms in a bowl of water, infused with the morning sun (or heated by fire, in the case of some of the English essences). The mother essence is generally preserved with brandy. This infusion is then further diluted to the *stock* level, and sometimes again to a *dosage* level. Generally it is the stock level of dilution which is available commercially from flower essence companies, although there are some pre-mixed combinations sold at the dosage level of dilution.

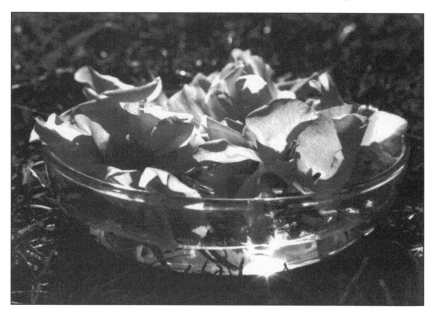

Making a mother essence: sun infusion of Sweet Pea flowers

Practical Directions for Administering Flower Essences

Using directly from stock

1. Flower essences can be taken directly from the stock bottle (the form in which most essences are sold).

2. Place four drops under the tongue, or in a little water. This dosage is most commonly taken four times daily.

Mixing the essences in a glass of water

1. Add four drops from each essence stock in your combination to a large cup or glass about three-quarters full of fresh water.

2. Stir the water for about a minute in a clockwise and counter-clockwise motion.

3. The essence combination can then be sipped several times throughout the day. Cover the glass to provide protection.

4. This mixture can be newly prepared after one to three days. In any case, it should be freshly stirred each day.

Preparing a dosage bottle

1. Fill a one-ounce (30 ml) glass dropper bottle nearly full of spring water or other fresh water.

2. Add a small amount of brandy (1/8 to 1/4 of the bottle) as a preservative. More brandy can be added if the dosage bottle is used over a number of months, or will be subject to high temperatures.

3. To the water and brandy mixture, add two to four drops of flower essences from the stock bottle of each essence selected.

4. After the essence stock has been added and before each subsequent use, you may want to rhythmically shake or lightly tap the bottle in order to keep the essences in a more potent or energized state.

5. Place four drops under the tongue, or in a bit of water. This dosage is most commonly taken four times daily. A 30 ml / 1 oz dosage bottle used in this manner will last approximately three weeks to one month.

6. The dosage bottle can be further diluted by adding four drops to a half-glass of water. Stir this mixture both clockwise and counter-clockwise, and sip slowly. This is one way to attenuate the taste of the brandy preservative.

Glass bottles and droppers are recommended, since plastic may adversely affect the subtle qualities of these natural plant remedies. It is best to use new bottles for new combinations of essences to ensure the cleanliness and clarity of the vibrational patterns.

Using a glass spray bottle or mister

1. Prepare as you would a dosage bottle.

2. Rather than taking the drops internally, spray the mixture around the body and in the environment.

3. Shake the bottle before each application to sustain potency.

Use in baths

1. Add about 20 drops of stock of each essence to a normal-sized bath tub of warm water.

2. Stir the water in a lemniscatory (figure-eight) motion for at least one minute to help potentize the remedies in the water.

3. Soak in this solution for approximately 20 minutes. Pat the skin gently dry, and then rest quietly or go to sleep to continue to absorb the subtle qualities of the essences.

Topical use

1. Add 6-10 drops of stock of each essence selected per 30 gm (1 oz) of creme, oil, or lotion.

2. Use on a daily basis either exclusively, or to supplement oral use.

3. Essence drops can also be applied directly on the body in conjunction with massage, acupressure or acupuncture, or chiropractic treatments.

Frequency and timing of dosage

Regular, rhythmic use of the flower remedies builds the strength of their catalytic action. Therefore, potency is increased not by taking more drops at one time, but by using them on a *frequent, consistent basis.* In most cases, the essences should be taken *four times daily,* although this may need to be increased in emergency or acute situations to once every hour, or even more often. On the other hand, children or other highly sensitive persons may need to *decrease the frequency* of use to once or twice daily.

The essences address the relationship between the body and soul, and therefore are most effective at the thresholds of *awakening* and *retiring,* since these are the times when the boundaries between body and soul shift. Other transition times of the day are also important, such as just before the noon or evening meals. Even when the essences are used in the midst of a hectic schedule, it is beneficial to allow a quiet moment of receptivity so that the messages of the flowers can be received at a subtle level. Many people find it helpful to remember to take the essences by keeping one bottle of their flower essence formula right on the bed-stand, and another one of the same combination in their purse, briefcase, or in the kitchen.

Although flower essences can be used on a short-term basis for acute situations, their ideal use is for long-term or deep-seated mental-emotional change. At this level, the most common cycle of essence use is four weeks or one month, a time interval which is strongly correlated to the emotional or astral body. Seven-day or 14-day cycles may also be of significance in the growth process. For particularly deep changes, a whole series of monthly cycles may need to be considered. However, in most cases changes will be noticed in about one month. At this interval there is usually the need to re-formulate or re-assess the flower essence combination. We recommend continuing to use a formula, or at least one or two key essences from the mix, for a period of time even after some change has been noticed. This allows a possibility for the essences to be "anchored" at deeper levels of consciousness.

Use with alcohol-sensitive persons

Many recovering alcoholics and other alcohol-sensitive persons have benefited greatly from the use of flower essences. Although flower remedies are preserved with brandy at the stock level, people have found much success in diluting the essences to the dosage level without the use of alcohol. Dilution methods insure that any alcohol ingested is chemically and physiologically insignificant, about one part in 600 when diluted in a one-ounce (30 ml) dosage bottle, or about one part in 4,800 in a eight-ounce glass of water. All of the following four methods have been reported to be effective:

1. Use two to four drops of stock in a large glass of water or juice, stir and sip slowly.

2. Prepare the essences in a dosage bottle, but fill it 1/4 to 1/3 full of apple cider vinegar as preservative, instead of brandy.

3. Prepare the essences in a dosage bottle, filled 1/3 to 1/2 full with vegetable glycerin. Vegetable glycerin is a derivative of coco-nut oil; it has a sweet taste and is used extensively to preserve herbal preparations.

4. The dosage bottle can also be prepared with no preservative if it is refrigerated, or used in a shorter period of time (several days to a week).

Enhancing Flower Essences

Amplification techniques

Because flower essences are vibrational in nature, it has been suggested that their effects can be further enhanced by such techniques as homeopathic potentization, or through the use of pyramids and crystals. Such methods may create new energy fields in or around the essences. However, we must ask whether they truly enhance the *process of soul development*, which is the ultimate goal of working with flower essences.

The desire to "amplify" flower essences often reflects the materialistic bias of our culture that "more is better." The gentle, gradual action of flower essences is generally the most appropriate way to work with soul development, for it allows us the freedom to choose and to change. In preparing the mother and stock levels of FES essences, we implement certain rhythmical procedures to stabilize their subtle properties. However, we have observed that if flower essences are subjected to repeated dilutions and successions in the classical homeopathic method, they may take on some of the coercive qualities of high potency homeopathic remedies, and incur the danger of provoking reactions if used incorrectly. Rather than attempting to obtain quicker results by magnifying the essence formula, *flower essence therapy aims to deepen the inner life*. In this way the subtle resonance between the flowering of the plant and unfoldment of the human soul can best be enhanced.

The importance of self-awareness practices

In the case studies collected by the Flower Essence Society, we have found that the most profound soul shifts occur when flower essence work is accompanied by practices which cultivate awareness of inner thoughts and feelings. Flower essence therapy is a journey of self-discovery. Whether through conscientious self-observation, dialogue with a support group or friends, or a therapeutic relationship with a professional counselor or health practitioner, it is important to have a way of consciously addressing the issues which are represented by the flower essences.

If our results with flower essences appear negligible and we wish to strengthen the effects of flower essences, we should look to the whole therapeutic process rather than just the essence itself. The following supportive practices can enhance the self-awareness and openness to inner change which the essences elicit.

Journal-keeping

Because of the materialistic bias of our culture, we can often be quite oblivious to the profound changes in our soul life engendered by the flower essences. In order to perceive shifts in consciousness, we must be prepared to lead ourselves and our clients into a much more intimate relationship with the life of the soul.

Keeping a journal while using the essences is one effective way of observing inner changes. Such mindfulness is particularly important because we are usually much less aware of the dynamics of our soul life than we are of bodily pain and sensation. It is especially helpful to keep a dream journal, since inner movement often comes to expression in dream life before surfacing to conscious awareness.

Affirmations

Another way of reinforcing the subtle message of the flowers is through the use of meditative thoughts, affirmations, or reflective prayer. By taking just a few minutes each day to work inwardly and consciously with the positive or "affirmative" changes toward which the flower essences point us, we can greatly increase their effect. The Flower Essence Society publishes a book, *Affirmations, The Messages of the Flowers in Transformative Words for the Soul*, which can provide guidance and suggestions for this work. Written and verbal affirmations can also be combined with inner images, visualization, or artistic work.

We should distinguish the transformative use of affirmations from the popular idea of positive thinking, which is frequently a part of "New Age" philosophy. If we use positive thoughts as a way of denying pain and suffering, or as a refusal to face our inner shadow, it creates distortion, imbalance, or illness rather than well-being. The wise use of affirmations with flower essences enables us to acknowledge pain and conflict, and steadfastly work toward transformation.

Artistic expression

Art is an expression *par excellence* of the soul. It can play a special role in flower essence therapy, both as a means of self-discovery, and as a transformational tool acting in synergy with the flower essences. A painting can be worth a thousand words about the soul, for its subtle language can often be expressed more clearly through form and color than through words. Many successful practitioners use some form of art with their clients to help assess their underlying issues. This is particularly important with children, who lack adult verbal and cognitive abilities.

In addition, art can be a very soul-satisfying way of expressing the growth which is experienced through flower essence therapy. The newly awakened feeling life may be more capable of revealing itself through a painting, song, poem, dance or movement, rather than through prosaic words. The goal is not necessarily to produce professional art, but to encourage expression of the richness and diversity of soul life which is evoked by flower essences.

Flower Essence Therapy
and Other Health Modalities

The holistic health movement

Flower essence therapy can be considered part of the *holistic health movement* a wide range of modalities both traditional and modern which support mind-body wellness. Included are such practices as herbology or phytotherapy, homeopathy, acupuncture, naturopathy, chiropractic, nutritional therapy, therapeutic massage, psychological and spiritual counseling, yoga, meditation, prayer, visualization, affirmations, various movement therapies, art and music therapy, flower essences, and many more. Furthermore, progressive medical doctors and nurses are expanding their practices to include a more holistic orientation.

Despite the fact that conventional scientists and medical practitioners remain generally skeptical about holistic health practices, they are receiving increasing public recognition. In the United States, a recent study by Dr. David Eisenberg in the prestigious *New England Journal of Medicine* showed that 37% of the U.S. adult population had used one or more holistic health practices, although about 70% of them had not told their physicians. In 1992 the United States National Institutes of Health set up an Office of Alternative Medicine to fund research in various alternative health modalities.

Although there are many political and scientific challenges remaining, it is clear that in one form or another, the holistic perspective will have an important role to play in the development of health care in our society. It is within this context that flower essence therapy will receive increasing recognition.

Flower essences in the spectrum of health care

The soul occupies a middle realm between body and spirit. Flower essence therapy is fundamentally a therapy of the soul; thus it must always take into account how change is grounded and stabilized in the body, and how it is freed and illumined through the spirit. Because of the soul's mediating relationship between body and spirit, flower essences combine very effectively with other modalities which address various aspects of body, soul, and spirit.

Health practitioners who work primarily with physical problems, for example, use flower essences to address some of the underlying emotional causes of these problems. Practitioners of deep-tissue therapeutic massage are principally concerned with the structure of muscles and connective tissue. Yet, muscle tension is often the result of emotional trauma and stress held in the body. Flower essences bring such issues into awareness, and allow for a mutual release of physical and emotional strain.   Many chiropractors report that their spinal adjustments last longer when flower essences are used to help their patients deal with stressful emotions.   Nutritional counselors use flower essences to enable their clients to overcome the emotional causes of eating disorders.   Progressive medical doctors use flower essences to address emotional issues connected with physical illness, as well as their patients' attitudes toward the healing process itself.

When used with other soul-oriented modalities, flower essences work in a complementary way.   For example, depth psychotherapy is an exceptional context for flower essence use, in which the essences can stimulate real breakthroughs in the developmental process.   Other soul work which is combined synergistically with flower essences includes art and music therapy, poetry, drama, and dream work.

Flower essences also have an important contribution to make to spiritual practice.   Many people following a spiritual path have difficulty coming to terms with the "shadow side" of emotional life, attempting to suppress these aspects of their being, rather than to acknowledge and transform them.   Flower essences are a vehicle for developing honest self-awareness, as well as releasing the vital forces often trapped in emotional repression.   In this way spiritual practices such as meditation can become truly integrated with moral and emotional development.

Flower essences in perspective

While flower essences have nearly universal application in a wide range of circumstances, they are neither a cure-all nor an answer for every problem.   Health and illness are multi-faceted experiences, involving many diverse factors.   While it is true that the state of the soul is reflected in the health of the body, it is also true that a body which is out of balance can negatively impact the soul.   For example, hypoglycemia (low blood sugar) can contribute to depression and anxiety by depriving the brain of proper nutrition.   These emotions will be difficult to overcome unless there is a change in diet to reduce or eliminate sweets.   At the same time, changing food habits may be difficult unless the emotional sources of food cravings are addressed.   In such situations a program combining nutritional counseling with flower essence therapy will be more effective than either modality by itself.

Those who use flower essences for themselves or others must know when to consult other professionals for assistance.   Flower essences work best when they are part of an overall program of health enhancement, which includes good nutrition, proper exercise, healthy relationships, involvement in work and community, artistic expression, and consultation with a variety of health practitioners and modalities, including medical care when appropriate.

Results of Flower Essence Therapy

Long-term and subtle effects

There is a full spectrum of responses to flower essences. Some people report immediate, discernible, and very dramatic results. Others appear to notice no differences at all, and may only slightly perceive shifts in well-being and in mental-emotional states after a considerable period of time. Most people typically respond to the essences somewhere in the middle of this range.

The effects of flower essences are subtle and cumulative. In other words, it is rare that someone will experience an immediate catharsis or total transformation. The essences work day by day, gradually from the inside out, by awakening forces of health and inner transformation. Patience, backed by consistency and regularity, is therefore crucial for flower essences to be effective.

Because the essences are used for transformation of the inner life, we may not experience them in a very direct way. We are more apt to observe their effect over a period of time, as we notice subtle shifts in the way we act, in the way we view ourselves and others, or even very real differences in our sense of physical well-being. Often it is others — friends, family, or work associates — who first notice and call to attention changes in our attitudes and patterns of behavior.

Unrealistic expectations about flower essences

We live in a culture that promotes quick answers and avoidance of pain. Advertising entices us with promises of instant symptom relief to enable us to cope with daily life. Because flower essences are liquids in glass dropper bottles, it is easy to approach them as if they are just another "quick-fix" remedy. This may lead to unrealistic expectations, and hinder our ability to experience their full benefits.

Flower essences are strengtheners of our own soul forces, enabling us to learn and grow from life's challenges. They invite us on a *healing journey*, and can be our allies and guides along the way. The essences are not intended to painlessly obliterate our problems, or provide instantaneous gratification. Such an expectation inevitably leads to impatience, disappointment, disillusion, or passivity. Most importantly, it results in an unwillingness to become an active participant in the healing process.

In situations of acute stress, emergency essence combinations such as the Five-Flower Formula may afford immediate relief and calming, providing an introduction to the "reality" of vibrational remedies. However, this is only a first step. Authentic flower essence therapy is an opportunity to explore foundational, long-term emotional issues, which cannot be effectively addressed by general emergency formulas.

For example, consider a person who leads a frenetic life and feels constant fatigue, to the point of creating health problems. Such a person may be tempted to take a flower essence combination with essences such as Olive and Nasturtium to feel more energized, without addressing the underlying causes of the stress and fatigue. A wiser approach would be to choose essences that deal with the ability to release tension and to examine fundamental lifestyle choices and underlying attitudes which lead to competitiveness, insecurity, workaholism, and other related syndromes.

In reading the flower essence descriptions in this *Repertory* and other publications, we may feel a desire to design a new personality for ourselves. It is easy to think that if we acquire the right list of desirable traits, we can become someone who will impress friends, family, or work associates. Such an attitude is a totally externalized perspective of ourselves, seeking to mold the soul's *persona* — the mask it wears to face the world — to fit the expectations and values of others.

Flower essences can indeed stimulate amazing personality changes by developing innate capacities which have been blocked or thwarted. Following the principle of resonance, the essences evoke only the potential already within us. They do not impose something from without (as do biochemical drugs), but catalyze what is an unrealized possibility, and help us to choose freely to fulfill our own purpose in life. We need to select essences to help address attitudes and emotions which are blocking realization of that purpose, as well as essences which activate those qualities which can help us fulfill our greater destiny.

Flower essences and inner development

Use of flower essences can enhance self-awareness practices such as meditation and, conversely, these practices deepen the effects of the essences. The essences are not substitutes for self-awareness and inner development, nor are they instant "consciousness in a bottle." Spiritual and psychic abilities emerge in a gradual way when we take an honest moral inventory of our shortcomings, strive to correct these faults, and work to fulfill our soul's destiny. As inner catalysts, flower essences stimulate our ability to respond, or take responsibility for our growth by deepening awareness of our feelings, underlying attitudes, and our spiritual Self.

This attitude of self-responsibility is especially important in our modern age, when many persons who pursue a path of inner development do so without the guidance of traditional religious authority or discipleship. Such a quest brings increased freedom, but it lacks the protection which spiritual community provided seekers in the past. This modern spiritual path challenges us to face the violence and confusion of the world without blocking the sensitivity and openness which spiritual unfoldment brings. In addition, because the modern seeker lives in the world rather than in the protection of ashrams and monasteries, there is an unprecedented opportunity to apply spiritual principles to the worldly challenges of family responsibility, money, desire, power, and relationships.

Flower essences help us come to terms with these challenges to the modern soul. They help us to maintain our spiritual sensitivity, and impart strength to meet adversity in the world. They insure that our spiritual awareness is physically and emotionally embodied. In this way spiritual seeking will not be a flight from the soul, but rather a way of enhancing our soul's capacity to be a bridge between the earthly and spiritual worlds.

Flower essences and physical conditions

Physical conditions can be important indicators for issues facing the soul. For example, a cold may indicate a disconnection with vital forces, for which Nasturtium essence would help. A sore throat may reveal constriction in self-expression for which an essence such as Larch may be chosen. Digestive problems may reveal emotional tension in the solar plexus for which Chamomile may be of assistance.

Because flower essences are soul remedies, they should not be used as are drugs or even herbal remedies for directly treating particular physical symptoms or illnesses. Nasturtium is not the flower essence for colds, nor is Larch the one for sore throats, nor Chamomile for all digestive problems. Essences are chosen according to the unique issues and experiences of the individual; those with the same physical symptoms may have quite different emotional patterns and life issues. Physical indications included in the *Repertory* are only guidelines for identifying the overall body-mind configuration which is the basis for essence selection.

While flower essences are not cures for particular physical ailments, the emotional and attitudinal shifts engendered by the flower essences can facilitate remarkable changes in physical health. Qualified medical practitioners report many cases in which flower essences play a key role in treatment programs for various diseases.

However, there are legal and ethical considerations concerning the use of flower essences for physical conditions by those who are not medical practitioners. First, there is the practical problem of not violating local laws specifying what licenses and qualifications are necessary for treating particular conditions. There are also important ethical issues, which would deserve attention even if there were no legal restrictions.

Particularly when working with severe conditions, health practitioners and home-care users of essences need to know the limits of their knowledge and skill. Using flower essences should not be an excuse to neglect medical help from a practitioner with the appropriate training and experience. Flower essences can be quite beneficial in such circumstances, but there also needs to be a qualified medical practitioner who can monitor any serious medical condition, and provide treatment if necessary.

The same caution applies to extreme psychological dysfunction, which may need the intervention of a trained counselor, psychologist, or psychiatrist.

Possible side-effects

What happens if the wrong flower essences are selected? Are there dangers or side effects associated with flower essence use? In general, flower essences are among the safest, most self-regulating health remedies available. If we take essences that are totally inappropriate and have little relationship to our real issues, then we will experience little effect.

Flower essences work by resonance; thus the wrong essences will not stimulate a "soul chord" within us. If we take too many essences, or essences which address only minor issues, they may be ineffective; substantive changes will not be achieved, or will take much longer to occur. Sometimes inappropriate or chaotic essence selections will stimulate confusion or a sense of uneasiness. Perhaps too many issues are "stirred up," or change happens faster than can be tolerated. On occasion, rapid psychological transformation — or our resistance to it — can produce unpleasant physical sensations such as fatigue, skin rashes, or headaches. Such reactions are generally short-lived, and may be an indication to re-formulate the flower essence combination, or to work with counseling and other practices to remove any psychological impediments to the therapeutic process.

The awareness crisis

One common experience reported by people using flower essences is an intensification of certain traits prior to experiencing a transformation. For example, someone taking Willow essence for resentment may have an acute awareness of resentment, before being able to let go and forgive. This seeming increase of an emotional trait has similarities to an "aggravation" produced by a homeopathic remedy, or a "healing crisis" stimulated by such cleansing practices as fasting.

We call this phenomenon an *awareness crisis*, because it is caused by bringing unconscious emotions and attitudes to the surface of awareness. Since they were previously hidden or disowned, these qualities seem more intense when brought to consciousness. Such experiences provide us with a clear opportunity to witness and acknowledge negative or dysfunctional aspects of ourselves.

Support from counseling, self-reflection, journal-writing, and other means of strengthening the "witnessing" aspect of consciousness can help create a smoother journey through the sometimes rough waters of this experience. If the awareness crisis becomes unusually intense (beyond a healthy level of discomfort), then one may reduce the frequency of dosage, or change the flower essence selection to ease the process.

With awareness comes the ability to understand and to change. It is difficult to let go of resentment and forgive if one is unaware or in denial of having any resentment. If self-awareness has already been cultivated, there often is no need for an awareness crisis; one is most likely to move directly into the transformative stage of the flower essence process.

Long-term changes possible with flower essence therapy

Although flower essences are typically chosen for specific emotional issues, profound soul growth can occur which goes beyond resolving the particular situation for which the essences were selected. Case studies and in-depth interviews with practitioners over a sixteen-year period have provided us with a comprehensive picture of seven major areas of soul development possible through long-term flower essence therapy.

These *meta-levels* of soul development are generally not envisioned at the commencement of the flower essence journey, but emerge as the soul opens with regular, sustained use of the flower essences and supportive practices. Together, these qualities give a beautiful picture of the soul in full blossom.

1. Emotional awareness and vitality is enhanced.

For the thousands of people who have experienced flower essence therapy, its most basic contribution has been to enhance the emotional life of the soul. Those who have felt emotionally numb or inhibited have developed new awareness of their issues, as well as an ability to experience and express a wider range of feelings. Those who have felt overwhelmed or drained by chaotic emotions have acquired a capacity for detached self-observation and mindfulness, thus maintaining a strong center of balance within emotional experiences.

The principle effect of the essences has been to enhance emotional flexibility and resilience, rather than simply to make people more — or less — emotional. Most people's soul repertoire is severely limited, often stuck in anger, depression, fear, or other habitual responses to life; others believe they must control or suppress their emotions altogether. Through flower essence therapy the soul becomes capable of experiencing the full spectrum of human emotional expression, including joy, grief, awe, anger, compassion, reverence, and so forth.

2. Awareness of the body is encouraged, with a greater sense of physical well-being.

Many people begin their healing journey with an awareness of discomfort or illness in the physical body. Practitioners report that flower essences lend support to programs of physical health by activating the vitalizing forces of the etheric body, bringing spiritual and soul forces into a closer relationship with the physical body, and generally mobilizing inner healing powers.

Furthermore, flower essence therapy often leads to a fundamentally new relationship with the physical body, an awareness of how the body is speaking through its physical symptoms. Instead of feeling *victimized* by illness, people begin to *take responsibility* for caring for their bodies, eliminating habits which are destructive to their health, and cultivating practices which nourish and strengthen the body. Moreover, they come to recognize that *the soul expresses itself through the physical body*, and that physical pains and tensions are frequently indications of anger, fear, overwhelm, depression, and other emotions which need to be addressed. It is a common experience that once underlying emotional issues are resolved, many physical symptoms can be released.

For those who suffer debilitating illness or injury, or who struggle with the effects of aging, flower essence therapy brings more acceptance of the body's condition, and an ability to honor the teachings of pain or limitation. At the same time, many generally healthy people report awakening to new possibilities for a vital, fulfilling life, without needing to compare themselves to the idealized images of youth, strength, and beauty promoted by our culture through its mass media.

For many sensitive souls, the journey from the expansive realms of spirit into the limited temporal and spatial dimensions of a physical body is inherently problematic. This often results in a desire to disown or deny the body, commonly manifesting in eating disorders and other destructive habits, or as a hesitation to become fully engaged in life. Flower essence therapy helps such individuals to overcome their fundamental ambivalence about the body by anchoring the soul in the physical world. They become more embodied physically and emotionally, and feel empowered to take an active role in their communities and society. In this way the soul is able to wholeheartedly accept its incarnation into physical matter, and enthusiastically experience life.

3. Attunement with Nature is developed.

One of the most remarkable experiences which practitioners regularly report is the awakening of a deep relationship with Nature, even on the part of those who have had little previous interest or connection with the natural world. Apartment dwellers may purchase a plant or start a window-sill garden. City residents will take walks in the park, or trips to the country side. They may remember a favorite flower or nature retreat from childhood, become motivated to take outdoor excursions more frequently, seek nature-oriented recreation, or plant a garden. There may be a deepened interest in ecological issues and protecting the Earth. Sometimes people using flower essences will even take an active interest in learning the botany and habitat of the flowers used in their healing.

Besides connecting us with the specific healing energies of particular flowers, the essences evoke the healing mantle of Natura, of *Nature as a living being*. We can then experience how Nature can nourish and protect us, and how our own healing is inseparable from our respect and care for the being of the Earth. In this way the individual soul finds a connection to the world soul of Nature.

4. Awareness of vocation in relationship to life purpose and world-service is clarified.

A fundamental soul issue which is addressed in flower essence therapy concerns the way in which people express themselves through their work. Many feel dissatisfaction with their job, or the lack of one. The first consequence of addressing this issue may be simply to raise deeper questions into awareness: "Am I working in this job only for survival needs or to fulfill others' expectations of me? Is my work truly a *vocation*, something I feel inwardly called to do as an expression of life purpose and service to others? Do I even know what I want to do with my life?"

Often such questioning has been repressed due to the painfulness of the likely answers. Flower essence therapy can lead to an honest self-examination, realistically addressing our capacities and untapped inner resources, as well as the passions and ideals which stir us. We learn to distinguish between the expectations of others, the demands of the personality for material success, and the true longing of our soul for a vocation which is authentically our own, an expression of our deepest desires. In the words of the contemporary poet David Whyte, "The soul prefers to fail at its own life, than succeed at someone else's."

It can be a daunting challenge to translate this new self-awareness into action in a world where economic constraints make choosing meaningful work difficult. Nonetheless, it is extraordinary just how many opportunities open up to someone who has made the commitment to act out of an inner sense of purpose. Whether it is transforming one's current job with a fresh attitude and a surge of creative energy, or finding a totally new situation, profound shifts in work and career are a remarkably frequent outcome of flower essence therapy. As people come into greater alignment with their life purpose, they also realize how their own development and personal destiny is inseparable from world destiny. They are then able to recognize that right livelihood necessarily involves world-service, facilitating the development of the individual soul within the larger world soul.

5. There is an awakening to the language of the soul.

As the soul life is awakened and emotional life harmonized, higher sensibilities become possible. Flower essence therapy facilitates an enhanced sense of the sacred and subtle dimension of life. Many people are inspired to create beauty in their environments; they also become more aware of soul symbols and inner meaning in daily activity and personal relationships.

Such an awareness allows the fecund world of dreams to enrich the waking life. Many people are surprised to find that dreams are greatly enlivened after using flower essences for several weeks or months. Dream recall is enhanced, and the dreams themselves become more vivid and pregnant with meaning. It is quite common for people to start dream journals, and to gain a sense of how their soul is speaking to them through the language of dreams.

As the soul awakens, it expresses itself most fully through the feeling life of the arts. Many people who have worked with flower essences report renewed appreciation and interest in the arts, discovering or re-discovering music, painting, sculpture, drama, writing, poetry, and other art forms — not necessarily to pursue as a career, but rather as an enrichment of their own soul life. Such artistic capacities develop profound sensitivity in the soul, which in its highest expression becomes an ability to serve others selflessly and with deep compassion.

6. A deeper understanding of relationships and karma is developed.

With the new self-understanding awakened by flower essence therapy, relationships with others also receive greater consideration. Often people realize the ways they have been hurt by others, including their family of origin. Flower essence therapy aids in acknowledging these feelings, and releasing them through forgiveness. Greater self-awareness also brings new responsibility. In further stages of flower essence therapy, people report being able to admit their own shortcomings, and make amends to those they have hurt — either family, friends, work associates, or the larger community.

Flower essences stimulate an enhanced perception of the deeper strands of experience and karma which link people with the lives of others. Those working with relationship issues gain a new appreciation of common purposes they share, and an increased understanding of unresolved issues from the past. These realizations often engender profound life changes. Many existing relationships which have been locked in destructive patterns for years can suddenly become intolerable to this newly sensitized awareness. As a result, new efforts may be made to heal a marriage, or a clear decision formed to end a harmful or dysfunctional relationship. Many people who have avoided relationships out of fear of being hurt find new courage to reach out to others, to seek intimacy, develop friendships, and participate in community life. The individual soul thus learns how its identity is woven together with other souls in the larger web of life.

7. There is a renewed commitment to spiritual seeking and expression.

The pre-eminent gift of flower essence therapy is to enable the soul to become a chalice to receive spiritual forces. People from a wide variety of religious and non-religious backgrounds report developing an interest in spiritual philosophy and ethics, even when this was not a conscious goal in their use of flower essences. Many persons awaken to the need to re-examine the religious, cultural, and spiritual roots of their childhood, while others find the courage to explore new dimensions of spirituality, or to find new forms of worship which are uniquely suited to their soul needs.

Questions such as "Who am I? Is there a purpose to life? Is there a life beyond the physical world?" assume a new importance. Many persons who first sought therapy for apparently physical problems or acute emotional stress are inspired to examine cultural and moral values — and ultimately the meaning of life itself — with renewed interest and dedication. This quest for meaning leads to a deeper experience of the Self beyond the confines of the day-to-day personality.

When flower essence therapy is carried to its full development, the Spiritual Self becomes the central organizing principle in the life of the soul. Just as the Sun shines its light on the many dimensions of soul life, awareness of the Self gives context and meaning to the other six *meta-levels* of soul development, involving our emotions, relationship with the body, attunement with Nature, vocation and life purpose, inner life and artistic development, and personal relationships and life karma. We come to realize that the awakening of the spiritual core within us, and its expression in all aspects of our lives, is the true goal of flower essence therapy and, indeed, of the healing quest.

Do we ever finish with flower essences?

If working with flower essences is a healing journey, do we ever arrive at the end? Is there a time when we have dealt with all our emotional issues and we no longer need flower essences? Such questions are based on an assumption that there is a static state of normality, health, happiness, perfection, bliss, or enlighten-ment that can be permanently achieved. In truth, as long as we are alive on this Earth our soul will always face challenges, and will always have the need to learn and evolve in the school of life. If we understand flower essences as catalysts for soul growth, rather than as remedies to fix our problems, they will always have the possibility of helping us. While there may be times we choose not to work with essences, or use other methods, flower essences can remain allies through many cycles and spirals of our soul's evolution.

References and Suggested Reading

The following is a partial list of titles which form a background to the concepts discussed in the overview.

Alchemy

Albertus, Frater. *Alchemists Handbook.* York Beach, ME: Samuel Weiser, 1974.

Fabricius, Johannes. *Alchemy: The Medieval Alchemists and their Royal Art.* Wellingsborough, England: The Aquarian Press, 1976.

Goodrick-Clarke, Nicholas, ed. *Paracelsus: Essential Readings.* Wellingsborough, England: Crucible, 1986.

Hall, Manly P. *The Mystical and Medical Philosophy of Paracelsus.* Los Angeles: Philosophical Research Society, 1964.

Hartmann, Franz, M.D. *Paracelsus: Life and Prophecies.* Blauvelt, NY: Steinerbooks, 1973.

Hartmann, Franz, M.D. *Jacob Boehme: Life and Doctrines.* Blauvelt, NY: Steinerbooks, 1977.

Holmyard, E.J. *Alchemy.* New York: Dover Publications, 1990.

Jacobi, Jolande, ed. *Paracelsus, Selected Writings.* Bollingen Series XXVIII. Princeton, NJ: Princeton University Press, 1988.

Jung, C.G. *Alchemical Studies.* Princeton, NJ: Princeton University Press, 1983.

Jung, C.G. *Mysterium Coniunctionis: An Inquiry into the Separation and Synthesis of Psychic Opposites in Alchemy.* Princeton, NJ: Princeton University Press, 1977.

Jung, C.G. *Psychology and Alchemy.* Princeton, NJ: Princeton University Press, 1980.

Junius, Manfred M. *Practical Handbook of Plant Alchemy.* New York: Inner Traditions, 1985.

McLean, Adam. *A Commentary on the Mutus Liber.* Grand Rapids, MI: Phanes Press, 1991.

Scott, Sir Walter, ed. *Hermetica: The ancient Greek and Latin writings which contain the religious or philosophical teachings ascribed to Hermes Trismegistus.* Boston: Shamballa, 1993.

von Franz, Marie-Louise. *Alchemy: An Introduction to the Symbolism and the Psychology.* Toronto, Canada: Inner City Books, 1980.

Waterfield, Robin. *Jacob Boehme: Essential Readings.* Wellingsborough, England: Crucible, 1986.

Anthroposophy and spiritual science

Hutchins, Eileen. *Parzival: An Introduction.* London: Temple Lodge Press, 1992.

Shepherd, A.P. *Rudolf Steiner: Scientist of the Invisible.* Rochester, VT: Inner Traditions International, 1954, 1987.

Steiner, Rudolf. *An Outline of Occult Science.* Spring Valley, NY: Anthroposophic Press, 1985.

Steiner, Rudolf. *How to Know Higher Worlds* (formerly *Knowledge of the Higher Worlds and its Attainment*). Hudson, NY: Anthroposophic Press, 1994.

Steiner, Rudolf. *Rosicrucianism and Modern Initiation.* London: Rudolf Steiner Press, 1982.

Steiner, Rudolf. *The Boundaries of Natural Science.* Spring Valley, NY: Anthroposophic Press, 1983.

Steiner, Rudolf. *The Philosophy of Freedom.* London: Rudolf Steiner Press, 1979.

Aromatherapy

Lavabre, Marcel. *Aromatherapy Workbook*. Rochester, VT: Healing Arts Press, 1990.

Tisserand, Robert B. *The Art of Aromatherapy*. Rochester, VT: Healing Arts Press, 1977.

Valnet, Jean, M.D. *The Practice of Aromatherapy*. Rochester, VT: Healing Arts Press, 1990.

Biodynamic agriculture

Biodynamics, published bi-monthly by the Bio-Dynamic Farming and Gardening Association, P.O. Box 550, Kimberton, PA 19442.

Klocek, Dennis. *A Bio-Dynamic Book of Moons*. Wyoming, RI: Bio-Dynamic Literature, 1983.

König, Karl. *Earth and Man*. Wyoming, RI: Bio-Dynamic Literature, 1982.

Steiner, Rudolf. *Agriculture*. London: Bio-Dynamic Agriculture Association, 1958.

Storl, Wolf D. *Culture and Horticulture*. Wyoming, RI: Bio-Dynamic Literature, 1979.

Cultural perspectives

Bohm, David, and Mark Edwards. *Changing Consciousness: Exploring the Hidden Source of the Social, Political, and Environmental Crises Facing our World*. New York: HarperCollins, 1991.

Merchant, Carolyn. *The Death of Nature: Women, Ecology, and the Scientific Revolution*. New York: HarperCollins, 1990.

Tarnas, Richard. *The Passion of the Western Mind: Understanding the Ideas That Have Shaped Our World View*. New York: Harmony Books, 1991.

Zoeteman, Kees. *Gaiasophy: The Wisdom of the Living Earth*. Hudson, NY: Lindsifarne Press, 1991.

Flower essences and Dr. Bach

Bach, Edward, M.D., and F.J. Wheeler, M.D. *The Bach Flower Remedies*. New Canaan, CT: Keats Publishing, 1979.

Bach, Edward, M.D. Julian Barnard, ed. *Collected Writings of Edward Bach*. Hereford, England: Flower Remedy Programme, 1987.

Barnard, Julian and Martine. *The Healing Herbs of Edward Bach, An Illustrated Guide to the Flower Remedies*. Bath, England: Ashgrove Press, 1988.

Barnard, Julian. *Patterns of Life Force*. Hereford, England: Flower Remedy Programme, 1987.

Chancellor, Philip M. *Handbook of the Bach Flower Remedies*. New Canaan, CT: Keats Publishing, 1980.

Cunningham, Donna. *Flower Remedies Handbook*. New York: Sterling Publishing, 1992.

Deroide, Philippe. *Les Elixirs Floraux: harmonisants de l'âme*. Barret-le-Bas, France: Le Souffle d'Or, 1992. (French)

Kaminski, Patricia. *Affirmations: The Messages of the Flowers in Transformative Words for the Soul*. Nevada City, CA: Flower Essence Society, 1994.

Scheffer, Mechthild. *Bach Flower Therapy*. Wellingsborough, England: Thorsons, 1986.

Weeks, Nora. *The Medical Discoveries of Edward Bach, Physician*. New Canaan, CT: Keats Publishing, 1979.

Wood, Matthew. *Seven Herbs: Plants as Teachers*. Berkeley, CA: North Atlantic Books, 1987.

Wright, Machaelle Small. *Flower Essences: Reordering Our Understanding and Approach to Illness and Health*. Jeffersonton, VA: Perelandra, 1988.

Goethean science and new scientific paradigms

Adams, George, and Olive Whicher. *The Plant Between Sun and Earth.* London: Rudolf Steiner Press, 1980.

Adams, George. *Nature Ever New.* Spring Valley, NY: Mercury Press, 1979.

Bockemühl, Jochen, ed. *Toward a Phenomenology of the Etheric World.* Spring Valley, NY: Anthroposophic Press, 1985.

Bohm, David. *Wholeness and the Implicate Order.* Boston: Routledge & Kegan Paul, 1982.

Bortoft, Henri. *Goethe's Scientific Consciousness.* Tunbridge Wells, Kent, England: Institute for Cultural Research, 1986.

Edelglass, Stephen, Georg Maier, Hans Gerbert, and John Davy. *Matter and Mind, Imaginative Participation in Science.* Hudson, NY: Lindsifarne Press, 1992.

Edwards, Lawrence. *The Field of Form: Research concerning the outer world of living forms and the inner world of geometrical imagination.* Edinburgh, Scotland: Floris Books, 1982.

Gleick, James. *Chaos: Making a New Science.* New York: Penguin, 1987.

Goethe, Johann Wolfgang von, and Rudolf Steiner. Herbert H. Koepf and Linda S. Jolly, eds. *Readings in Goethean Science.* Wyoming, RI: Bio-Dynamic Farming and Gardening Association, 1978.

Goethe, Johann Wolfgang von. Douglas Miller, ed. *Goethe: Scientific Studies.* New York: Suhrkamp Publishers, 1988.

Goethe, Johann Wolfgang von. Frederick Ungar, ed. *Goethe's World View, Presented in His Reflections and Maxims.* New York: Frederick Ungar Publishing Co., 1963.

Grohmann, Gerbert. *The Plant, Vols. 1 & 2.* Kimberton, PA: Bio-Dynamic Literature, 1989.

Hauschka, Rudolf. *The Nature of Substance.* London: Rudolf Steiner Press, 1983.

Iovine, John. *Kirlian Photography: A Hands-On Guide.* Blue Ridge Summit, PA: TAB Books (McGraw-Hill), 1993.

Kolisko, Eugen and Lilly. *Agriculture of Tomorrow.* Bournemouth, England: Kolisko Archives Publications, 1939, 1978.

Lehrs, Ernst. *Man or Matter: Introduction to a Spiritual Understanding of Nature on the Basis of Goethe's Method of Training Observation and Thought.* London: Rudolf Steiner Press, 1985.

Pelikan, Wilhelm. *Healing Plants.* London: *The British Homoeopathic Journal*, 1970-71. (out of print), partial translation of *Heilpflanzenkunde.* Dornach, Switzerland: Philosophisch-Anthroposophischer Verlag am Goetheanum, 1963.

Pelikan, Wilhelm. *L'Homme et les Plantes Médicinales, Tome 1-3.* Paris: Editions du Centre Triades, 1986. (French translation of *Heilpflanzenkunde*)

Pfeiffer, Ehrenfried. *Sensitive Crystallization Processes.* Spring Valley, NY: Anthroposophic Press, 1936, 1975.

Schwenk, Theodor. *Sensitive Chaos.* London: Rudolf Steiner Press, 1965.

Schwenk, Theodor, and Wolfram Schwenk. *Water — The Element of Life.* Hudson, NY: Anthroposophic Press, 1989.

Schwenk, Theodor. *The Basis of Potentization Research.* Spring Valley, NY: Mercury Press, 1988.

Selawry, Alla. *Ehrenfried Pfeiffer: Pioneer of Spiritual Research and Practice.* Spring Valley, NY: Mercury Press, 1992.

Sheldrake, Rupert. *A New Science of Life: The Hypothesis of Formative Causation.* Los Angeles: J.P. Tarcher, 1981.

Steiner, Rudolf. *Goethe's World View.* Spring Valley, NY: Mercury Press., 1985.

Steiner, Rudolf. *Goethean Science.* Spring Valley, NY: Mercury Press, 1988.

Steiner, Rudolf. *Man as Symphony of the Creative Word.* Sussex, England: Rudolf Steiner Press, 1991.

Thompson, William Irwin, ed. *Gaia 2: Emergence: The New Science of Becoming.* Hudson, NY: Lindsifarne Press, 1991.

Watson, E.L. Grant. *The Mystery of Physical Life.* Hudson, NY: Lindsifarne Press, 1992.

Whicher, Olive. *Sun Space: Science at a Threshold of Spiritual Understanding.* London: Rudolf Steiner Press. 1989.

Wilber, Ken, ed. *The Holographic Paradigm and other Paradoxes.* Boulder, CO; Shamballa, 1982.

Zajonc, Arthur. *Catching the Light: The Entwined History of Light and Mind.* New York: Bantam Books, 1993.

Herbology and botany

Bailey, Liberty Hyde, Ethel Zoe Bailey, and the staff of the Liberty Hyde Bailey Hortorium. *Hortus Third: A Concise Dictionary of Plants Cultivated in the United States and Canada.* New York: MacMillan Publishing, 1976.

Balls, Edward K. *Early Uses of California Plants.* Berkeley, CA: University of California Press, 1962.

Baumgardt, John Philip. *How to Identify Flowering Plant Families.* Portland, OR: Timber Press, 1991.

Culpeper, Nicholas. *Culpeper's Complete Herbal.* London: W. Foulsham, undated.

Foster, Steven, and James A. Duke. *A Field Guide to Medicinal Plants: Eastern and Central North America.* Peterson Field Guide Series #40. Boston: Houghton Mifflin, 1990.

Gerard, John. *The Herbal, or General History of Plants: The Complete 1633 Edition as Revised and Enlarged by Thomas Johnson.* New York: Dover Publications, 1975.

Grieve, M. *A Modern Herbal, Vols. I & II.* New York: Dover Publications, 1971.

Hickman, James C., ed. *The Jepson Manual: Higher Plants of California.* Berkeley and Los Angeles, CA: University of California Press, 1993.

Hoffman, David. *The Holistic Herbal.* Forres, Scotland: Findhorn Press, 1986.

Millspaugh, Charles. *American Medicinal Plants.* New York: Dover Publications, 1974.

Moore, Michael. *Medicinal Plants of the Mountain West.* Santa Fe, NM: Museum of New Mexico Press, 1979.

Moore, Michael. *Medicinal Plants of the Pacific West.* Santa Fe, NM: Red Crane Books, 1993.

Niehaus, Theodore F., and Charles L. Ripper. *Pacific States Wildflowers.* Peterson Field Guides #22. New York: Houghton Mifflin Company, 1976.

Parsons, Mary Elizabeth. *The Wildflowers of California.* New York: Dover Publications, 1966.

Schauenberg, Paul, and Ferdinand Paris. *Guide to Medicinal Plants.* New Canaan, CT: Keats Publishing, 1990.

Smith, James Payne, Jr. *Vascular Plant Families.* Eureka, CA: Mad River Press, 1977.

Stark, Raymond. *Guide to Indian Herbs.* Blaine, WA: Hancock House, 1981.

Strehlow, Dr. Wighard, and Gottfried Hertzka, M.D. *Hildegard of Bingen's Medicine.* Santa Fe, NM: Bear and Company, 1988.

Homeopathy

Cook, Trevor M. *Samuel Hahnemann: The Founder of Homoeopathic Medicine.* Wellingsborough, England: Thorsons, 1981.

Coulter, Harris L. *Homoeopathic Science and Modern Medicine: The Physics of Healing with Microdoses.* Richmond, CA: North Atlantic Books, 1981.

Danciger, Elizabeth. *Homeopathy: From Alchemy to Medicine.* Rochester, VT: Healing Arts Press, 1988.

Kent, James Tyler, M.D. *Lectures on Homoeopathic Philosophy.* Richmond, CA: North Atlantic Books, 1981.

Shepherd, Dr. Dorothy. *A Physician's Posy.* Devon, England: Health Sciences Press, 1969.

Ullman, Dana. *Discovering Homeopathy.* New York: Grove Press, 1980.

Vithoulkas, George. *The Science of Homeopathy.* Berkeley, CA: North Atlantic Books, 1993.

Whitmont, Edward C., M.D. *Psyche and Substance: Essays on Homeopathy in the Light of Jungian Psychology.* Richmond, CA: North Atlantic Books, 1980.

Whitmont, Edward C., M.D. *The Alchemy of Healing: Psyche and Soma.* Berkeley, CA: North Atlantic Books, 1993.

Medical and holistic paradigms of health

Advances: The Journal of Mind-Body Health, published quarterly by the Fetzer Institute, 9292 West KL Avenue, Kalamazoo, MI 49009.

Bott, Victor. *Anthroposophical Medicine, An Extension of the Art of Healing.* London: Rudolf Steiner Press, 1972.

Dossey, Larry, M.D. *Healing Words: The Power of Prayer and the Practice of Medicine.* New York: HarperCollins, 1991.

Dossey, Larry, M.D. *Medicine and Meaning.* New York: Bantam, 1992.

Dossey, Larry, M.D. *Recovering the Soul.* New York: Bantam, 1989.

Evans, Dr. Michael, and Iain Rodger. *Anthroposophical Medicine: Healing for Body, Soul, and Spirit.* London: Thorsons, 1992.

Friedman, Dr. Howard S. *The Self-Healing Personality.* New York: Penguin Books, 1992.

Laughlin, Tom, with James P. Moran, M.D. *The Mind and Cancer: Six Psychological Factors that May Lead to Cancer.* Malibu, CA: Panarion Press, 1990.

Leviton, Richard. *Anthroposophic Medicine Today.* Hudson, NY: Anthroposophic Press, 1988.

Mees, L.F.C., M.D. *Blessed by Illness.* Spring Valley, NY: Anthroposophic Press, 1990.

Moyers, Bill. *Healing and the Mind.* New York: Doubleday, 1993.

Murphy, Michael. *The Future of the Body.* Los Angeles: Jeremy P. Tarcher, 1992.

Ornish, Dean, M.D. *Dr. Dean Ornish's Program for Reversing Heart Disease.* New York: Ballentine Books, 1991.

Poole, William, with the Institute of Noetic Sciences. *The Heart of Healing.* Atlanta, GA: Turner Publishing, 1993.

Simonton, O. Carl, M.D., Stephanie Simonton, and James Creighton. *Getting Well Again.* New York: Bantam, 1992.

Steiner, Rudolf. *Health and Illness, Vols. 1 & 2.* Spring Valley, NY: Anthroposophic Press, 1983.

Temoshok, Lydia, and Henry Dreher. *The Type C Connection: The Behavior Links to Cancer and Your Health.* New York: Random House, 1992.

Twentyman, Ralph, M.D. *The Science and Art of Healing.* Edinburgh, Scotland: Floris Books, 1989.

Wood, Matthew. *The Magical Staff, The Vitalist Tradition in Western Medicine.* Berkeley, CA: North Atlantic Books, 1992.

Psychotherapy and soul care

Assagioli, Roberto, M.D. *Psychosynthesis: A Collection of Basic Writings.* New York: Penguin Books, 1986.

Barasch, Marc Ian. *The Healing Path: A Soul Approach to Illness.* New York: Tarcher/Putnam, 1993.

Bittleston, Adam. *Counselling and Spiritual Development.* Edinburgh, Scotland: Floris Books, 1988.

Bragdon, Emma. *The Call of Spiritual Emergency: From Personal Crisis to Personal Transformation.* New York: Harper and Row, 1990.

Bryant, William. *The Veiled Pulse of Time: An Introduction to Biographical Cycles and Destiny.* Hudson, NY: Anthroposophic Press, 1993.

Campbell, Joseph, ed. *The Portable Jung.* New York: Penguin Books, 1986.

Cousineau, Phil, ed. *Soul: An Anthology. Readings from Socrates to Ray Charles.* New York: HarperCollins, 1994.

Gill, Eric. *A Holy Tradition of Working.* West Stockbridge, MA: Lindsifarne Press, 1983.

Grof, Stanislav, M.D., and Christina Grof, eds. *Spiritual Emergency: When Personal Transformation Becomes a Crisis.* Los Angeles: Jeremey Tarcher, 1989.

Jung, C.G. *Man and His Symbols.* New York: Dell, 1968.

Jung, C.G. *Memories, Dreams, and Reflections.* New York: Vintage, 1989.

Hillman, James. *Re-visioning Psychology.* New York: HarperCollins, 1976, 1992.

Hillman, James. *The Thought of the Heart & the Soul of the World.* Dallas, TX: Spring Publications, 1992.

Hoffman, Bob. *No One Is to Blame: Getting a Loving Divorce from Mom & Dad.* Palo Alto, CA: Science and Behavior Books, 1979.

Kühlewind, Georg. *From Normal to Health: Paths to the Liberation of Consciousness.* Great Barrington, MA: Lindsifarne Press, 1988.

Lievegoed, Bernard. *Man on the Threshold: The Challenge of Inner Development.* Stroud, England: Hawthorne Press, 1985.

McNiff, Shaun. *Art as Medicine: Creating a Therapy of the Imagination.* Boston: Shamballa, 1992.

Moore, Thomas. *Care of the Soul: A Guide for Cultivating Depth and Sacredness in Everyday Life.* New York: HarperCollins, 1992.

Nelson, John E., M.D. *Healing the Split: Madness or Transcendence?* Los Angeles: Jeremy P. Tarcher, 1990.

Progoff, Ira. *At a Journal Workshop.* New York, NY: Dialogue House Library, 1988.

Roszak, Theodore. *The Voice of the Earth.* New York: Simon & Schuster, 1992.

Sardello, Robert. *Facing the World with Soul.* Hudson, NY: Lindsifarne Press, 1991.

Walsh, Roger, M.D., Ph.D., and Frances Vaughn, Ph.D. *Paths Beyond Ego: The Transpersonal Vision.* Los Angeles: Jeremy Tarcher, 1993.

Ward, Keith. *Defending the Soul.* Oxford, England: Oneworld Publications Ltd., 1992.

Whyte, David. *The Heart Aroused: Poetry and the Preservation of Soul in Corporate America.* New York: Doubleday, 1994.

Zweig, Connie, and Jeremiah Abrams, eds. *Meeting the Shadow: The Hidden Power of the Dark Side of Human Nature.* Los Angeles: Jeremy Tarcher, 1991.

The Flower Essence Society

The Flower Essence Society was founded in 1979 by Richard Katz, and incorporated as part of the non-profit organization Earth-Spirit in 1982. Since 1980 the Society has been co-directed by Patricia Kaminski and Richard Katz, who are married and professional partners. There are three major purposes of the Society: 1) to promote plant research and empirical clinical research on the therapeutic effects of flower essences; 2) to conduct training and certification programs for active flower essence practitioners, as well as public classes and seminars throughout the world; and 3) to provide a communication and referral network for those who are teaching, researching, or practicing in the field of flower essence therapy.

Tax-deductible donations or memberships to the Flower Essence Society to help sustain its educational and research programs are greatly appreciated. Case studies and practitioner reports are actively encouraged and warmly welcomed. Please write or call the Flower Essence Society for further information on our research program, membership rates, discounts, class schedules, newsletters and announcements, books, and other educational resources.

Wild Iris

Flower Essence Society, P.O. Box 459, Nevada City, CA 95959 USA.
telephone: 800-548-0075 or 916-265-9163; fax: 916-265-6467

Part II

Soul Issues:
Categories and
Themes

Categories and Cross References

Abandonment

(See also Abuse, Loneliness, Rejection)

Angelica — feeling abandoned by the spiritual world; to make a connection with spiritual guidance and support

Baby Blue Eyes — feeling rejected and abandoned by one's father

Bleeding Heart — feeling abandoned in relationships; need for more detachment and emotional self-sufficiency

Chicory — feelings of rejection or abandonment resulting in excessively needy or manipulative behavior

Evening Primrose — feeling rejected by one's mother in early infancy or in utero; cold or detached feelings toward others due to experience of abandonment and rejection

Holly — feeling unloved and rejected by others; using hostility toward others to mask feelings of emotional abandonment; feeling of isolation or alienation which stifles the heart

Mallow — difficulty making social contact with others, leading to feelings of abandonment

Mariposa Lily — feeling abandoned due to lack of bonding with one's mother; promotes connection with divine feminine principal; ability to nurture and feel nurtured

Oregon Grape — expecting rejection, abandonment from others; paranoia

Pink Monkeyflower — fearing abandonment and rejection, accompanied by a deep feeling of shame

Sweet Chestnut — despair of the soul, feeling abandoned by God

Sweet Pea — social alienation and isolation; not feeling at home or finding social roots

Abuse

(See also Addiction, Destructiveness)

Black Cohosh — entanglement in abusive or addictive relationships; difficulty in breaking from patterns of violence and destruction

Black-Eyed Susan — avoidance or lack of acknowledgment of prior abuse or exploitation; unconsciously repeating abusive pattern toward oneself or others

Centaury — for those who accept abuse and exploitation from others, usually in the role of serving or placating others

Dogwood — for those beaten or physically violated during childhood, lacking in gracefulness and gentleness in physical/etheric bodies

Echinacea — suffering extreme abuse and exploitation, need to restore and reclaim essential dignity

Evening Primrose — physical, sexual or emotional abuse when it is absorbed unconsciously in utero or during infancy, often leading to emotional and sexual repression

Golden Ear Drops — ability to make emotional contact with prior abuse, to feel pain which may have been numbed or blotted out

Hibiscus — inability to feel sexual warmth or vitality, often due to prior abusive or exploitative relationships

Impatiens — anger and intolerance toward others which is easily aroused, sometimes leading to violence or abuse

Mariposa Lily — abuse and abandonment from mother, leading to childhood trauma and emotional wounding

Pine — emotional self-abuse or neglect, due to prior guilt, shaming or abusive circumstances

Pink Monkeyflower — abuse or exploitation as a child or as sex partner; shame and guilt feelings

Pink Yarrow — absorbing emotional violence of others, psychic toxicity and congestion

Pretty Face — for those beaten, violated, shamed or made to feel ugly or unwanted

Purple Monkeyflower — occult or ritual abuse which predisposes the soul to fear of the spiritual world

Rosemary — physical abuse which leads to disconnection with the physical body; inability to feel warm and secure in one's physical body

Snapdragon — tendency to be verbally abusive, with biting or derogatory comments

Star Of Bethlehem — to soothe the trauma of abuse; can also be used when memories of past abuse are brought to one's awareness

Sweet Chestnut — abuse which is so severe, one feels life is no longer worth living; deepest despair and anguish

Vine — compulsion to control or exploit others, often through emotional or physical abuse

Acceptance

(See also Denial, Tolerance)

Agrimony — accepting painful feelings which are hidden by a mask of cheerfulness

Alpine Lily — acceptance of the female body, especially of the reproductive organs

Baby Blue Eyes — knowing the innate goodness of others and the world, especially when prone to cynicism or bitterness

Beech — accepting differences in others when there is a tendency to be critical or judgmental

Bleeding Heart — acknowledging the need of others to be free in relationships

Buttercup — accepting one's own self-worth, especially when there is a tendency to be self-effacing

Calendula — perceiving the inner meaning of what others say; true listening

Calla Lily — accepting one's sexual identity, when confused or ambivalent

Chrysanthemum — accepting one's own mortality, or any painful loss or death process in one's life

Crab Apple — learning to live with imperfection and impurity in oneself or others

Fairy Lantern — accepting the responsibilities of adulthood

Fawn Lily — full participation and acceptance of the mundane world, of its imperfection and daily stress, especially when there is a desire within the soul to retreat or hold back

Forget-Me-Not — being at peace about the death of loved one; transforming an earthly relationship into a spiritual one

Fuchsia — acceptance of deep, repressed emotions which need to be honestly expressed

Holly — to develop compassion and understanding, especially when there is a tendency to be hostile or jealous

Impatiens — allowing others to have their own pace; accepting the unfolding of life events

Love-Lies-Bleeding — acceptance of profound pain or suffering; ability of the soul to follow the path of suffering to spiritual transformation or self-sacrifice

Mustard — accepting dark, painful emotions; working through depression and darkness

Oak — knowing one's limits; knowing when to let go of the struggle

Penstemon — inner strength to accept adverse or difficult personal circumstances

Pine — self-acceptance; releasing guilt and self-blame

Pink Monkeyflower — fear that others will not accept one's deepest feelings or soul qualities

Sage — understanding and acceptance of life experience; reflecting and learning from experience

Saguaro — openness to the value of legitimate authority or the wisdom of elders

Scotch Broom — accepting obstacles as opportunities for growth and service; especially helpful when there is a sense of world doom

Action

(See also Manifestation)

Aloe Vera — heartfelt actions; letting the heart guide outer activity; especially when too much activity leads to burnout

Blackberry — putting ideas into action; when forces of will are stymied; overcoming inertia

Cayenne — bringing a fiery impetus to slow-moving situations

Golden Yarrow — ability to be active and outgoing, despite extreme sensitivity and vulnerability to one's environment or to the feelings of others

Hornbeam — overcoming resistance to daily responsibilities

Indian Pink — attraction to lifestyle with too much activity; ability to center oneself

Iris — when creative forces are stagnant; inability to fully express the soul's feeling for beauty

Mountain Pride — courageous action; taking a stand for one's beliefs

Sunflower — removing blockages to positive action resulting from a damaged masculine self-image or damaged relationship with one's father

Tansy — taking decisive action; cutting through lethargy

Addiction

Agrimony — abuse of drugs to create a cheerful persona; hiding true feelings

Angelica — especially useful during drug withdrawal, to help soul realign with benevolent spiritual guides

Arnica — repairing shock and trauma from drug abuse, especially when physical/etheric integrity of nervous system has been damaged

Aspen — use of drugs to cover fear of the unknown, to dampen sensitivity

Baby Blue Eyes — submerging oneself in drugs due to feeling that the world is too harsh, no longer trusting in the goodness of people or events

Basil — obsessive sexual promiscuity or fascination with pornography; addiction to sexual relationships or sexual stimulation

Black Cohosh — getting caught in relationships which are abusive or addictive; entrapped by addictive lifestyle of oneself or others

California Poppy — dream-like glamour or tendency toward escapism; hallucinogenic drugs

Canyon Dudleya — attachment to psychic experiences, compulsive seeking of spiritual or psychic highs

Chamomile — nervousness, hyperactivity, or irritability associated with drug withdrawal; calming and stabilizing

Chaparral — cleansing of accumulated psychic toxins from drug abuse

Chestnut Bud — breaking repetitive patterns of addiction or strong habits which encourage addictive behavior

Chrysanthemum — use of drugs, especially alcohol, to escape confrontation with psychic pain and loss; deep fear of death and dying

Clematis — use of drugs to escape from body and from present time, particularly psychedelic drugs

Fairy Lantern — addiction as a form of escapism; especially the need to use drugs to escape responsibilities and pressures of adulthood

Five-Flower Formula — initial treatment of addiction, to stabilize the body-mind; also helpful in treating drug overdose

Golden Yarrow — using drugs as a social buffer to dull sensitivity

Lavender — sedating nerves frayed from drug use, especially stimulants

Milkweed — using drugs which stupefy or sedate the consciousness (opiates and sedatives); inability of soul to cope with ego or individuated Self

Morning Glory — breaking free of addictive habits, especially the need for stimulants

Mountain Pennyroyal — drug or alcohol use which makes one susceptible to psychic aberration or contamination from astral entities

Nicotiana — addiction to smoking tobacco, or use of any drugs which numb the sensitivity and sever one from true feelings of the heart

Olive — depletion of mind and body from long-term use of drugs and other stimulants

Peppermint — promoting a more awake state without stimulant drugs

Pink Monkeyflower — using drugs to anesthetize intolerable emotional pain or sensitivity; drug addiction as a mask to cover soul shame and pain

Rosemary — using drugs to sever connection with the body; insecure in physical body

Sagebrush — letting go of old habit patterns and lifestyles which may contribute to drug use; also, feelings of emptiness or anxiety during drug withdrawal

Scarlet Monkeyflower — use of drugs to blot out true feelings, especially anger and powerlessness

Self-Heal — overall healing support for addiction therapy; confidence in one's inner resources to overcome addiction

Star Of Bethlehem — physical and psychic burnout from drug abuse

Star Tulip — for true connection to spiritual Self, especially when drugs are used to stimulate false psychic states

Sunflower — low self-esteem associated with drug usage; to develop a healthy self-image

Adolescence

Alpine Lily — healthy relationship to menstrual period and breast development; harmonizing feelings about one's female body with emotions and feelings in the heart

Angelica — protecting soul sheaths during times of searching or experimentation

Baby Blue Eyes — cynicism; feeling loss of innocence, pain of awakening to adulthood; disturbances with male figures

Basil — attraction to pornography or sexual conquest; inability to integrate emerging sexual identity with core Self

Bleeding Heart — for "crushes," brokenheartedness in relationships

California Poppy — fascination with drugs, escapism

California Wild Rose — cynicism, apathy, deep-seated alienation; possible suicidal feelings

Calla Lily — delayed puberty; when child has mixed messages or feelings about sexual identity

Chamomile — rapid mood swings; emotional instability

Crab Apple — self-disgust about acne or other feelings of ugliness or impurity

Fairy Lantern — delayed puberty; irregular or delayed menstruation in girls; overly feminine tendencies or delayed maturity in boys; anorexic tendencies, psychological need to remain childlike

Gentian — discouragement after academic, athletic or social setback

Golden Yarrow — providing protection for shy or sensitive individuals, encouraging greater social participation

Goldenrod — false social persona in group; inability to be true to oneself; easily influenced by group pressure

Heather — preoccupation with oneself; tendency to withdraw; excessive masturbation

Holly — pent-up emotions expressed negatively in family and school; feelings of jealousy, envy, rivalry at home and school

Larch — positive integration of creative forces with sexual forces; associated with voice change in boys; overall confidence

Mallow — feelings of social insecurity and group pressures; trouble making and keeping friends

Manzanita — dis-identification with the body; obsessive dieting; anorexia nervosa or bulimia

Mariposa Lily — stormy periods with mother or other female figures; too-early onset of puberty in girls or boys, hardening of childhood forces

Mustard — deep despair suffered in silence, often a precursor to suicide; depressed mood which can overwhelm the adolescent soul

Penstemon — feelings of being "not good enough," challenges in athletic or scholastic events

Pink Monkeyflower — fear of expressing or exposing true feelings, extreme sense of vulnerability

Pomegranate — balanced development of creative forces in teenage girls; promoting a healthy attitude toward onset of menstruation

Pretty Face — feelings of ugliness or rejection; wanting to be seen as beautiful as a form of social acceptance

Sagebrush — breaking free of old habits and personality traits which are no longer appropriate; emotional maturation; positive acceptance of feelings of aloneness and individuation

Saguaro — extreme feelings of rebelliousness; resistance to authority figures

Sticky Monkeyflower — awkwardness of sexual feelings; fears of intimacy which lead to sexual aggression or extreme inhibition and isolation

Sunflower — conflict with one's father; development of the masculine Self, positive individuality in boys or girls

Sweet Pea — social alienation, conflicts with family, feeling disconnected from community; seeking social roots and bonds; helps those with destructive social ties (such as gangs) to find a healthier sense of community

Walnut — having the courage to follow one's own convictions despite peer pressures or societal judgments

Wild Oat — confusion about goals in life; to find life direction and purpose

Willow — resentment and bitterness; a feeling that life is "not fair," blaming parents, authority figures, society

Aggressiveness

Impatiens — tendency toward impatience and bossiness

Larkspur — positive leadership; balancing a tendency toward self-aggrandizement

Mountain Pride — positive strength and assertiveness in the face of adversary forces; warrior-like qualities

Nicotiana — physical toughness or "macho" qualities, numbing the feeling life in order to appear strong

Oregon Grape — meeting others with hostility; expecting aggression from others

Poison Oak — tendency to "fight" rather than "flight," coping with sensitivity by warding off others

Snapdragon — aggressiveness in the use of the spoken word, verbal abuse and angry outpouring of energy

Sunflower — balancing aggressive traits by developing positive masculine identity; counteracting excessive egotism

Tiger Lily — tendency toward over-assertiveness, forced masculinity; bringing feminine balance

Trillium — overcoming greed or lust for power

Trumpet Vine — healthy assertiveness, especially when speaking

Vine — putting one's own wishes before those of others; compulsion to be in control

Aging

Angel's Trumpet — appropriate and balanced acknowledgment of aging process, especially physical deterioration and dying; surrender to spiritualization of the body

Angelica — protection when crossing the threshold of death; during surgery or life-threatening illness; providing protection for the loosening of the subtle bodies which occurs during aging

Baby Blue Eyes — bitterness or cynicism about the world; integrating worldly experience with childlike trust

Beech — being overly critical, inability to "forgive and forget"

Bleeding Heart — losing a husband, wife, or friend; letting go of a past relationship so one can go on with life

Buttercup — diminished self-esteem, feelings of unworthiness or that one's contribution has no value

California Wild Rose — feeling connected to the Earth during the aging process; for those who may be prematurely occupied with the "other side"

Centaury — sense of dignity and strength of individuality, often compromised when physically dependent as in nursing homes

Chicory — tendency to be needy, demanding, reverting to childish behavior

Chrysanthemum — confrontation with one's own mortality at any stage of life, especially mid-life crisis; shift to higher spiritual identity as source of true immortality

Clematis — dreaminess, awareness moving in and out of body

Gentian — overcoming pessimism and despair in the face of setbacks in physical health or loss of physical faculties

Heather — preoccupation with problems and worries, over-concern with oneself

Hibiscus — to maintain sexual warmth and responsiveness during aging process

Holly — opening the heart, letting go of hostility; making peace in all relationships which need healing, so that the soul may depart with a sense of completion

Honeysuckle — tendency to dwell in the past, excessive nostalgia

Lavender — calming and soothing when agitated; difficulty in sleeping

Madia — inability to concentrate or focus on details

Mimulus — numerous small fears related to daily living; for the "shut-in" who does not take risks

Penstemon — courage to face obstacles, impediments, and physical handicaps

Peppermint — brings mental alertness when the mind is foggy; energizes thinking faculties

Pretty Face — over-identification with youthful appearance; helps in accepting aging process and allowing inner beauty to radiate

Purple Monkeyflower — feeling uneasy or afraid due to out-of-body states or other spiritual experiences; accepting aging as a process of spiritualization

Queen Anne's Lace — blurred vision, especially when the soul is seeking to change from physical to metaphysical vision

Rosemary — difficulty inhabiting the body; forgetful, tendency toward drowsiness, cold in extremities

Sage — discovering the inner wisdom of life experiences; insight and peace about the meaning of one's life; inner serenity

Saint John's Wort — grounding and protection as one begins losing connection with the physical body and losing control of bodily functions; disturbed sleep and dreams

Self-Heal — instilling confidence in one's own healing forces, counteracting over-dependence on medical staff or family

Star Tulip — failing eyesight and hearing; helping transition from physical sight and sound to spiritual listening and perception; stimulating the shift from physical to spiritual awareness as a natural process of aging

White Chestnut — calming the chattering mind; breaking the hold of obsessive thinking and worrying

Willow — feelings of blame or bitterness about life; tendency toward stiffness or hardening as in arthritis

Alienation

Alpine Lily — feeling estranged from the female body and deeper feminine Self, especially from the experience of menstrual period and other reproductive or biological functions

Baby Blue Eyes — feeling that the world is harsh; no longer trusting in the innate goodness of people, feeling cut off from spiritual world

Buttercup — not feeling "worthy" to others, or by worldly standards

California Wild Rose — apathy and indifference to life; possible suicidal tendencies

Calla Lily — alienation from sexual identity; not feeling at home in one's male or female body

Chrysanthemum — inability to accept death or dying process, deep soul conflict about the transitory nature of earthly life

Evening Primrose — emotional distancing, lack of emotional presence due to unconscious absorption of toxic emotions in utero and in infancy; feeling rejected and unwanted

Fairy Lantern — fear of facing adulthood; *puer eterna*, or eternal child

Fawn Lily — for a reclusive soul who suffers in a challenging world, overly needy of perfection and an insulated environment

Golden Ear Drops — contacting painful feelings from childhood, which may have been bottled up inside

Lady's Slipper — separation from one's own inner authority and destiny, self-doubt accompanied by nervous depletion and sexual exhaustion

Manzanita — aversion to the physical body and physical world

Mariposa Lily — estrangement from one's mother or from the feminine; feeling unloved and unwanted

Milkweed — separation or estrangement from core Self, inability to cope with core identity

Poison Oak — discomfort with others, needs distance and space

Pretty Face — feeling cut off from one's own inner sense of what is beautiful and harmonious; alienated from the physical Self

Saguaro — hostility toward authority figures; rebelliousness

Shooting Star — profound alienation; not feeling at home on Earth

Sunflower — disturbed relationship with one's father or father archetype in others

Sweet Pea — not feeling connected with family, community or land; fear of social commitment

Violet — feeling as if one is an outsider or a stranger to others; helpful when moving to a new area

Water Violet — distancing oneself from others; seeing others as unworthy of one's attention

Aloofness

Baby Blue Eyes — aloofness with tendency to cynicism

California Wild Rose — aloofness as a form of apathy, lack of involvement or enthusiasm

Fawn Lily — tendency to hold soul forces back due to fear of contamination or stress

Mallow — opening to others, overcoming self-created barriers to friendship or lack of social warmth

Nicotiana — for the "loner" who is emotionally unavailable or distant

Pink Monkeyflower — holding back from emotional participation due to fear that deepest Self will be rejected

Tansy — appearing aloof or nonchalant, especially when accompanied by lack of vitality

Violet — openness to others, especially in groups

Water Violet — feeling separate from others, especially with a sense of disdain or pride

Altruism

(See also Service)

California Wild Rose — ability to be motivated, to care about others and the Earth

Chicory — helping others without the need of getting something back; developing selfless giving; counteracting emotional neediness

Elm — to balance heroic tendencies; for those who assume responsibility but feel overwhelmed and frustrated

Larkspur — joyful leadership for the good of all

Tiger Lily — overcoming aggressiveness in work with others

Trillium — overcoming selfishness or greed; working for the common good

Ambition

Aloe Vera — workaholic tendencies; feeling burned out, depleted

Elm — taking on too many responsibilities, resulting in overwhelm or despondency

Larkspur — self-aggrandizement in leadership roles

Oak — strong forces of will and achievement goals, which press the body to the limits of endurance

Tiger Lily — overly masculine striving; strong competitive attitude

Trillium — over-concern with acquiring power and possessions

Vine — obsession with wielding power over others

Ambivalence

(See also Conflict, Hesitation, Indecision)

Alpine Lily — for women, difficulty accepting female body

California Wild Rose — lack of commitment; indifference to life and life destiny

Calla Lily — confusion about sexual identity, or the expression of sexuality

Easter Lily — uncertainty about sexuality, feeling it may be impure

Evening Primrose — ambivalence about parenting and about commitment in relationship due to traumatic rejection

Fairy Lantern — inner conflict about growing up, emotional conflict between child's feelings and adult responsibilities

Fawn Lily — conflict about how to use soul forces; inner peacefulness versus worldly involvement

Golden Yarrow — desire to be a part of social or artistic experiences, but feeling too sensitive

Manzanita — aversion to the physical body and physical world; ambivalence about being incarnated in a body

Pomegranate — confused about choice of career and/or family life

Saguaro — conflict regarding authority figures; rebellion

Scleranthus — difficulty in decision-making, wavering between choices

Self-Heal — uncertainty about one's power to get well

Shooting Star — not fully accepting being on Earth or being a part of humanity

Violet — wanting to join with others but afraid of losing oneself in the group; shy, yet seeking social warmth

Anger

(See also Hostility, Resentment)

Black-Eyed Susan — repressed anger which needs to be brought to awareness

Chamomile — restoring calm when emotionally upset

Fuchsia — deep-seated anger that needs to be released, especially when false or hyper-emotionality is expressed

Holly — anger when love is thwarted or denied

Impatiens — quick to anger

Poison Oak — easily irritated, coping with hypersensitivity by showing anger or hostility

Scarlet Monkeyflower — fear of anger; recognizing and transforming anger

Snapdragon — inappropriate expressions of anger, especially directed as verbal abuse

Willow — deeply held anger leading to bitterness and resentment

Animals and Animal Care

Arnica — shock, trauma, illness, injury, surgery

Aspen — unknown fear or terror in an animal; especially indicated when treating wild or nervous animals

Bleeding Heart — breaking undue emotional attachments to the caretaker, such as whining cats or moping dogs waiting for the owner to return

Borage — lifting the spirit of an animal that may be depressed because of illness or old age

Chamomile — for barking dogs; emotional upset accompanied by stomach distress such as gas or vomiting

Cherry Plum — extreme tension or stress, such as a terrified animal that is trapped

Chestnut Bud — instilling effective learning patterns during training; to stimulate the animal's emotional memory and ability to retain training, not repeat mistakes

Chicory — especially indicated for younger animals such as whining puppies or kittens; also indicated when the illness may be psychosomatic or to get attention

Cosmos — to encourage interspecies communication; helpful where different animals are gathered; useful when training animals, or establishing psychic bonds in one-on-one relationships; indicated for both animal and caretaker

Dill — overwhelm or confusion such as during travel or upset of schedule

Five-Flower Formula — for any form of stress or emergency, or when uncertain of which remedy to give

Holly — jealous pets, especially when jealousy involves another pet vying for the attention of the caretaker

Impatiens — for nervous, "high-strung," impulsive animals

Love-Lies-Bleeding — wounded or deeply suffering animal which may not live

Mariposa Lily — assisting mother-infant bonding, especially if the animal is being introduced to a surrogate mother; also good for young animals in a new home

Mimulus — nervous conditions in animals; good for jittery horses or shy animals who hide from people

Penstemon — illness or trauma; gives inner strength during adverse circumstances

Pink Yarrow — pets who take on or mirror the emotions of their human caretakers

Quaking Grass — helping animals living together in a group or herd to adjust; especially important when a new animal has been introduced

Red Clover — calming to hysterical animals, particularly cats; can be used effectively when taking an animal to a veterinarian for treatment

Self-Heal — add to almost any combination to stimulate inner healing forces of an animal, awaken vitality and will to live

Snapdragon — for animals who bite; especially indicated for aggressive tendencies in horses such as biting and sucking

Star Of Bethlehem — abused animals, or any animal who has suffered injury or trauma

Tiger Lily — for hostile or aggressive cats or dogs

Vervain — for hyperactive, overly tense animals

Vine — for animals which dominate younger or weaker animals

Walnut — before and after a major move; to help break links to old places of residence; also good for animals giving birth

Wild Rose — for apathetic, listless animals

Anxiety

Aspen — anxiety that has no known reason

Cerato — excessive anxiety about failure, thus depending on others for advice

Chamomile — calming overly anxious states

Chrysanthemum — morbid thoughts of one's own death, or deep suppression of such thoughts

Elm — overstriving for perfection; fear that one will let down or disappoint others

Filaree — worry and concern about trivial problems of daily life

Garlic — chronic anxiety and worry; ghostly countenance

Golden Yarrow — performance anxiety, especially when felt in solar plexus

Goldenrod — needing social approval; unsure of one's own values

Larch — fear of failure, paralyzed by anxiety

Mimulus — excessive anxiety and nervousness about daily life; *everyday fears*; fretful, timid attitude

Mustard — free-floating anxiety, especially when accompanied by depression

Nicotiana — coping with anxiety by anesthetizing emotions; showing a "cool" exterior

Pink Monkeyflower — inability to trust that others will accept one; shame or guilt

Pretty Face — anxiety about personal appearance; wanting to be acceptable to others by appearing physically pleasing

Trumpet Vine — speaking with greater expressiveness, despite fears; anxiety which blocks natural soul warmth and color

Apathy

(See also Involvement)

California Wild Rose — indifference to life; building stronger forces of enthusiasm

Gorse — to encourage hope in those who have given up all hope

Peppermint — apathetic thinking; mental sluggishness

Tansy — apparent laziness, stagnant energy, overly phlegmatic

Wild Rose — lacking motivation to get well, especially with lingering illness

Appreciation

Buttercup — recognizing one's self-worth, and the gifts one has to share with others

Calendula — perceiving the inner meaning of what others say

California Wild Rose — joy of life, deep appreciation and gratitude for being on Earth

Holly — ability to feel joy and happiness for others

Manzanita — knowing the value of the physical body and world; deep appreciation for the body as the "temple of the spirit"

Oregon Grape — ability to see the goodhearted intentions of others

Quaking Grass — appreciation for the worth of others in group work

Sage — appreciating the lessons of life, learning and growing from life experience

Attachment

Angel's Trumpet — for the soul which is too attached to body during the dying process; surrendering to the spiritual transition of death

Bleeding Heart — holding on to others, emotional possessiveness

Canyon Dudleya — attachment to extraordinary experiences, inflating or exaggerating ordinary events of daily life

Chicory — obsessive need to get attention in relationships, particularly in negative ways

Chrysanthemum — over-identification with mundane personality, with worldly fame and fortune; inability to accept death or transitory nature of earthly life

Love-Lies-Bleeding — over-personalization of one's pain or suffering; to develop a more transpersonal level of understanding

Morning Glory — holding on to destructive habit patterns, addictions

Oak — holding on to struggle, not knowing when to let go; identified with a heroic struggle

Red Chestnut — bringing calm but caring detachment when others are in need; counteracting over-concern and obsessive worry for others

Sage — appropriate detachment as part of aging process, ability to gain larger soul perspective

Sagebrush — holding on to false identity and life circumstances which are no longer appropriate

Trillium — greedy attachment to possessions and/or power

Attention

(See also Concentration and Focus)

Chicory — need to receive excessive attention from others

Clematis — being in the here-and-now

Heather — drawing attention to oneself by talking about one's problems

Madia — to focus attention and concentration

Pink Monkeyflower — avoiding social attention, wanting to hide or cover up

Queen Anne's Lace — to focus and clarify psychic forces, especially as they relate to vision and perception

Rabbitbrush — attention to many details while maintaining an overview of the "big picture"

Authority

Centaury — over-dependence on the authority of others; for the subservient "doormat" who needs validation from outside authority

Cerato — accepting inner knowingness and authority; for those who rely on the authority of others to decide what is true

Fairy Lantern — childlike dependence on the authority of others; feigning helplessness or dependency

Lady's Slipper — estrangement from one's inner authority, inability to integrate higher spiritual purpose with real life and work on Earth; imbalances between the crown and root chakras

Purple Monkeyflower — fear of spiritual authority or those in positions of spiritual power

Sage — elder wisdom, using life wisdom to guide and help others, inner authority based on actual experience

Saguaro — conflict or rebellion against authority; respect for true spiritual authority

Snapdragon — verbal bullying and threatening behavior, controlling others especially through verbal abuse

Sunflower — conflict involving feelings about father or father figures

Vine — overly imposing one's authority on others

Walnut — independence from the authority of others; charting one's own path in life free from the hindering influences of others

Avoidance

(See also Denial, Escapism, Procrastination, Resistance)

Agrimony — wearing a cheerful mask which hides painful emotions

Black-Eyed Susan — not looking at or acknowledging dark emotions, hidden or threatening parts of the Self

Canyon Dudleya — wishing to escape mundane states of consciousness; connecting to daily events and ordinary reality

Chrysanthemum — denial or avoidance of one's mortality; overemphasis on temporal identity; to develop awareness of the spiritual Self

Clematis — escape from the present by dwelling in more pleasant daydreams of the future

Evening Primrose — deep sexual or emotional repression due to abuse and rejection in early childhood

Fairy Lantern — avoiding full adult identity and responsibilities

Fawn Lily — not wanting to face stressful or challenging situations

Fuchsia — repressing awareness of basic emotions, often covered with superficial emotionality

Honeysuckle — escaping the present by dwelling in more pleasant feelings of the past

Nicotiana — avoidance of real feelings by developing a false persona of strength or toughness, especially through a numbing or deadening of the soul life

Pink Monkeyflower — fear of one's deepest feelings and of sharing these with others; profound feelings of shame

Poison Oak — creating distance from others by erecting barriers which are hostile or offensive

Scarlet Monkeyflower — fear of dealing with or experiencing anger and strong emotions

Water Violet — refraining from social contact out of a feeling of superiority; aloofness

Awakeness

Chestnut Bud — to observe one's experience clearly and learn from it

Clematis — ability to be fully present and wakeful, especially when tendency is to float or drift away

Cosmos — to stimulate mercurial qualities of the mind; ability to integrate thoughts with speech, to speak and think with clarity

Dill — absorption of many sensations and experiences, leading to nervous overwhelm

Milkweed — inability to cope with awake states of consciousness, desire of soul to return to unconsciousness

Morning Glory — vitality and freshness; overcoming energy-sapping addictive habits; awakening life energy without the need for stimulants

Peppermint — stimulates healthy mental alertness; overcoming mental sluggishness and lethargy

Rabbitbrush — ability to handle many diverse activities with clear attention

Rosemary — inability to be fully present in one's body, or to receive information through one's physical vehicle; tendency to drowsiness or forgetfulness

Saint John's Wort — for those who are overly expanded into a dream-like consciousness, inability to come properly into body consciousness

Awareness

(See also Clarity, Insight, Wisdom)

Angelica — attunement to higher worlds, especially for guidance and protection

Black-Eyed Susan — penetrating insight into emotions

Calendula — sensitivity to the meaning of what others say

Chaparral — psychic cleansing of disturbing images; awareness through dreams and meditation

Chestnut Bud — recognizing the lessons of past experience; not repeating mistakes

Cosmos — ability to bring higher thought into spoken word; higher mental awareness

Forget-Me-Not — understanding the karmic dimension in personal relationships; recognizing one's connection with those in the spiritual world; deep mindfulness of subtle realms

Fuchsia — bringing repressed emotions to the surface of consciousness

Golden Ear Drops — to bring understanding by re-experiencing hidden traumas, usually from childhood

Love-Lies-Bleeding — extending awareness of one's suffering; seeing one's personal experience within a larger human and cosmic context

Madia — mental clarity and concentration

Manzanita — embodiment, awareness of the physical body and world

Mugwort — awareness during dreaming and experiences of the spiritual threshold; greater psychic sensitivity

Queen Anne's Lace — balanced psychic awareness, especially when sexual or emotional feelings distort clarity

Rabbitbrush — seeing the big picture, an overview of the details of a situation

Sage — inner wisdom of life experiences, understanding the meaning of life

Scarlet Monkeyflower — integrating the "shadow," awareness of powerful emotions, anger

Shasta Daisy — synthesizing many diverse ideas into a unified whole; awareness of underlying relationships or patterns

Star Tulip — greater receptivity to subtle states of awareness, especially in meditation and dreams

Yerba Santa — recognition of deeply repressed emotions, especially emotional pain within the heart

Awkwardness

(See also Body)

Dogwood — emotional trauma stored within the body, leading to physical awkwardness; often with a history of physical abuse

Mallow — discomfort in social situations, fear of reaching out to others

Manzanita — alienation from the physical body and physical world; not feeling at home in the body

Pink Monkeyflower — social insecurity due to feelings of shame, fear of exposure

Pretty Face — feeling awkward due to concern about physical appearance

Shooting Star — feeling alien and out of place; not fully in touch with one's humanity ·

Sticky Monkeyflower — unease or awkwardness regarding one's sexuality, leading to avoidance or aggression

Violet — feeling uncomfortable in group situations; fear of submerging one's individual identity in a group

Balance

California Poppy — balance in inner development; not seeking false spiritual "highs" or illusory glamour

Calla Lily — balancing one's male and female aspects

Corn — spirituality which relates to both Heaven and Earth, and both the physical body and psychic awareness

Fawn Lily — balance between inner spirituality and outer commitment

Goldenrod — balance between social "group" consciousness and individual awareness

Lotus — balanced spirituality; to bring right relationship between crown chakra and other energy centers

Morning Glory — balance and regularity in daily habits and life-style

Mugwort — to balance the psychic life, especially harmonizing transitions between daytime and nighttime consciousness

Nasturtium — to bring intellectual forces into balance and integration with metabolic processes; to renew life forces which are drained due to overworry and intense mental activity

Nicotiana — to balance the heart forces, especially to integrate the feeling life with bodily strength; to feel earthly forces of strength in consonance with the inner life of the soul

Pomegranate — to balance female creativity, both inner and outer, creative and procreative

Queen Anne's Lace — to harmonize emerging psychic faculties, especially when distorted by lower emotional or sexual projections

Quince — balancing the soul's need to express both power and love; to integrate nurturing feelings within a role which also requires authority and responsibility

Scleranthus — extreme instability and imbalance; restlessness and confusion, especially when unable to make clear, firm decisions

Sunflower — imbalanced ego identity, vacillating between self-effacement and self-aggrandizement

Vervain — to bring inner equanimity and moderation; extreme intensity or passionate idealism which often leads to nervous depletion

Barriers

Evening Primrose — lack of emotional presence; inability to form deep relationships due to traumatic rejection in infancy

Fawn Lily — naturally reclusive, protecting oneself from too much social contact

Goldenrod — creating barriers to others by antisocial or obnoxious behavior

Mallow — creating barriers to friendships with others; increasing warmth and trust in social contacts

Penstemon — strength and courage to overcome obstacles

Pink Monkeyflower — creating barriers out of feelings of shame, unworthiness or vulnerability; highly sensitive and not wanting exposure

Poison Oak — fear of intimate contact with others, coping with sensitivity by not allowing contact, especially through hostility or anger; needing to understand the meaning of boundaries or limits

Rock Water — extreme rigidity, self-discipline or asceticism that creates barriers to flowing contact

Star Tulip — feeling a barrier in relation to the Higher Self; building more receptivity in listening

Walnut — breaking through limits from past associations and influences

Water Violet — feeling distant and aloof from others, especially when due to pride

Blame

(See also Resentment)

Baby Blue Eyes — blame when tinged with cynicism

Beech — blame with critical judgment of others

Larch — self-blame when making errors, often leading to inability to take risks

Oregon Grape — expecting blame or negativity from others

Pine — self-blame; being hard on oneself; filled with guilt feelings

Pink Yarrow — tendency to absorb others' feelings of blame; emotional projection

Sage — blaming others or circumstances for life destiny; gaining a higher perspective

Saguaro — blaming authority figures for personal and world problems

Snapdragon — verbal criticism and abuse of others

Willow — finding fault with others or with one's situation; deeply held feelings of resentment, toxic bitterness

Body

(See also Awkwardness, Eating Disorders, Feminine Consciousness, Immune Disturbances, Instinctual Self, Masculine Consciousness, Psychosomatic Illness, Sexuality)

Aloe Vera — burnout or exhaustion, especially from overstriving or overuse of creative forces; balance and renewal of life forces

Alpine Lily — disturbance in or rejection of the female organs; alienated from bodily experience of female Self

Arnica — trauma, especially from physical injury; deep shock which disassociates spiritual forces from body

Borage — a feeling of heaviness in the body, especially around the heart

California Pitcher Plant — tendency to suffer weak digestion; tumor-prone; tendency to develop waterlogged or mucous conditions; promoting greater physical vigor

California Wild Rose — weak, apathetic or listless; poor progress in healing due to lack of interest in life

Clematis — embodiment, becoming fully present in the body, for those who are pale, devitalized, and seem to be "elsewhere"

Corn — ability to feel grounded and in touch with the Earth, especially in urban environments

Crab Apple — obsession with bodily impurities and imperfections; also to enhance dietary cleansing programs, fasting or detoxification

Dandelion — releasing emotional tension in body; good adjunct to therapeutic bodywork

Dogwood — tendency to be accident-prone, ungraceful

Fairy Lantern — desire to stay in prepubescent stage; unable to identify with mature sexuality or adult body type

Fawn Lily — fragile, delicate temperament, easily fatigued; highly developed spirituality which needs to find greater connection to the physical dimension

Five-Flower Formula — to help body to stabilize during extreme trauma, surgery or shock

Fuchsia — physical distress due to emotional repression, often manifested as headaches

Garlic — ghostly or pale-looking, drained, poor immune response; tendency to parasites or infections, especially when accompanied by nervous fear

Golden Yarrow — tension in solar plexus; oversensitive but struggles to be outgoing

Hibiscus — integration of libido and sexuality with soul warmth

Hound's Tongue — overweight accompanied by overly materialistic attitude toward life; heavy or dull bodily awareness, need for levity

Indian Paintbrush — ability to use vital forces to energize one's creative and artistic expression

Iris — sense of weight or pressure in the neck, unable to experience or receive inspired thoughts

Love-Lies-Bleeding — intense physical suffering through wounding or disease; finding inner meaning and acceptance of intense pain; to stimulate the immune system

Manzanita — appreciation of the body as the "Temple of the Spirit;" tendency to bodily abuse or denial (e.g. anorexia nervosa or bulimia)

Nasturtium — lack of physical and etheric vitality due to excessive study and other intellectual activities

Nicotiana — false grounding of the body by numbing or deadening the feeling life; appearance of strength or toughness, devoid of feelings

Olive — extreme fatigue and exhaustion, especially after a long-term illness or stressful situation

Penstemon — ability to endure and accept physical hardships or handicaps

Peppermint — when bodily processes overwhelm the thinking function

Pink Monkeyflower — shame about sexual organs, often due to prior abuse or exploitation

Pomegranate — conflict about creative and procreative forces in women, leading to PMS or other reproductive disorders

Pretty Face — over-identification with outer image of body or cosmetic or health image; inability to radiate true inner beauty; also a hidden feeling that the body is inherently ugly and must be decorated or masked in order to appear beautiful

Purple Monkeyflower — physical symptoms arising from extreme tension and fear of spiritual experiences below the level of conscious understanding; also, feeling of intense pressure in crown or brow due to fearful psychic experiences

Queen Anne's Lace — distortions of physical sight; emergent psychic vision which needs integration

Rosemary — for those who feel incompletely incarnated in their body; insecurity in physical expression of the body; poor circulation and cold extremities

Self-Heal — to arouse recuperative powers of the body; integrating body and mind in healing process

Shooting Star — deep-set alienation from the Earth or human life; disassociated from the physical world

Snapdragon — extreme tension in jaw and mouth, TMJ symptoms, grinding teeth, disturbed metabolic function, need to direct energy to lower metabolism when misplaced as anger and verbal abuse

Star Of Bethlehem — to release trauma from particular parts of the body, often stored from the past; can be applied topically to the appropriate area

Tansy — tendency to be lethargic, heavyset

Vervain — pronounced tension from overenthusiasm, tendency to fanaticism or extremism; uses nerves and will to push the body

Yerba Santa — deterioration, wasting away, especially with symptoms involving congestion of the chest, heart and lungs

Breakthrough

(See also Avoidance, Catharsis, Inertia, Resistance, Transition)

Black-Eyed Susan — opening up awareness of hidden areas of the Self; breakthrough of self-awareness

Blackberry — ability to put thoughts into action; manifestation

Cayenne — to catalyze the will to overcome inertia and move decisively to one's next step

Five-Flower Formula — ability to call on deep inner resources in times of great stress

Fuchsia — bringing repressed emotions to awareness, especially when false emotions have been used to cover deeper feelings; also when emotional repression leads to psychosomatic symptoms

Indian Paintbrush — ability to rouse vital forces for creative work

Iris — to overcome creative blocks when lacking inspiration

Morning Glory — overcoming depleting habit patterns, catalyzing fresh forces of vitality

Mountain Pride — ability to rally courage and strength when faced with overwhelming challenges

Sagebrush — letting go of old "baggage," of identifications and attachments which no longer serve one; able to take the next step

Scarlet Monkeyflower — to bring repressed emotions to awareness, especially when there has been a fear of powerful emotions such as anger

Scleranthus — to come to a decision after wavering between alternatives

Tansy — decisive action; overcoming lethargy and procrastination

Walnut — freedom from the influences of the past, from the ideas of others; setting out on one's own path

Brokenheartedness

(See also Personal Relationships)

Angelica — transcending personal relationships as the only source of emotional fulfillment; feeling the presence of benevolent spiritual beings

Bleeding Heart — emotional detachment and acceptance when ending a relationship

Borage — to bring cheerful courage and upliftment; to ease pain, constriction or grief which weighs down the heart

California Wild Rose — acceptance of painful feelings in the heart, especially when there is a tendency to avoid pain or real life experience

Chamomile — calming emotional trauma or argumentativeness in relationships

Forget-Me-Not — to open the heart to spiritual realms, especially to transcend personal grief for one who has died; to instill a spiritual recognition of the departed soul

Holly — opening the heart to true love and acceptance; compassion

Honeysuckle — dwelling on past relationships; living in the past, inability to cope with present reality

Love-Lies-Bleeding — physical or emotional pain which stretches the boundaries of the heart; ability to learn compassion through personal suffering

Pink Monkeyflower — to retain trust and vulnerability despite previous heartbreak or trauma

Sweet Chestnut — feeling that one's heart is being split open; great and intense anguish that is often transpersonal or spiritual; "dark night of the soul"

Yerba Santa — accumulation of psychic toxins within the heart; deep-seated pain and trauma which blocks the heart from full expression

Calm

Agrimony — false outer calm, hiding inner conflict

Angel's Trumpet — deep peacefulness in the soul, ability to experience death or spiritual initiation with equanimity

Canyon Dudleya — overexcitement, tendency to dramatize emotional life or create intense emotional and psychic experiences

Chamomile — fretful, fussy emotions; tension, particularly in the stomach region

Cosmos — to harmonize an overly active mind, when many ideas flood in simultaneously

Filaree — letting go of worries and anxieties that tend to unnecessarily limit one's free participation in life

Five-Flower Formula — immediate calm in accidents or life-threatening situations

Garlic — release of nervous fears and insecurities that weaken life forces

Indian Pink — remaining calm and centered in the midst of intense activity

Larch — confidence in one's creative ability; for those who are fearful of making a mistake

Lavender — soothing frayed, overstimulated nerves

Mimulus — calming when nervous, fretful, or overly anxious about small events of daily life

Nicotiana — false appearance of calm when in reality the emotions are numb and unresponsive; using tobacco addiction to calm nerves

Pink Yarrow — tendency to be an emotional sponge; absorbing emotional qualities of others, leading to emotional oversensitivity

Purple Monkeyflower — to bring calm objectivity to spiritual experiences, especially when there is fear of the occult

Red Chestnut — sending positive, healing thoughts to others; releasing worry or over-concern for others

Red Clover — to bring calm to situations of panic and group hysteria; keeping one's individual awareness and clarity

Star Of Bethlehem — to soothe and harmonize the effects of shock or trauma

White Chestnut — constant churning and overactivity of the mind

Catalyst

Black-Eyed Susan — insight into emotions when there has been a lack of emotional awareness

Blackberry — putting thoughts into action; ability to manifest and act upon intentions

Cayenne — mobilizing the will, overcoming inertia, particularly when feeling stuck

Indian Paintbrush — bringing forces of vitality to the creative process; expressing creative inspiration

Tansy — overcoming sluggishness or indecisiveness, especially when vitality has been suppressed

Catharsis

(See also Breakthrough, Purification, Release)

Black Cohosh — ability to confront abusive or destructive forces; taking hold of and transforming threatening circumstances

Black-Eyed Susan — release of hidden emotions by bringing the light of understanding and insight

Cayenne — promoting catharsis by bringing more fiery stimulus to stagnant situations

Chaparral — psychic cleansing often through disturbing dreams or meditation; to release negative or violent images absorbed from mass media, drugs or other experiences

Evening Primrose — ability to heal trauma from in utero and early infancy experiences, particularly when unwanted or rejected

Fuchsia — release of repressed emotions, which may be covered by superficial emotionality or psychosomatic symptoms

Golden Ear Drops — release of painful childhood memories, often expressed in deep crying

Holly — release of hostility or anger; often used when not sure of underlying issues

Love-Lies-Bleeding — intense pain or suffering which impels the soul toward transcendence and spiritual insight

Scarlet Monkeyflower — release of powerful emotions, especially anger; overcoming fear of strong emotions

Willow — release of anger, blame, resentment

Centeredness

(See also Calm, Daydreaming, Groundedness)

Angelica — to move and act with awareness of subtle realities; spiritual centeredness

Canyon Dudleya — lack of grounding in ordinary physical experience, tendency toward hysteria and psychic inflation

Corn — centeredness in crowded environments such as cities; grounded spirituality related to the Earth; finding one's spiritual roots

Five-Flower Formula — immediate centering and clarity during stress or trauma

Golden Yarrow — ability to set aside personal anxiety or sensitivity when needing to focus on outer activity

Goldenrod — centeredness in social situations; keeping aware of true identity when there is a tendency to create a false persona

Indian Pink — keeping a still center in the midst of intense activity or pressure

Red Clover — keeping calm and centered in the midst of group hysteria and panic

Rosemary — inability to center in body or feel body as a physical anchor

Certainty

(See also Confidence, Clarity, Decisiveness, Doubt)

Angelica — ability to feel presence and guidance of higher realms, especially angelic realms

Cerato — following one's inner knowing, especially when overly reliant on others' advice

Forget-Me-Not — acting with greater conviction in relationships, by acknowledging spiritual and karmic factors

Goldenrod — knowing the inner Self; finding one's own values despite group pressure

Mullein — finding inner conviction, sorting out moral values

Saint John's Wort — knowing the power of one's inner light, of divine protection; especially for fears related to psychic vulnerability

Scleranthus — acting from the certainty of inner knowing; decisiveness

Vervain — rigid certainty about one's beliefs; fanaticism

Wild Oat — knowing one's life purpose and vocation

Challenge

(See also Stress)

Blackberry — strength of will to overcome inertia; manifestation

California Wild Rose — strength to take hold of life when it is particularly challenging; overcoming the tendency to retreat from life in the face of adversity; suicidal tendencies

Elm — confidence to meet challenging and demanding responsibilities; overcoming feelings of overwhelm in the face of challenges

Five-Flower Formula — centering and restoring balance when under great stress

Gentian — perseverance in the face of challenge; to counteract despondency and the tendency to give up after a setback

Hornbeam — energy and enthusiasm to meet the challenges of everyday life; involvement in daily work

Love-Lies-Bleeding — ability to endure suffering or pain, especially to discover deeper meaning in the experience

Mountain Pride — strength to meet the challenges from adverse forces; the spiritual warrior

Penstemon — inner strength to meet adversity, especially harsh and extreme circumstances in the physical world

Red Clover — keeping calm and centered in the midst of challenging circumstances, especially when others are emotionally upset and unbalanced

Rock Rose — self-transcending courage when faced with a severe or life-threatening test

Scotch Broom — seeing challenges as opportunities for growth and service

Sweet Chestnut — ultimate spiritual test, subjecting the soul to deep anguish and loneliness

Wild Rose — tendency to give up; apathetic when faced with a challenge to one's health

Cheerfulness

Agrimony — false cheer which hides inner conflict from oneself and others

Borage — cheerful courage in the face of challenges, especially when feeling weighed down

California Wild Rose — zest for living, interest in Earthly affairs

Hornbeam — tendency to approach life as a dull routine; need for more cheerful involvement in life's tasks

Larkspur — cheerfulness in leadership, especially when overly dutiful or grim

Mustard — moving through darkness to awareness of light and inner joy

Zinnia — to encourage childlike humor, lightness of heart

Children

(See also Father and Fathering, Inner Child, Mother and Mothering, Pregnancy)

Angelica — to protect a child, to instill a connection with guardian angel and other spiritual sources of protection

Aspen — fear of the unknown, nightmares

Baby Blue Eyes — feeling divorced from childlike innocence and trust; hardening of soul forces due to bitter life experiences, especially abandonment or abuse by father

Beech — conflict with siblings and peers; intolerant and judgmental attitude

Black Cohosh — abusive, exploitative or incestuous childhood relationships and experiences which still have a dark, psychic hold on the soul

Blackberry — developing more interest and involvement in tasks at school and home

Buttercup — low self-esteem in a child, especially when child feels diminished in family constellation

California Wild Rose — poor appetite, insufficient interest in the physical world

Calla Lily — mixed emotional signals about one's sexual identity as a child; for those whose parents desired a child of a different sex

Centaury — for the "pleaser," the compulsively good child who may try to be the peacemaker in a dysfunctional family, neglecting his/her own needs and feelings

Chamomile — calming emotional tension or hyperactivity in children; fussiness; colicky babies; insomnia

Chestnut Bud — for children who have difficulty with learning experiences, who often need to repeat learning or who lag behind others

Chicory — emotional neediness; creating temper tantrums; demanding excessive attention, usually by negative behavior; clinging tendency

Clematis — for the daydreamer, whose attention is elsewhere

Dogwood — hardening of body and emotions due to trauma, especially emotional or physical abuse; lacking innocence and ease of childhood; disturbances in the etheric body; awkwardness

Echinacea — severe trauma or abuse; to reclaim self-esteem and self-respect

Elm — for the child who takes on adult responsibilities in a dysfunctional or broken family

Evening Primrose — to heal deeply traumatic wounds of the adopted or unwanted child, who has unconsciously absorbed feelings of rejection and abandonment

Fairy Lantern — unresolved issues around childhood, inappropriate clinging to childlike role or identity beyond normal maturation cycle

Fawn Lily — unable to experience physical warmth in childhood surroundings, tendency to develop highly articulated inner world, cut off from others

Five-Flower Formula — accidents, or extreme situations when child is totally out of control, either physically or emotionally

Golden Yarrow — to help overly sensitive children, to encourage involvement while providing protection

Holly — sibling rivalry and jealousy; feeling that there is not enough love to go around

Impatiens — to help overly hasty, impulsive or restless children, who can become easily frustrated

Iris — building and sustaining artistic and soulful sensitivities in child's development; helpful for children whose creativity has been suppressed by parents, school or society

Larch — self-confidence in creative expression and speech; overcoming the fear of ridicule by others; free-flowing spontaneity

Mallow — to develop social impulses, warmth and sharing

Manzanita — to help the young child to incarnate, to come more fully into the body, especially with disturbed birth or birth trauma

Mariposa Lily — lack of parental bonding, especially with the mother; nurturing and bonding; instills warmth and positive childhood forces; abuse, abandonment, divorce, birth trauma

Mimulus — timidity, shyness; everyday fears such as fear of the dark

Penstemon — difficulty in experiencing the body; especially for challenges to physical development such as injury, weakness or deformity

Pink Monkeyflower — abuse or exploitation as a child, extreme shame and fear of exposure, emotional introversion

Pink Yarrow — oversensitivity in family situations; internalizing family trauma-drama

Purple Monkeyflower — for children who are subjected to ritual abuse; exposure to spiritual experiences which create fear and rob the child of feeling protected and nurtured

Rock Rose — terrifying nightmares and deep-set fears

Saint John's Wort — fear of the dark and other sleep-related traumas (e.g. bedwetting); for children who are fair-skinned and sensitive

Self-Heal — self-confidence and self-reliance; helping child to draw on his/her own forces to become well

Shasta Daisy — integration of the emerging identity of the child; rebuilding a sense of wholeness after traumatic experiences

Shooting Star — for children who feel alien, that they do not belong; often associated with trauma at birth, difficulty incarnating

Star Of Bethlehem — deep shock or trauma such as divorce, death of a family member, accident, severe illness

Sunflower — to develop a healthy sense of Self, especially when relationship to one's father is disturbed

Trumpet Vine — shyness in speech; instills vitality and strength in verbal expression

Vine — strong-willed children, the "bully"

Violet — painful shyness, learning how to share oneself with others

White Chestnut — insomnia, when the mind is full of concerns from the day

Wild Rose — listlessness or apathy, especially after a lingering illness

Yarrow — for very psychic and sensitive children, who need extra protection in their etheric sheaths

Yerba Santa — gentle release of internalized trauma, especially with tendency to respiratory disturbance; melancholia or wistfulness; often associated with family stress such as divorce or death

Choice

(See also Certainty, Decisiveness)

California Wild Rose — to be fully incarnated, to accept the challenges of life on Earth

Cerato — trusting one's inner knowledge in making decisions, rather than relying on the advice of others

Mullein — listening and following inner guidance when in conflict about moral values

Pomegranate — conflict between choosing family or career as an expression of feminine creativity

Scleranthus — to act decisively from inner knowingness, rather than vacillating between alternatives

Shooting Star — to accept life on the Earth; for those who feel alien, who don't fit in

Wild Oat — clarity about life direction, life work; having a strong inner sense of purpose and life destiny

City Life

(See also Earth Healing and Nature Awareness, Environment)

Chaparral — cleansing the subconscious of images of violence and degradation

Corn — feeling disoriented, ungrounded in crowded urban environments

Dill — overwhelmed by the fast pace of urban life; excess sensory stimulation

Fawn Lily — unable to cope with stress and challenge due to need for perfection and peace

Golden Yarrow — ability to perform or create in very intense environments, despite sensitivity

Indian Pink — keeping still in the midst of intense activity; centeredness

Nicotiana — mechanization and hardening of the body due to urban stress; numbing of finer sensibilities, especially when accompanied by attraction to addictive substances

Oregon Grape — expecting hostility from others; mistrust and fear of others; feeling a need to protect oneself by taking a hostile or aggressive stance

Pink Yarrow — tendency to absorb the feelings of crowds; too-porous aura; oversensitive

Tiger Lily — tendency toward aggressive behavior

Yarrow — depletion due to oversensitivity to the frenetic pace of city life, to the cacophony of sensory and psychic forces

Yarrow Special Formula — protection from environmental pollution and disharmony

Clarity

(See also Awareness, Certainty, Decisiveness)

Deerbrush — purity and clarity of motivation, especially affecting the heart center; integration of inner feeling with outer action

Dill — confusion from the intensity of too many experiences

Forget-Me-Not — greater spaciousness and mindfulness; in touch with how spirit permeates the physical world

Madia — focus and clarity of thought; overcoming distractions

Mountain Pennyroyal — strength and clarity of thoughts; especially the need to purge negative or foreign thought-forms

Peppermint — mental alertness; able to activate mental forces

Queen Anne's Lace — distinguishing psychic impressions from subjective emotions; objective clairvoyance

Star Tulip — ability to contact higher realms

White Chestnut — to achieve mental clarity by cultivating inner quiet

Wild Oat — clarity about one's life purpose and vocation

Cleansing

(See also Purification)

Chaparral — emotional cleansing, especially during dreams; cleansing of subconscious; often related to psychic or drug abuse

Crab Apple — releasing emotional and/or physical impurities, especially where there is a strong sense of uncleanness, whether real or imagined

Deerbrush — gentle cleanser of the heart; purifying motivation and intention

Easter Lily — purification of sexual desires and sexual organs

Evening Primrose — release of toxic emotions unconsciously absorbed from parents, often stemming from emotional and physical abuse

Golden Ear Drops — release of traumatic childhood memories, especially through tears

Holly — releasing negative emotions such as jealousy, envy, hostility

Mountain Pennyroyal — clearing the mind of negative thoughts taken on from others

Sagebrush — shedding of false identity; letting go of old lifestyles or personal identity that is no longer needed; emptying

Self-Heal — overall balance and regeneration during cleansing and healing process

Yerba Santa — release of deep and hidden emotional toxins, especially those emotions which cloud the heart and breathing

Co-Dependence

Agrimony — hiding true feelings, especially using an outer mask of cheerfulness to be socially agreeable

Black Cohosh — confronting and transforming abusive, violent or destructive relationships; especially for those who have a pattern of abusive relationships

Bleeding Heart — overly possessive and clinging in relationships; letting go of emotional dependence on others

Buttercup — low self-esteem; inability to feel one's own self-worth in social relationships; self-deprecating attitudes

Centaury — unhealthy need to serve or please others; unbalanced giving which weakens and depletes the true Self; accepting exploitation from others

Cerato — overly reliant on the advice of others; inability to make clear and firm decisions for oneself

Chicory — emotional neediness, especially the tendency to manipulate others for self-benefit; possessiveness

Elm — attempting to secure affection by being the hero; afraid to let others down

Fairy Lantern — feigning helplessness or over-dependence in relationships; inappropriate need to be seen as a child, or to receive approval for childlike behavior

Goldenrod — dependence on social approval of others; inability to clarify one's own values

Mariposa Lily — feeling of abandonment and insecurity from childhood which distorts current relationships

Milkweed — extreme dependence; lack of ego strength; needing to be cared for

Pine — internalizing guilt; taking on blame or accepting responsibility for others' faults

Pink Monkeyflower — masking inner feelings, especially feelings of vulnerability; unable to be emotionally authentic

Pink Yarrow — enmeshed in others' feelings; inability to identify the source of one's own emotions; inappropriate merging with others

Quince — to balance polarities of love and power; integration of receptive and assertive qualities

Red Chestnut — over-identification with the problems of others; excessive worry and concern for others

Red Clover — living in psychic aura of family blood ties; unable to act for oneself

Sunflower — developing a healthy sense of ego; ability to feel more radiant and assertive

Tansy — suppressing energetic response; holding back real capacities out of desire to placate family system

Walnut — dysfunctional ties to family system or social standards which prevent full actualization of goals and life destiny

Willow — seeing oneself as a victim; not taking responsibility for emotions

Communication

(See also Self-Expression, Speaking)

Calendula — sensitivity to the meaning of the other person's words; warmth and healing in interpersonal communications

Cosmos — ability to convey higher thoughts in an articulate, clear way; harmonization of thinking with speech

Deerbrush — conveying one's true intentions; purity of motivation

Dogwood — grace and emotional ease in relating to others

Forget-Me-Not — connection with spiritual guides; remembering those who live beyond the physical realm

Larch — blocked expression due to lack of self-confidence

Pink Monkeyflower — fear of expressing real feelings; fear of censure or judgment

Pretty Face — holding back from being too visible; to allow one's real Self to shine

Quaking Grass — ability to listen and work with others in group situations

Scarlet Monkeyflower — to communicate true feelings, especially powerful emotions

Snapdragon — tendency to be angry and argumentative in communications with others

Trumpet Vine — to give vitality and dynamism to verbal expression

Violet — tendency to hold back in communication; shyness

Water Violet — aloofness, not wanting to share thoughts with others

Community Life and Group Experience

(See also Cooperation, Prejudice)

Agrimony — difficulty in reading personality in group, appearing cheerful and easy going, but often filled with inner torment

Beech — blames or criticizes others; needs to become less rigid

Blackberry — able to generate ideas or philosophical overview, but difficulty engaging will in group projects

Calendula — for poor listeners, with difficulty in being receptive to what others are saying; argumentative

California Poppy — seeking group experiences which offer escape, glamour or spiritual glory; easily influenced by charlatans, hustlers or gurus

California Wild Rose — lack of involvement in group or community, wanting others to do the work

Canyon Dudleya — attraction to charismatic or psychic experiences in group settings; inflating or creating emotional energy and drama

Elm — taking on too much responsibility, "hero complex," tendency to feel overwhelmed and alone

Fawn Lily — difficulty becoming involved in group settings, overly delicate and spiritual, preferring to retreat rather than face conflict or strife

Filaree — focusing on petty details or worries, often destroying enthusiasm of group

Golden Yarrow — ability to work in groups, to express oneself or to take a public stand, despite inherent sensitivity

Goldenrod — concern about status or social approval in group; responds more out of peer pressure than true inner values

Heather — turning energy toward oneself, excessive need to draw attention to one's personal problems

Holly — jealousy and envy toward others; developing compassionate acceptance and joy for others

Impatiens — too impatient for group involvement, often becoming a loner because of intolerance for others and for slow process of group work

Lady's Slipper — holds back from giving help or sharing talents with others; inability to contact true power and capability

Larkspur — positive leadership and charisma, not feeling burdened or overdutiful

Love-Lies-Bleeding — personal suffering or pain which drives soul inward; finding a bridge from personal experience to shared human experience; ability to receive therapeutic support through group work

Mallow — ability to develop friendships, to bring soul warmth to group settings; to form bonds rather than barriers in relationships

Milkweed — over-dependence on family care or institutionalized care; needing to have another direct and decide for oneself

Mountain Pride — ability to take a stand, to be assertive, to make changes in community; political risk-taking

Oregon Grape — social paranoia, expecting hostility from others or misperceiving others' intentions

Pink Monkeyflower — holding back from sharing; profound reserve and inner anguish, guilt and shame about sharing real feelings

Pink Yarrow — absorbing emotions and feelings of others in group; no longer in touch with one's own feelings or boundaries; overly sympathetic

Purple Monkeyflower — healing the soul of coercive, threatening or exploitative experiences in religious groups, often leading to fear or distrust of anything spiritual

Quaking Grass — ability to harmonize with group, to see self-identity within larger matrix of group identity

Sage — to bring a more detached perspective to group decision-making, seeing the larger view and long-term needs; also, cultivation of respect for the wisdom of elders in community

Shasta Daisy — ability to unify and synthesize many ideas and contributions in group setting; to bring all parts together into a greater wholeness

Snapdragon — tendency to make biting or sarcastic comments, verbally aggressive

Star Thistle — difficulty giving of oneself, or of one's time or money to group; difficulty in sharing due to fear of lack

Sweet Pea — for the traveler or wanderer; inability to establish roots in community, or to commit oneself to larger community needs

Tiger Lily — combativeness which overrides ability to work cooperatively

Vine — controlling others; using personal will to adversely influence will of others

Violet — holding back from sharing with others; shy, fear of losing oneself in group

Water Violet — avoiding working with others; feelings of superiority or disdain; tendency to classism or racism

Willow — blaming others for hurts real or imagined; finding it difficult to forgive and let go

Yellow Star Tulip — developing empathy for others; receptivity to the feelings and experiences of others

Compassion

Bleeding Heart — learning to love another in freedom

Calendula — ability to listen and understand; especially in verbal communication

Centaury — misdirected compassion, overly servile and lacking in true individuality; trying to please others rather than serving true needs

Fawn Lily — unthawing spiritual Self, allowing one's spiritual forces to flow to others

Heather — understanding the sufferings of others; overcoming preoccupation with one's own problems

Holly — recognizing the suffering and needs of others; compassionate presence

Love-Lies-Bleeding — moving beyond personal experience to more universal compassion; especially when pain or suffering is involved

Mallow — ability to feel warm and caring with others; ability to form social bonds

Mariposa Lily — nurturing with warmth; mothering

Pink Yarrow — to distinguish compassion from overly sympathetic identification; learning objective love for others

Poison Oak — fear of being seen as compassionate; fear of merging, especially when expressed as a hostile warrior-like stance

Sunflower — warm sun-like forces; radiant compassion

Water Violet — difficulty showing compassion for others; remaining aloof

Yellow Star Tulip — developing perceptive and empathetic capacities; sensitivity to suffering of others

Competitiveness

Golden Yarrow — for those who are inherently shy and non-competitive, but nevertheless need to put themselves forward

Holly — competitiveness as a form of insecurity; working against others; rivalry or envy

Impatiens — tendency to take over for others, especially when feeling they are too slow

Mountain Pride — courage and strength to challenge adversaries; positive aspects of being a spiritual warrior

Oak — pushing oneself hard for success; high achievement goals which need balance and limits

Penstemon — inner competitiveness; strength to meet challenges despite setbacks

Tiger Lily — overly aggressive competition, transformed into positive social action

Trillium — overcoming aggressive greed and acquisitiveness

Concentration and Focus

(See also Attention, Learning Difficulties, Scatteredness, Study)

Clematis — tendency for awareness to float out of the body

Cosmos — inability to focus; being flooded by too much information, especially when speaking; integration of thinking and speech

Filaree — obsession with details, losing the larger view

Honeysuckle — being in the present time, rather than dwelling in the past

Indian Pink — holding focus when surrounded by intense activity

Madia — attention to detail, focus on a single aspect; overcoming tendency to be distracted

Peppermint — greater mental attention and wakefulness

Pink Yarrow — losing focus due to emotional blurring and merging with others

Queen Anne's Lace — focus of psychic forces, when confused or blurred; concentration of "third eye"

Rabbitbrush — ability to handle many different details or activities at one time; mental flexibility and alertness

Rosemary — poor memory; inability of thinking function to work through physical vehicle

Shasta Daisy — ability to bring many diverse ideas into a whole; seeing an integrated picture uniting various parts

Walnut — focusing on life goals in spite of social or family expectations; ability to abide by one's convictions

White Chestnut — stilling the thoughts of an overactive mind

Wild Oat — clarity in life direction and vocation; choosing and committing to a life goal

Confidence

(See also Certainty, Decisiveness)

Buttercup — knowing self-worth, especially with regard to vocation and lifestyle

Cerato — relying on one's inner knowing, rather than another's advice

Elm — knowing one is capable of fulfilling one's obligations without anxiety

Fairy Lantern — moving forward to next stage of life, no longer clinging to the past; ability to accept adult responsibilities

Garlic — overcoming fears and insecurities that drain and weaken; greater resistance and overall strength

Golden Yarrow — confidence that one can perform despite anxiety or oversensitivity

Larch — confidence in self-expression or public performance, especially with tendency to doubt abilities

Mimulus — confidence to face daily challenges and fears, for those with a phobic personality

Mountain Pride — confidence in one's power to challenge or confront adversity

Penstemon — strength in the face of adversity or misfortune; knowing one is able to sustain and endure

Pretty Face — confidence in one's inner beauty, especially when tormented by concerns about one's personal appearance

Purple Monkeyflower — following one's own spiritual guidance, especially when fear or repression may have stymied soul's inner sense of spiritual truth

Saint John's Wort — facing the world by the strength and protection of one's inner light

Scleranthus — confident decision-making, especially when there has been a tendency to vacillate

Self-Heal — trusting one's self-healing abilities, especially with tendency to seek many outer modes of healing

Sunflower — radiant expression of individuality; positive, confident ego

Trumpet Vine — self-confidence when speaking, being able to project oneself, greater vitality

Conflict

(See also Ambivalence)

Agrimony — inner torment and conflict, hidden from others

Alpine Lily — conflict about one's feminine aspects, especially between the earthly feminine and spiritual feminine

Basil — relationship conflict, tension between sexual and spiritual aspects; secretiveness about sexuality in relationship

Calendula — communication problems in relationship, leading to conflict, arguments

Easter Lily — inner conflict between polarities of sexuality and purity

Fawn Lily — inability to cope with conflict, desire to retreat or insulate oneself

Holly — jealousy or envy of others, not feeling loved

Lady's Slipper — plagued by self-doubt, especially when feeling a higher destiny and calling which one is not able to integrate in daily life

Pomegranate — conflict between career and family, particularly in women

Quaking Grass — personality conflict in group situations; harmonizing of individuals in a group

Quince — conflict between showing strength and emotional warmth and nurturing

Saguaro — conflict about authority or in relation to male power

Scleranthus — inner conflict when making decisions; wavering between alternatives

Self-Heal — confusion about wellness or health program; unable to contact inner source of healing

Sunflower — inner conflict about father image, or relation to masculine aspect of oneself

Sweet Pea — conflict with others in community or family

Wild Oat — confusion about life purpose, career choices

Cooperation

(See also Community Life and Group Experience)

Holly — ability to feel loving; inclusion of others

Quaking Grass — bending and blending of individual egos for a common purpose

Tiger Lily — working with others cooperatively; overcoming aggressive tendencies

Trillium — ability to work for the common good; overcoming greed and unbalanced desire for personal power

Courage

Aspen — courageously facing the unknown, confronting hidden fears

Black Cohosh — courage to confront rather than shrink from abusive or threatening situations

Black-Eyed Susan — courage to encounter dark or unknown parts of the psyche

Borage — cheerful courage; uplifting the heart to face challenges; buoyancy

Chrysanthemum — courage to contemplate one's own death and shift identification away from physical Self

Evening Primrose — ability to face feelings of rejection and abandonment from experiences in early childhood, to encounter core emotions of such trauma

Fawn Lily — strength to give oneself to the world, despite innate desire to retreat

Garlic — courage to overcome fright or nervousness by developing strength

Golden Yarrow — courage to put oneself forward despite sensitivity

Larch — confidence in one's creativity; overcoming doubt of one's abilities

Mimulus — ability to face the challenges of daily life, especially everyday fears and worries

Mountain Pride — confronting darkness or evil in the world; becoming a dynamic spiritual warrior

Mustard — courage to confront darkness, to go through depression

Penstemon — inner strength to face personal adversity

Pink Monkeyflower — willingness to let others see one's true feelings, to overcome shame and guilt

Rock Rose — self-transcending courage, especially in terrifying situations

Scarlet Monkeyflower — courage to face negative or powerful emotions

Creativity

Aloe Vera — burned-out feeling from intense activity, overuse of creative forces; integration and centering of creativity in the heart

Blackberry — creative power of thought; motivation of the will; manifestation of one's ideas in the world

Buttercup — knowing the worth of one's creative contributions

Cosmos — flooding of nervous system with creative thoughts or inspiration, which need organization and synthesis; integration of higher mental bodies with emotional Self

Dogwood — especially for movement artists; allowing body to experience inner harmony and grace; resolving emotional feelings of awkwardness

Golden Yarrow — especially for performing artists; protection for highly developed sensitivity

Hound's Tongue — combining thinking and imagination, reason and reverence; creativity which employs both the right and left hemispheres of the brain

Indian Paintbrush — bringing vitality to creative expression, especially from earthly forces; replenishing the life forces which flow into the creative will

Iris — creative inspiration, especially from higher realms; artistic expression, transcending feelings of limitation regarding creativity

Larch — allowing spontaneous creative expression for those who stifle themselves

Nasturtium — bringing more vitality; for those who tend to be too intellectual or dry

Pomegranate — conflicting creative desires, especially in the expression of the feminine part of Self; conflict whether to create biologically through the body, or through artistic or career expression

Queen Anne's Lace — to balance and harmonize emerging clairvoyance or psychic abilities; especially when they may distort or harm the creative process

Sagebrush — to cleanse the perception; stereotypical or fixed concepts which prevent truly fresh or original perception

Shasta Daisy — ability to synthesize; creative thinking which allows parts to form a meaningful whole

Snapdragon — re-channeling power and creative energy which may be misdirected into aggression

Star Tulip — to become sensitive and receptive, to allow oneself to become a container for higher expression

Trumpet Vine — bringing greater liveliness to verbal expression, especially for dramatic artists; stage presence, dramatic flair

Yellow Star Tulip — stimulating forces of empathy and compassion; allowing artistic expressions to represent the real feelings of others

Zinnia — bringing greater spontaneity, especially childlike originality and inventiveness

Criticism

Beech — criticizing the faults of others; judgmental attitude

Crab Apple — self criticism, obsession with one's imperfections

Filaree — being overly fastidious, "picky;" obsession with insignificant problems

Pine — self-criticism which includes self-blame and guilt

Rock Water — being extremely hard on oneself, with overly strict standards

Saguaro — excessive criticism of authority figures out of a spirit of rebellion

Snapdragon — verbal criticism and abuse, misplaced aggression

Cynicism

Baby Blue Eyes — mistrust, holding back energy; cynical detachment

California Wild Rose — lack of interest or enthusiasm for living; excessive detachment or apathy

Holly — cynical hatred or mistrust of others

Hound's Tongue — cynicism due to inability to contact spiritual realms or activate higher thought

Mountain Pride — transforming feelings of dissatisfaction into positive energy for change

Nicotiana — tough "macho" stance which hides or blunts deeper feelings

Oregon Grape — expecting the worst from others; projecting hostility

Pink Monkeyflower — cutting off true feelings; emotional coldness or distance as a mask to hide deeper, more vulnerable feelings

Sage — tendency to see life as ill-fated or undeserved; inability to perceive higher purpose and meaning in life events

Star Thistle — tendency to hold back from sharing; inability to open oneself to others due to fear of lack, or feeling that others want too much

Willow — bitter and resentful about life events; inability to forgive and forget

Darkness

(See also Gloom)

Black Cohosh — brooding, powerful sense of darkness both within oneself and within one's environment, usually characterized by violent or destructive elements in one's lifestyle

Black-Eyed Susan — avoidance or repression of traumatic experiences and negative emotions; bringing insight and awareness to darker areas of the psyche

Gorse — soul darkness which is characterized by personal despair and hopelessness, including psychic attachment to darkness and suffering

Mustard — depressive states, or experience of darkness characterized by isolation and despair; when depression descends suddenly and for unknown reasons

Pretty Face — to bring more inner radiance when the countenance or body seems darkened or masked

Saint John's Wort — fear of physical darkness; disturbed sleep and dream states; depression related to seasonal darkness

Scotch Broom — feelings of overwhelm and burden which darken the psyche, especially the feeling of impending doom or apocalypse which paralyzes the positive forces of the soul

Sweet Chestnut — for "the dark night of the soul" — intense personal anguish and suffering which presses the soul to the breaking point; suicidal tendencies

Daydreaming

(See also Centeredness, Groundedness)

Clematis — excessive daydreaming or fantasizing, often as a form of escape from present circumstances

Fawn Lily — tendency to create highly articulated inner life, without ability to integrate daily challenges in work or home

Honeysuckle — escape from the present with thoughts of the past; reliving old memories

Madia — tendency to distraction; lack of concentration

Mugwort — to develop more awareness of moving between different states of consciousness; greater psychic sensitivity

Saint John's Wort — feeling lost in the world of dreams, or in out-of-body states

Death and Dying

(See also Grief)

Angel's Trumpet — appropriate surrender to death, ability of soul to prepare for crossing into spiritual world

Angelica — ministering to one crossing the threshold of death; helping the soul find protection and benevolence from the angelic realm

Black Cohosh — life-threatening situations characterized not by physical illness but violence, murder or revenge; confronting and transforming death and violence

Black-Eyed Susan — for those in denial or avoidance of a terminal illness; developing the courage to look at one's true situation, and the insight to understand it

Bleeding Heart — letting go, releasing attachment to those who can no longer be with us

Borage — overcoming grief or heavy-hearted feelings from the death or impending death of a loved one

Chrysanthemum — deep sense of despair about one's own mortality, inability to accept transitory nature of earthly life, shifting awareness from lower Self to higher Self

Five-Flower Formula — extreme pain or shock in situations of death and dying, helping the soul to register consciousness

Forget-Me-Not — ability to forge telepathic link with loved one who has died, to hold consciousness of another who lives beyond earthly realm

Holly — bringing calm and acceptance to the heart, forgiving others, making peace with worldly relationships before death

Love-Lies-Bleeding — profound pain or suffering which moves one beyond the limits of self-identity; soul and spiritual transcendence

Mariposa Lily — resolving conflicts with one's mother or other female figures; attunement with the Divine Feminine as a loving force

Mountain Pride — courage to fight negative thought-forms about death; seeing death or terminal illness as a challenge or initiation for the soul

Penstemon — extreme physical hardship and suffering associated with terminal illness; courage to accept and endure suffering

Pink Yarrow — oversensitivity to the thoughts and fears of others around the issues of death

Purple Monkeyflower — extreme fear of dying due to inability to trust oneself as a purely spiritual being; fear-based religious beliefs which impede the dying process

Red Clover — dealing with charged family situations at times of death or terminal illness; group hysteria and other emotional extremes

Rock Rose — fear of death, especially the fear that the ego will be utterly annihilated or destroyed

Sage — surveying life experience, realizing lessons learned, reflecting and accepting life and death as a larger soul-process of evolution

Sagebrush — ability to let go, to experience inner emptiness and nothingness as a pre-condition of spiritual birth

Saint John's Wort — fear of out-of-body states; anchoring inner light and awareness as the soul expands beyond the physical world

Scarlet Monkeyflower — anger about death; for the encounter with the double or shadow side at death

Star Of Bethlehem — to soothe shock resulting from hearing of death or learning of an impending death

Star Tulip — to increase receptive awareness of subtle states of consciousness; to shift awareness from physical to metaphysical seeing and hearing

Sunflower — resolving conflicts with one's father, making peace with one's inner masculine Self

Sweet Chestnut — extreme mental anguish and sense of isolation within the soul; a feeling that one is cut off from God

Walnut — making transitions; breaking links, especially when others may hold on too tightly and not allow the release of the departing soul

Willow — releasing bitterness and resentment toward family, friends or others; taking responsibility for the events of one's life; ability to forgive

Decisiveness

(See also Certainty, Choice, Clarity, Indecision)

Blackberry — bringing ideals into action, stimulating forces of will

Cayenne — cutting through stagnation or indecision

Cerato — overcoming inward uncertainty; knowing from within rather than seeking the advice of others

Madia — clarity of purpose; ability to focus intentions

Mountain Pride — taking a decided public stand for one's beliefs

Mullein — acting on moral values; following inner guidance

Pomegranate — making a decision when torn between feminine ideals of personal mothering and world-creative mother

Scleranthus — feeling torn between two choices; generally restless and indecisive

Tansy — tendency to procrastination and lethargy

Wild Oat — decisiveness about career and service in the world

Denial

(See also Acceptance, Avoidance, Resistance, True to Self)

Agrimony — denial of emotional pain, hiding emotions with a mask of cheerfulness; using pain-numbing or euphoric drugs to cover anxiety and pain

Angel's Trumpet — not accepting the dying process

Angelica — not accepting the reality of the spiritual world or higher guidance and presence

Black-Eyed Susan — not acknowledging deep and hidden emotions; denial of the "shadow" aspect of the personality

California Poppy — psychic "highs" or euphoria stimulated by drugs, especially when used to avoid facing oneself honestly

Chestnut Bud — ignoring the lessons of past experience

Chrysanthemum — denial of aging process by trying to create a youthful appearance or by holding on to fame, status or material possessions as if these conditions were permanent

Deerbrush — denial of true motives; not acknowledging hidden feelings behind one's actions

Forget-Me-Not — denying the reality of life after death and life before birth; strengthening one's awareness of karmic bonds with beings in the spiritual world

Hound's Tongue — denial of spiritual beings or processes, resulting in intellectual materialism

Milkweed — blotting out pain with drugs, alcohol, food, sleep, or other consciousness-numbing experiences

Mullein — tendency to self-deception; inability to be honest with oneself and others

Nicotiana — denial of real feelings, especially those of the heart; blunting of raw emotional experience, often accompanied by addiction to tobacco or related substances

Queen Anne's Lace — suppression of one's inner sight to avoid seeing what is uncomfortable and painful

Scarlet Monkeyflower — emotional repression out of fear of powerful emotions

Self-Heal — not recognizing one's own inner healing power

Star Tulip — rejection of the reality of one's inner life; denial of inner guidance, of the spiritual realm

Willow — not taking responsibility for one's actions; blaming others, resentment

Depression and Despair

Baby Blue Eyes — despair when beset by cynicism, no longer trusting in goodness of the world

Borage — discouragement, especially grief or heavy-heartedness

California Wild Rose — alienation from life; not accepting difficulty or challenge

Chamomile — to stabilize the emotions; calming and soothing

Chrysanthemum — deep soul angst about one's own life and death; inability of soul to accept death and dying as a larger spiritual process

Elm — despair about one's ability to fulfill responsibilities and expectations

Gentian — doubt and discouragement from setbacks; lack of faith

Gorse — hopelessness; expectation of suffering

Hornbeam — depression when facing the tasks of daily life, such as work

Love-Lies-Bleeding — pain and suffering which drives soul too deeply inward; to experience one's pain within a larger human context

Milkweed — deeply depressed state, inability to cope with daily affairs, desire to obliterate consciousness

Mustard — feeling overwhelmed by a "black cloud" for unknown reasons; wide mood swings

Olive — depression stemming from physical exhaustion

Pine — despair and anxiety about one's own faults and mistakes

Sagebrush — feelings of personal devastation, a feeling that one has reached rock bottom; ability to accept emptiness and loss

Scotch Broom — discouragement in the face of obstacles, especially feelings of world doom

Sweet Chestnut — extreme anguish; the "dark night of the soul"

Wild Oat — dissatisfaction with one's work, despair over finding life's work or direction

Wild Rose — apathy and resignation when faced with illness or other challenges in life

Yerba Santa — internalized sadness, especially when held in the chest region; emotional pain

Desire

(See also Greed, Sexuality)

Basil — clandestine sexual desire which undermines relationships; need to integrate sexual desire and spirituality

Blackberry — bringing desires into manifestation

Bleeding Heart — possessiveness in relationships; desire to hold on to the other person, attachment to the experience of "being in love"

California Pitcher Plant — suppression of instinctual desires such as hunger and sex

California Poppy — craving stimulating experiences through drugs or psychic "highs"

Centaury — weak sense of personal desire; neglecting what one wants for the desires of others

Deerbrush — unconscious desires; unclear motivations

Easter Lily — conflicts about sexual desire; feeling sexuality is impure

Hibiscus — repression of sexual desire; to stimulate sexual warmth and responsiveness

Lady's Slipper — lack of sexual desire due to nervous exhaustion and depletion

Manzanita — denial of physical desire due to estrangement from physical body and physical world

Milkweed — craving for experiences which dull consciousness, such as drugs, alcohol, excessive food

Quaking Grass — altruistic sacrifice of individual desires and preferences for the good of the larger group

Rock Water — repression of desires out of a too-strict sense of discipline, asceticism

Sagebrush — release of desires and cravings which hinder one's growth

Scleranthus — confusion about what one wants, leading to indecision

Sticky Monkeyflower — repression or inappropriate acting out of sexual desire; split between heart feelings and sexual desire

Tansy — catalyzing a stagnant will; acting on one's desires

Trillium — greed and lust for possessions and power; inability to sacrifice personal desire for the common good

Walnut — courage to follow one's heart despite the judgments of others

Wild Oat — confusion about what one wants to do in life; lack of a consuming passion or vocation; developing a desire to do world service

Destructiveness

(See also Abuse)

Beech — lashing out critically at others

Black Cohosh — involvement in or attraction to destructive or violent relationship or lifestyle

Bleeding Heart — trying to hold on and manipulate others in order to feel wanted, with a destructive effect on the relationship

Calendula — hurting others with one's use of words, lack of warmth in communication

Cherry Plum — being destructive or losing control when under extreme stress or pressure; also for fear of doing so

Crab Apple — self-destructive attitude by obsessing on imperfections and impurities

Dogwood — tendency to abuse oneself; accident-prone; ungraceful

Holly — strong negative emotions for others; hatred, jealousy or rivalry

Impatiens — over-impulsive behavior; quick to anger, can throw or break things on impulse

Manzanita — lack of connection or respect for physical body, resulting in self-destructive behavior

Morning Glory — harmful personal habits and erratic lifestyle; drug abuse

Mustard — self-destructive behavior when feeling depressed (e.g. not eating or sleeping properly)

Pine — hard on oneself; condemning of one's past; emotionally self-destructive

Saguaro — delinquent or destructive behavior motivated by rebellion against authority

Scarlet Monkeyflower — tendency to sudden or blind rage, extreme anger, often held back and then suddenly released

Snapdragon — destructive tendencies, especially verbal abuse and biting sarcasm

Detail

Beech — preoccupied with small details or faults of others; highly critical

Crab Apple — obsession with details and faults, especially with regard to personal cleanliness and health

Filaree — excessive worry about details and trivialities without proper perspective

Madia — focusing attention to detail, especially when there is a tendency to become distracted or sidetracked

Rabbitbrush — active grasp of detail; alert awareness; coordinating different activities simultaneously

Shasta Daisy — ability to combine or synthesize many different details into a large picture; imaginative perception

Devitalization

(See also Rejuvenation, Vitality)

Aloe Vera — feeling drained and depleted of vitality due to overuse of creative forces

Fawn Lily — living too much in the spiritual world, inability to draw strength from physical world

Garlic — lack of vitality due to fear, nervousness or parasitic entities

Hibiscus — loss of sexual responsiveness; inability to experience sexuality as an expression of soul warmth

Hornbeam — weariness due to lack of interest in work or other daily tasks

Indian Paintbrush — depletion of vital forces from creative expression; dry, overly abstract expression

Morning Glory — low energy from destructive or abusive habits; addiction

Nasturtium — tendency toward dry intellectualism; lack of life-force

Nicotiana — mechanization of the body, tendency to see one's body as a machine; suppression of emotions, leading to reduced life forces or vitality

Olive — depletion of physical vitality after a long illness or struggle

Pink Yarrow — feeling drained of energy from absorbing the negative emotions of others

Rosemary — lack of physical warmth and presence; cold extremities and poor circulation

Saint John's Wort — living too much at the periphery of consciousness; expanded state of consciousness which drains vital forces

Yarrow — feeling drained of energy due to harsh environment or negative/hostile thoughts of others

Yarrow Special Formula — loss of energy from disharmonious environmental energies such as radiation, electrical fields, allergens

Zinnia — tendency toward overseriousness; feeling dull and lifeless

Discouragement

(See also Depression and Despair)

Borage — feeling disheartened or heavy-hearted, low-spirited

Gentian — discouragement after a setback; lacking faith in the unfolding of life events

Gorse — hopelessness, expectation of suffering; morose disposition

Larch — giving up after failure; lacking inner confidence to try again

Mustard — feeling overcome by a mood of hopelessness and helplessness

Penstemon — discouragement because of handicap or other personal misfortune; need to persevere

Scotch Broom — discouragement particularly about the world situation; feeling "What's the use?"

Dislike

(See also Criticism, Hate)

Beech — criticism of others due to high standards of perfection

Buttercup — negation of one's vocation or lot in life

Crab Apple — disgust with imperfections and impurities

Holly — jealousy, hostility toward others, often out of a feeling of being unloved, or not included in love

Manzanita — aversion to the physical body; viewing the body as "unspiritual"

Oregon Grape — views others with distrust; suspicious

Willow — dislike of others, feeling bitter and resentful

Disorientation

Clematis — tendency for awareness to float in and out of the body; dreaminess

Corn — confusion in crowded urban areas, feeling a lack of grounding or connection with the Earth

Cosmos — disoriented speech which is rapid or inarticulate

Five-Flower Formula — immediate centering when disoriented by extreme stress or trauma

Indian Pink — disorientation when surrounded by intense activity

Madia — inability to focus thoughts, becoming distracted or scattered

Milkweed — tendency to blot out consciousness through drugs, accidents, illness or inappropriate spiritual practices

Queen Anne's Lace — foggy or blurred vision, confused psychic impressions

Red Clover — tendency to hysteria and panic, especially in a group situation

Rosemary — feelings of sleepiness and memory loss; not feeling fully anchored in physical body

Doubt

(See also Certainty)

Buttercup — doubting one's true worth or vocation

Cerato — invalidating one's own decision-making abilities

Gorse — lack of faith that things will work out, that there is a meaning to life events

Larch — uncertainty about one's creative expression or ability to perform in front of others

Penstemon — questioning one's ability to meet difficulties

Red Chestnut — questioning the ability of others to handle a crisis; negative concern for others

Scleranthus — confusion about one's feelings and thoughts; indecision

Scotch Broom — questioning one's ability to meet difficulties, with a sense of world doom

Self-Heal — denying one's own self-healing abilities, relying solely on outside support

Dreams and Sleep

Angelica — receptivity of soul to spiritual guidance in dream life

Black-Eyed Susan — needing to examine disturbing or recurrent dreams; insight into repressed or buried parts of oneself

Chaparral — disturbed or chaotic dreams; release of trauma, sometimes through catharsis; cleansing of psyche

Clematis — dreamy, sleepy disposition; integration of dream life into daily life

Evening Primrose — stimulation of memories of life before birth or early infancy, often through dreams

Forget-Me-Not — to facilitate communication and connection with spirit guides or departed souls in dreams and sleep

Hornbeam — desire to sleep as avoidance of daily tasks and responsibilities

Lavender — nervous disposition, causing difficulty sleeping or sleep which is not restful

Milkweed — profound desire to sleep as a way of escape; dependence on sedatives, sleeping pills

Morning Glory — disturbed rhythms in sleep, poor dream recall, difficulty awakening in morning

Mugwort — awareness across the threshold; greater activity and consciousness in dreams; integration of dream life and psychic awareness with ordinary reality

Rosemary — sleepiness and forgetfulness in daytime due to poor incarnation in body, developing greater wakefulness and vitality

Saint John's Wort — disturbed, fearful dreams; fear of the dark or of going to sleep, traumatic nightmares; out-of-body experiences

Star Tulip — greater receptivity and awareness of dream symbolism and dream recall; more awareness of subtle realms

White Chestnut — restless, fitful sleep due to anxious feelings or repetitive mental chatter

Dryness

Aloe Vera — feeling of being burned out, overuse of creative forces

Golden Ear Drops — releasing repressed tears; contacting core emotions

Hibiscus — warm, moist soul forces in sexual expression

Indian Paintbrush — lacking vitality or earthiness in creative expression

Iris — lack of flowing creative expression; developing higher inspiration

Nasturtium — overly dry intellectualism, not integrated with life forces

Trumpet Vine — expressing more color and soul vitality when speaking

Zinnia — lack of humor, overseriousness

Dullness

Baby Blue Eyes — numbing of emotions due to harsh life experiences, violence or abuse as a child

California Wild Rose — apathy, lack of interest in life; to develop enthusiasm

Cosmos — stimulating mental clarity, especially more lively and thoughtful speech

Forget-Me-Not — lack of awareness of spiritual beings and processes; developing greater mindfulness of the spirit world

Hornbeam — experiencing life's tasks as a dull duty

Hound's Tongue — dullness of thought life through pre-occupation with material awareness; need for more levity

Iris — lack of creativity or imaginative perspective

Morning Glory — dull and unresponsive in the morning; difficulty waking up or feeling refreshed from sleep

Peppermint — developing greater mental alertness when thinking is dull

Star Tulip — lack of awareness of spiritual realms; to develop psychic receptivity

Yellow Star Tulip — oblivious to the needs of others; dull or numb awareness; to develop greater social sensitivity

Zinnia — overwork or serious approach which dulls the consciousness

Dutifulness

Centaury — excessive obligation to the needs of others

Elm — taking on too much responsibility, then feeling overwhelmed

Hornbeam — lack of energy for work, seeing life's tasks as joyless burdens and duties

Larkspur — experiencing leadership as a burdensome duty

Mountain Pride — transforming dutifulness to passionate commitment and involvement in life's challenges

Rock Water — too narrow a sense of duty, leading to self-denial or rigidity

Walnut — dutifulness to family values or societal standards; inability to break free from a limiting sense of duty

Zinnia — bringing a more playful attitude in one's activities, especially when burdened by a joyless sense of duty in work and family life

Earth Healing and Nature Awareness

(See also City Life)

California Wild Rose — loving and serving the Earth, real interest and care for the world of Nature; stewardship

Clematis — other-worldly attitude, lack of interest in physical world; escapist tendencies

Corn — feeling fully present on Earth, especially through hands and feet; to allow one's consciousness of the Earth to fully permeate one's body

Crab Apple — tendency to see the Earth as unclean, "dirty" or "soiled;" not wanting to be contaminated, indoor lifestyle

Deerbrush — to cleanse impurities in the heart which block attunement and sensitivity to Nature

Dill — overwhelming of senses due to machines, noise, and other technological stimuli; ability to be nourished by the quiet beauty and simplicity of Nature

Echinacea — subjection to extreme geopathic stress in the Earth, where natural forces have been shattered or annihilated

Hound's Tongue — inability to bring spiritual perception to the natural world; tendency to see Nature as an object, or conglomeration of physical forces

Impatiens — inability to slow down, to sense the natural time cycles and seasonal expressions of Nature; being too busy to relate to Earth as a living being

Iris — relating to the natural world as source of joy and inspiration; to see the "iridescence" of Nature, to be sensitive to natural beauty

Manzanita — estrangement from the earthly world and from the physical body; to help the soul develop reverence and respect for physical experience

Morning Glory — being out of rhythm with natural cycles; inability to feel that eating, sleeping and daily habits are connected to larger rhythms within Nature

Mountain Pride — warrior-like courage to take a stand for the Earth, and for values greater than one's own self-interest, despite opposition or controversy

Nasturtium — preponderance of intellectual activity which estranges one from Earth; disconnection from physical body and larger physical body of Earth

Nicotiana — integration of the finer etheric sensibilities of heart with the etheric sheaths of the Earth; shift of consciousness from exploiting or striving against the Earth, to feeling nurtured and sustained by earthly forces

Poison Oak — relating to Nature through sports or other activities that conquer or subdue; unconsciously creating barriers to real experience of Nature; perception of Nature as an engulfing or annihilating force

Scotch Broom — pessimism or despair about the fate of the Earth which stymies one's ability to serve; to move beyond personal despair to greater vision and hope

Shooting Star — unbalanced interest in other-worldly or extraterrestrial phenomena; profound sense of alienation from Earth, need for soul to understand why it is incarnated on Earth

Sweet Pea — inability to feel rooted, lacking a sense of place on Earth; urban and suburban living conditions which have denied the soul's interest and connection to the Earth and Earth-centered community

Tiger Lily — aggressive tendencies which can lead to exploitation of the Earth or natural resources

Vine — compulsion to control animals and other living beings of Earth; seeing oneself as hierarchically dominant and superior to other species

Yellow Star Tulip — to develop empathic forces; to experience other living beings of the Earth in a soulful, compassionate manner

Zinnia — childlike joy and interest in Nature; to contact a sense of wonder and joy for Earth and all living things

Eating Disorders

(See also Body)

Agrimony — using food as a way of escaping or masking real feelings

Black-Eyed Susan — patterns of denial related to eating; to consciously face one's eating behaviors, such as bingeing, eating forbidden food, hiding or stealing food

California Pitcher Plant — tendency to weak digestion; difficulty breaking down foreign elements in food; physical vigor and strength through harnessing instinctive forces

California Wild Rose — poor appetite, low vitality, lack of interest in food and in the physical world

Cerato — ability to determine and act upon one's own nutritional needs, especially when overly reliant upon others' advice, or on nutritional programs or fad diets

Chamomile — tension-created digestive disturbances in the stomach area; flatulence

Cherry Plum — feeling out of control about eating; binge/purge cycles as in bulimia or anorexia

Chestnut Bud — eating out of habit; to break repetitive patterns of eating that are counterproductive

Crab Apple — exaggerated fear of impurities in food or of body toxins; excessive need for cleansing diets or purgatives; also to promote release of toxins during fasting or cleansing programs

Dill — overstimulation in life leading to digestive disorders; taking in too many varied sensory experiences, leading to indigestion

Evening Primrose — prone to overeating, tendency to have an expanded stomach as though pregnant; seldom feeling full or nourished by food even when large amounts are eaten

Fairy Lantern — emphasis on thinness or anorexic tendencies so that body will continue to look childlike

Fawn Lily — general lack of interest in food or physical substance, due to overly spiritual lifestyle

Golden Yarrow — digestive problems or emotional tension in the solar plexus and stomach, due to conflict between sensitivity and involvement in the world

Goldenrod — overweight used to hide one's true Self, creating social barriers to others; obnoxious or repulsive eating habits to get negative attention from others

Hound's Tongue — overweight when due to overly materialistic attitude toward life; need for more levity, upliftment; need to spiritualize relationship to matter

Impatiens — tendency to eat too fast, not chewing, savoring or enjoying food

Iris — craving for sweets and general hypoglycemic tendencies, especially as a way to deny or repress true creative needs of the soul; using food to feel high or elevated, rather than using forces of inspiration

Manzanita — inability to love physical body; tendency to starve or abuse the body as in anorexia nervosa and bulimia

Mariposa Lily — lack of feeling nurtured as a child, overeating or denying food as a result; using food as an emotional crutch or "mother" substitute

Milkweed — blotting out consciousness with food, often eating to the point of stupefaction

Morning Glory — addiction to junk food, erratic eating patterns; late night bingeing; desire for stimulants such as caffeine

Nicotiana — craving for food when in withdrawal from tobacco or related substances; desire to eat as a way of numbing the intensity of emotional experience

Peppermint — sleepiness after eating, inability to use mental forces; lack of integration of metabolism with thinking forces

Pink Monkeyflower — obesity as a way of masking and protecting the body, as a shield for shame; fear that others will see body as it really is

Pink Yarrow — using food as a buffer for emotional oversensitivity; stuffing oneself to "dull out" or numb feelings

Pretty Face — seeing oneself as ugly, creating image of extreme fatness or thinness because of inability to find true source of inner beauty

Rock Water — excessive strictness in diet, ascetic approach; harsh physical regimen; views body as a machine

Rosemary — poor metabolic response to food, stagnant digestion, inability to transform physical matter due to poor relationship of soul to the body

Self-Heal — confidence in body's ability to digest and assimilate food; being nourished and energized by what one eats

Snapdragon — desire to experience oral activity; continuous biting, crunching and chewing as a sublimation for feelings of misplaced libido or unexpressed anger

Tansy — tendency to create a heavy-set body or overweight due to sluggishness, lethargy

Walnut — to break habitual ties to old patterns of eating and develop new relationship to nourishing foods; moving away from social or cultural ties to food or food rituals

Yarrow — using body weight as a shield or armor of protection from psychic oversensitivity

Egotism

(See also Pride, Self-Aggrandizement)

Angelica — instilling greater awareness of spiritual activity, beyond daily life and mundane ego

Canyon Dudleya — tendency to psychic inflation; desire to attach importance to oneself by creating intense psychic experiences

Chicory — needy and demanding of personal attention; never getting enough love and attention; "emotional tyrant"

Chrysanthemum — attachment to ego identity, psychological need to establish one's personality in the material world as a protection against death and mortality

Goldenrod — false social persona to gain acceptance from others

Holly — envy and jealousy toward others due to emotional insecurity; wanting to feel important due to an inner sense of being unloved

Larkspur — exaggerated sense of self-importance in leaders

Lotus — seeing oneself as spiritually advanced; spiritual pride

Oak — inability to surrender or yield; compulsion to be the hero

Quaking Grass — insensitivity to the needs of others in a group situation

Sagebrush — letting go of previously held images of oneself, experiencing "no-Self" as a precondition of change and transition

Sunflower — lack of true self-esteem expressed as bombastic egotism; overcompensating expression of individuality; to develop balanced ego awareness

Vine — overpowering the will of others with one's own will

Water Violet — keeping one's distance from others; feelings of disdain, elitism, classism, racism or cultural bias

Emergency

(See also Spiritual Emergency and Opening)

Angel's Trumpet — for wartime and natural disasters; to assist peaceful transition in dying process, conscious transition of soul out of body

Angelica — protection and guidance from the spiritual realms, especially for those who have opened up their psychic centers too quickly

Arnica — easing shock and trauma, especially with physical injuries; re-uniting soul and spirit with the body

Canyon Dudleya — inability to cope in emergency, tendency to hysteria and overwhelm

Chamomile — to calm distraught emotions

Cherry Plum — out of control, hysterical, suicidal or destructive due to extreme stress

Crab Apple — mental and physical cleansing; for wounds and toxins

Dill — nervous overwhelm due to assault on the senses through noise, light, air, smoke, etc.

Echinacea — experiences which disintegrate the sense of Self; deeply shattering experiences destructive to the core Self

Five-Flower Formula — for all cases of emergency or first aid, for immediate calming and centering

Golden Yarrow — ability to cope and to help others despite one's sensitivity

Indian Pink — keeping centered amidst intense activity; leadership in crisis

Lavender — restoring calm after nervous burnout

Love-Lies-Bleeding — wounded, bleeding or dying; extreme pain which pushes soul beyond its limits

Purple Monkeyflower — extreme fear or hysteria of a psychic or occult origin

Queen Anne's Lace — for blows to the head, especially when vision is distorted

Red Clover — calm and centered despite group panic; dispels hysteria; promotes leadership in crisis situations

Rock Rose — profound fear of imminent death, destruction or annihilation

Saint John's Wort — spiritual protection in injury or life-threatening situations; to restore inner light; protection during out-of-body states

Self-Heal — recuperation and rejuvenation; wholeness of etheric forces to counteract physical stress

Star Of Bethlehem — soothing and balancing in cases of shock and extreme trauma; restores harmony and peace

Yarrow — protecting against physical or psychic negativity in the environment

Yarrow Special Formula — resistance to radiation or other environmental toxins; geopathic stress

Energetic Patterns

Aloe Vera — lack of energy; feeling burned out by overuse of physical and vital forces

Arnica — blocking life energy due to past shock and trauma which prevents full response to healing

Blackberry — igniting and manifesting one's forces of will; directing energy from head to limbs

California Wild Rose — apathy, with a dulled response to life; to develop more enthusiasm

Canyon Dudleya — calming overly excited states tending toward hysteria

Cayenne — breaking up stagnant energy patterns; adding more fire; transforming energy into action

Chestnut Bud — stuck energetic patterns, particularly repetitive cycles with no transformation or learning

Five-Flower Formula — harmonizing severely disturbed or traumatized energy

Fuchsia — emotional catharsis; shifting from hyper-emotionality to deeper feelings

Hornbeam — listless energy, appearing tired for no apparent reason

Indian Paintbrush — blocked creative expression; feeling dull and inexpressive in creative endeavors; having inspiration, but lacking vital, earthy forces

Lady's Slipper — nervous exhaustion and sexual depletion, integration of root and crown chakras

Lavender — keyed-up energy, as though one is in a tight ball; extreme nervous tension, difficulty relaxing

Morning Glory — erratic energy patterns, especially dull and unresponsive in the morning, hyperactive in evening; using stimulants to increase energy

Nasturtium — lacking in vitality, dry and drained; depletion of metabolic forces through overly intellectual activity

Nicotiana — rousing the heart through tobacco or other stimulants; to awaken the heart through authentic feelings rather than physical substances

Olive — profound fatigue and exhaustion after a taxing ordeal or illness

Peppermint — mental sluggishness especially after eating; metabolic imbalance which drains mental-thinking forces

Pink Yarrow — absorbing too much energy from others, leading to negativity and sense of overwhelm

Rosemary — lack of warmth, cold extremities and lowered vitality; lack of body awareness

Self-Heal — full energetic engagement; ability to tap inner reserves of strength and healing potential

Tansy — acting slow, lethargic and sluggish; procrastinating; avoiding energetic involvement

Yarrow — drained and depleted from absorbing negative thoughts of others, or by one's social or physical environment

Yarrow Special Formula — vital energy depleted by radiation or other environmental toxins

Enthusiasm

Blackberry — involvement of one's will forces in the world; physical manifestation

California Wild Rose — increased enthusiasm for life, for earthly destiny; counteracting apathy with positive forces of caring

Cayenne — igniting the will; fiery action that cuts through stagnation

Larkspur — charismatic, joyful leadership, especially when there is a tendency toward grim dutifulness

Vervain — extreme idealism which leads to nervous tension; an overbearing and fanatical attitude

Zinnia — to encourage exuberance; joyful involvement in life

Environment

(See also City Life, Earth Healing and Nature Awareness, Immune Disturbances)

Angelica — extended awareness of environment, perception of subtle forces at work in auric environment

Beech — over-identification with environment; compulsion to have everything perfect, leading to a critical nature

Corn — discomfort in crowded environments, such as large cities

Crab Apple — oversensitivity to environment, especially to impurities or imperfections

Indian Pink — calm and clarity in the midst of intense outer activity

Iris — ability to bring beauty, artistry, and a sense of soul warmth to home, workplace, and community

Madia — scattered and confused environment; inability to organize or focus

Pink Yarrow — over-dependence on the "perfect" environment as an emotional buffer; emotional oversensitivity to social and psychic environment; for those who are a "psychic sponge"

Poison Oak — to learn boundaries and limits between Self and Nature, as well as with others; erecting negative boundaries through hostility

Shooting Star — not feeling at home in one's environment; profound alienation, or sense of being "out of place"

Star Tulip — increasing awareness of more subtle influences and energies in the environment

Sweet Pea — inability to bond with physical environment or social community; wanderer

Yarrow — oversensitivity to negativity, disharmony, pollution, noxious influences; often manifest as allergic reactions

Yarrow Special Formula — susceptibility to negative energies in the environment, such as radiation, electrical fields, allergens, pollution

Yellow Star Tulip — sensitive awareness of subtle forces in Nature and in other living beings

Envy

Buttercup — feeling lack of self-worth, leading to envy of others

Calla Lily — wishing to be of the opposite sex

Goldenrod — comparing oneself with others; over-concern with social position

Holly — envying the good fortunes of others; jealousy over what others have; feeling left out, unloved

Honeysuckle — feeling those of a past time had it better; nostalgia

Pretty Face — envious of the physical appearance of others; making unfavorable comparisons with others with regard to physical beauty

Trillium — coveting the power or possessions of others; greed

Erratic Behavior

Dogwood — accident-prone or ungraceful

Impatiens — overly impulsive or impatient behavior

Indian Pink — inability to remain centered; overly nervous response to intense activity

Morning Glory — irregular habits and life energy; erratic sleep patterns, relying on stimulants

Scleranthus — inconsistent thoughts and actions; tendency to vacillate from one choice to another

Escapism

(See also Avoidance, Denial)

Agrimony — escaping emotional involvement behind a mask of cheerfulness

Basil — escaping commitment in relationship by deceptive or secretive sexual behavior

Black-Eyed Susan — fear of looking at repressed emotions; bringing the light of conscious awareness to life situations

Blackberry — not fully engaging one's will, living in ideas but evading manifestation

California Poppy — attraction to glamour, spiritual highs or drugs, looking outside rather than within for enlightenment; fascination with psychic phenomena

California Wild Rose — apathy or social alienation; to arouse one's heart and will forces

Canyon Dudleya — escaping by living in extreme emotions, fanatical causes, or psychic superstructures; lack of presence in daily and practical life

Chestnut Bud — repeating experiences rather than confronting real issues and lessons

Chrysanthemum — avoiding consideration of one's own mortality; solely involved in earthly fame and fortune

Clematis — preferring quiet fantasy and inner life rather than active involvement with others

Deerbrush — avoiding honest confrontation with oneself, especially examining underlying motives for one's behavior

Evening Primrose — avoiding commitment or emotional involvement; emotionally unavailable due to early childhood trauma and abandonment

Fairy Lantern — preferring to live in psycho-emotional matrix of family patterns derived from childhood; avoiding adult responsibility

Fawn Lily — protecting oneself; preferring a more monastic or reclusive lifestyle; difficulty in sharing one's spirituality with others

Filaree — focusing on inessential or unimportant concerns which sap true life purpose, not breaking through to major transformation or understanding

Forget-Me-Not — cutting off awareness of spiritual realms, especially of loved ones who have died or seek to be reborn

Fuchsia — tendency toward hyperemotionality or psychosomatic illness; to penetrate to one's core pain and suffering

Gentian — lack of effort due to discouragement over failure

Honeysuckle — preferring to dwell in memory of better times, rather than face the pain and challenge of the present

Love-Lies-Bleeding — using one's handicap or suffering as a crutch or excuse; finding social connection or shared human experience

Milkweed — escaping core identity and ego awareness, often through soporific drugs

Mimulus — avoiding or escaping real challenges in daily life due to fear; pronounced timidity

Morning Glory — escaping through drugs and stimulants, cutting off connection to feeling life within body and within Nature

Mountain Pride — inability to take a personal stand in worldly or community affairs, escaping from risk-taking or confrontation

Mullein — inability to follow inner guidance or to discriminate and adhere to moral values

Nicotiana — appearing "in control," especially over one's feeling life; escaping from the raw pain of the feelings

Pink Monkeyflower — avoidance of intimate relationships; fear of revealing true feelings for fear of rejection; hiding or veiling feelings

Poison Oak — avoidance of intimacy by projecting a hostile barrier

Scarlet Monkeyflower — fear of raw emotions or powerful expressions; lack of contact with core levels of anger or rage

Scleranthus — avoidance of making choices in life; compromising integrity by trying to be all things to all people

Self-Heal — not confronting healing from inner level; escaping responsibility for own healing by dependence on therapists and therapies

Shooting Star — not being fully present for human life and human community; fascination for extraterrestrial or out-of-body experiences

Sticky Monkeyflower — fear of intimacy; escaping vulnerability and commitment, especially in sexual relationships

Sweet Pea — being the endless wanderer and traveler; inability to establish roots in a community, to find sense of place

Violet — holding back from participation in group life or community affairs; fear of losing one's identity in social situations

Walnut — feeling bound by current influences and standards; inability to make a transition toward one's true destiny

Water Violet — feeling disdain for others; holding back involvement out of a sense of superiority

Wild Oat — endless seeking or experimentation, avoiding commitment to life purpose or work goals

Exhaustion and Fatigue

(See also Energetic Patterns)

Aloe Vera — overuse of creative forces; feeling burned out; bringing life forces to heart center

California Wild Rose — resistance to the course of one's life, blocking the flow of life-force

Echinacea — complete breakdown; feeling oneself as utterly annihilated and shattered

Elm — taking on too much responsibility; overwhelmed by tasks assumed

Hornbeam — feeling too tired to face the tasks of the day, largely due to inner resistance

Impatiens — impatient or overly tense attitude toward life, leading to exhaustion

Indian Paintbrush — blockage of vitality in creativity; fatigue and lackluster performance

Lady's Slipper — nervous exhaustion often accompanied by sexual depletion, lack of integration between crown and root chakras

Lavender — nervous tension leading to depletion and exhaustion

Morning Glory — overreliance on stimulants; erratic sleeping and eating patterns which destroy natural vitality; difficulty arising in the morning

Nasturtium — hyperactivity of mental forces leading to extreme fatigue

Oak — pushing oneself even when exhausted

Olive — complete depletion of mind and body; fatigue from overwork, physical stress, or illness

Peppermint — mental fatigue; lethargy in the thinking process

Self-Heal — inability to contact inner healing forces

Vervain — nervous exhaustion from extreme or fanatical lifestyle

White Chestnut — repetitive, circular thoughts; worries which drain energies and deprive one of sleep

Wild Rose — resignation due to a long, lingering illness

Yerba Santa — deep melancholia which invades the body, feeling of wasting away; deterioration

Failure

(See also Confidence, Manifestation, Perseverance, Rejection)

Buttercup — feeling that one's vocation or contribution doesn't count

Elm — feeling that one is a failure or is letting others down; overanxious striving leading to a sense of falling short

Gentian — undue doubt and discouragement from setback or failure

Larch — fear and anticipation of failure due to poor self-image; often giving up even before trying

Oak — resistance to failure; attachment to "hero" role

Penstemon — overcoming failure with increased strength and determination

Faith

(See also Trust)

Angelica — trusting in the angelic realm, in higher guidance

Aspen — faith when facing the unknown

Baby Blue Eyes — trusting in life, especially when soul forces are hardened or jaded

Borage — upliftment and buoyant courage; faith that life will work out despite challenges

California Wild Rose — trust in the value and meaning of life on Earth

Cherry Plum — ability to sense and trust higher forces of spiritual help, despite intense stress

Forget-Me-Not — knowing that there is life beyond the physical realm; ability to discern and perceive the activity of spiritual beings, especially those with whom there is a karmic bond

Mimulus — faith that one can meet the small challenges of everyday life; overcoming timidity

Oregon Grape — accepting the goodwill of others, especially when there is a tendency toward mistrust

Sage — faith in the meaning and working of destiny; able to see and learn from the unfolding events of one's life

Scotch Broom — seeing societal obstacles or global problems as opportunities for growth and service in the world

Self-Heal — trusting one's own self-healing powers

Sweet Chestnut — restoring faith when stretched beyond all limits; extreme mental isolation and anguish

False Persona

(See also Honesty, True to Self)

Agrimony — hiding true feelings under a mask of cheerfulness; outward display of happiness despite emotional pain and anguish

Calla Lily — false identification with opposite sex; accepting one's true sexuality

Canyon Dudleya — attachment to overly spiritual or psychic persona, inability to accept ordinary or daily reality

Chrysanthemum — attachment of lower Self to wealth, social standing and physical body, due to a deep fear of death and mortality

Fairy Lantern — presenting a demeanor of helplessness, dependency; childlike persona

Goldenrod — creation of false persona in group situations to win social approval

Lotus — spiritual egotism; resistance to seeing "lower" or shadow aspects of one's character

Nicotiana — "macho" personality, appearing grounded and in control by numbing or suppressing real feelings

Pink Monkeyflower — fear of exposing true feelings, inability to open up

Pretty Face — obsessive personal grooming in order to appear outwardly beautiful or handsome

Purple Monkeyflower — false religious identity or allegiance, due to fear of censure or criticism

Sagebrush — false or dysfunctional self-image; finding essential Self and letting go of unnecessary identifications; inner purification

Sunflower — false or unbalanced egotism; false desire to appear important to others

Fanaticism

California Poppy — susceptibility to fanatical or extreme causes and movements

Canyon Dudleya — "stirred up" or extreme emotions, tending to hysteria

Vervain — trying to convert others to one's beliefs; intense enthusiasm of the true believer

Vine — imposing one's will on others; tyrannical disregard for the autonomy of others

Father and Fathering

(See also Masculine Consciousness, Home and Lifestyle)

Baby Blue Eyes — disturbed relationship to father, often involving abuse or abandonment; unable to trust in goodness of the world due to lack of guidance or protection from father

Chrysanthemum — drive to accumulate material wealth, status or power which overshadows the interpersonal values of family and children

Elm — assuming responsibility for role of provider but later feeling overwhelmed and despondent; very helpful for new fathers

Fairy Lantern — difficulty assuming fatherly responsibilities due to arrested emotional development in childhood; resentment of wife's motherly attention to children, wants attention for oneself

Fawn Lily — remaining aloof from family and role as father due to preoccupation with other-worldly spiritual values; bringing more warmth and love into family life

Larch — difficulty conveying confidence or authority in father role; doubting own capacities

Pine — internalizing much guilt and self-blame due to overly strict or harsh father; self-deprecation which prevents full realization of own fathering capacities

Pink Monkeyflower — unresolved psychological wounds or abuse from own childhood which prevents emotional expression or vulnerability; emotionally unavailable in father role

Quince — internal conflict about role of father, especially in balancing strength and love; vacillating between strict disciplinarian or permissive father

Sage — realizing elder wisdom in one's father or other important male figures; ability to reflect and learn from own experience as a father

Saguaro — conflict with or abuse from father, grandfather or other males in family lineage, resulting in alienation from father role; healing one's relationship with ancestral family and elders

Scarlet Monkeyflower — episodes of rage or power battles with child; feeling powerless as father due to own unresolved issues about anger and power

Sunflower — general remedy for healing relationship with one's father and self-image internalized from father

Sweet Pea — difficulty in making a commitment to family, community and living environment; fathers who are absent, travel often, or frequently relocate or uproot family

Vine — exerting harsh or extreme control over children; feeling a need to be dominant in father role

Zinnia — relating to children in a playful way by contacting one's own childlike nature; to counterbalance workaholism or other ways of avoiding children and one's inner child

Fear

(See also Paranoia)

Angelica — overcoming fear by connecting with higher realms as a source of spiritual guardianship and protection

Aspen — vague anxieties, unconscious fears

Black Cohosh — fear of threatening, violent or abusive relationships; overly intense, congested psychic energy which attracts fear-based relationships

Black-Eyed Susan — fear of powerful emotions; bringing the light of awareness into darker emotions

California Pitcher Plant — fear of the instinctual aspects of the Self; repelled by the instinctual functions of the body as "lower"

Cherry Plum — fear of losing control or becoming destructive; nervous breakdown or insanity

Chrysanthemum — fear of death and dying; unbalanced attachment to earthly life

Fairy Lantern — fear of growing up, of adult identity

Fawn Lily — deep soul fear of contamination by physical world; wanting to stay "spiritual"

Filaree — petty worries and anxieties, especially with a tendency to compulsive or obsessive behavior

Five-Flower Formula — to calm extreme fears when no other remedy can be determined; for immediate benefit

Garlic — nervous fear, weakness and devitalization; stage fright

Golden Yarrow — performance anxiety; wanting to project oneself but overly anxious and sensitive

Holly — fear that others will receive more love and attention

Larch — fearful anticipation of others' judgment of what one says or does; fear of failure; lack of confidence in one's own ability

Mimulus — worries of daily life; specific and known fears; timidity

Mountain Pride — fear of the adverse forces of our time; developing a positive sense of spiritual warriorship

Oregon Grape — prone to expecting emotional hostility from others; paranoia

Pink Monkeyflower — concern about exposing and expressing true feelings; fear of being exposed by others

Poison Oak — fear of intimate contact with others, of being vulnerable; protecting against fear by developing an angry or hostile persona

Red Chestnut — concern and worry for others; excessive fear for safety of others

Rock Rose — terror at possible loss of Self, death or ego-death

Saint John's Wort — fear during dreams or out-of-body traumas; fear of spiritual adversaries

Scarlet Monkeyflower — fear of powerful emotions, especially anger

Star Thistle — worry about lack, leading to stinginess

Sticky Monkeyflower — conflict and fear about intimacy, especially sexual; fear of being vulnerable in relationships

Sweet Pea — fear of social commitment in family and community

Violet — fear of losing one's individuality in a group situation; tendency to shyness or retreat

Feminine Consciousness

(See also Mother and Mothering, Pregnancy, Sexuality)

Alpine Lily — integration of the feminine with female sexual and biological Self

Baby Blue Eyes — wounding from father or male figures, resulting in distrust and hostility toward others, especially men

Black Cohosh — tension in reproductive organs; congested menses; overly intense psychic energy

Bleeding Heart — tendency toward codependent relationships; developing strength in the heart; ability to love others based upon freedom and self-respect

Buttercup — low self-esteem; seeing women's traditional roles as inferior; developing authentic assessment of one's true worth, apart from societal standards

Calla Lily — family pressure or inner desire to be male although born female; finding true sexual identity and inner balance of masculine and feminine

Canyon Dudleya — hysteria or out-of-body states of consciousness; unbalanced attachment to psychic states of consciousness, need to cultivate more masculine objectivity

Corn — archetype of Earth Mother, integration of feminine identity with Earth consciousness; nurturing strength

Easter Lily — difficulty integrating female sexual identity; vacillating between extremes of prudish or promiscuous behavior

Evening Primrose — deep wounding to feminine identity transmitted from mother during infancy or while in utero; emotional coldness or sexual unresponsiveness due to disturbed early relationship with mother

Fairy Lantern — desire to remain a little girl, helpless and dependent; holding on to childish qualities, limited sexual development; delayed or irregular menstruation

Fawn Lily — for the "ice princess": profound beauty and aloof spirituality which needs to flow more into the Earth and humanity

Hibiscus — warmth and responsiveness in sexuality; integration of sexuality with heart feelings

Iris — attunement to feminine muses; inspiration; ability to create a chalice or container for soul creativity

Lady's Slipper — nervous depletion which interferes with sexual vitality

Love-Lies-Bleeding — unusual or heavy bleeding during menses, especially when accompanied by intense physical suffering or mental anguish

Mariposa Lily — receptivity to human love, maternal nurturing; ability to mother and be mothered

Mugwort — enhancing and balancing moon-like, receptive qualities of the psyche; to assist all flowing processes in the body, such as menstruation

Pink Monkeyflower — feelings of extreme vulnerability and shame, often from sexual exploitation or abuse

Pink Yarrow — overly feminine merging; sympathetic forces confused with compassion; to develop emotional objectivity and appropriate boundaries

Poison Oak — fear of being engulfed in feminine, fear of intimacy

Pomegranate — creative expression of the feminine aspect of the Self, both in procreation and in worldly creativity; often an underlying emotional cause of PMS symptoms

Pretty Face — excessive preoccupation with external standards of beauty; inability to contact inner feminine qualities of beauty and grace

Quince — developing the strength of love, feminine power; especially when strength and love are seen as polarities

Saguaro — to address issues of wounding or abuse in ancestral history; extreme alienation or rebellion to persons in authority, especially men; finding positive archetypes of elder or wise person

Snapdragon — powerful forces of libido or sexual energy which have been culturally repressed due to feminine stereotype, especially with tendency of these to manifest as verbal anger, criticism or jaw and mouth tension

Star Tulip — spiritual receptivity, opening the feminine aspect of the Self to higher worlds; inner listening or telepathic attunement, especially meditation or dreams

Sunflower — integrating positive masculine animus; healing relationship with father and other male figures; radiant individuality and self-esteem

Tiger Lily — balance of the feminine forces when tending toward overly masculine assertiveness; also for transition to menopause, re-orienting feminine forces

Willow — "victim" consciousness, toxic levels of resentment and anger, blaming others for unpleasant or exploitative life experiences

Yellow Star Tulip — developing feminine forces of listening and attunement in social situations; greater sensitivity to others, empathy

Flexibility

(See also Spontaneity, Tolerance)

Dogwood — gracefulness and ease in life, especially when emotions and bodily movements are harsh, cold or rigid

Oak — developing more flexibility in struggle, knowing one's limits, knowing when to let go of the struggle

Quaking Grass — flexibility in group situations; seeing all sides of an issue, all points of view

Rabbitbrush — ability to maintain multifaceted consciousness; assimilation of simultaneous events

Rock Water — developing a flowing attitude toward life; easing overly strict self-imposed standards

Willow — accepting and forgiving others; letting go of resentment

Forgiveness

Baby Blue Eyes — to heal cynicism or other forms of "soul hardness," through forgiveness and acceptance of past trauma

Beech — forgiving faults in others; overcoming tendency to be critical

Golden Ear Drops — letting go of and healing childhood trauma

Holly — seeing others as part of the human family; ability to drop feelings of separateness

Mariposa Lily — making peace with one's childhood, especially with one's mother

Pine — self-forgiveness for one's own errors and faults, for not being perfect

Sage — making peace with life, especially as part of aging process; accepting and learning from life events, letting go of emotional attachment

Willow — forgiving the errors of others; overcoming tendency to bitterness, resentment or blame

Freedom

Bleeding Heart — emotional nonattachment in relationships; respecting the freedom of the other

Centaury — freedom from unwarranted domination by others

Chestnut Bud — to break habits which bind and limit; freedom from needless repetition in life experience

Fairy Lantern — confusion of freedom and responsibility; childishness or escapism as an inappropriate expression of freedom

Iris — transcending a sense of limitation or weight; winged creativity

Morning Glory — freedom from erratic or devitalizing habit patterns or addictions

Pink Monkeyflower — emotional freedom to express true feelings, when emotions are imprisoned due to shame and fear

Purple Monkeyflower — creating own spiritual identity and values, especially if conforming to false values due to fear

Sagebrush — letting go, emptying and freeing oneself from excess attachment in life and surroundings

Scarlet Monkeyflower — freedom to express one's powerful emotions openly and honestly

Trumpet Vine — freedom to speak clearly and forcefully without holding back

Walnut — breaking free of limiting influences, especially from past circumstances

Wild Oat — overattachment to freedom, leading to lack of direction or purpose in life

Frustration

Blackberry — inability to manifest intentions in actions; frustration of the will

Gentian — disappointment and frustration by setback or delay

Impatiens — frustration with the slowness of others and of life

Indian Paintbrush — difficulty bringing vitality to creative expression

Iris — frustration in creative expression due to lack of inspiration; feeling limited or "dried up"

Penstemon — frustration with adversity, unexpected challenges

Gloom

(See also Darkness, Depression and Despair)

Baby Blue Eyes — feelings of gloom tinged with cynicism

Black Cohosh — profoundly dark states of mind, characterized by suspicion and incessant brooding

Gorse — despair and hopelessness about one's personal affairs

Mustard — gloom in the form of a personal black cloud; sudden and unexpected feeling of gloom

Red Clover — easily influenced by projections of gloom and doom, group panic

Scotch Broom — depression about disasters and tragedies in the world

Grace

Angel's Trumpet — ability of the soul to leave the physical body peacefully and gracefully when dying; any profound soul transition

Angelica — feeling in touch with the grace of the angelic realm

Calendula — graceful receptivity to others; feminine forces of listening and receiving

Deerbrush — purity of feelings within the heart

Dogwood — gentleness and grace of expression flowing from a balanced emotional life; restoring innocence and grace lost in previous traumatic situations

Holly — ability to extend grace and forgiveness to others

Lotus — spiritual harmony, feeling of wholeness

Pine — ability to forgive oneself; to feel grace as a spiritual gift

Star Tulip — being in touch with the anima, the more gentle feminine aspects of Self

Vervain — extreme intensity, fervency of feelings which rob one of grace and ease

Greed

(See also Desire, Materialism and Money, Selfishness)

Chrysanthemum — trying to establish monetary power as a protection against mortality; materialistic consciousness

Goldenrod — wanting material possessions to insure social status

Sagebrush — holding on too tightly, over-identification with possessions or lifestyle as a psychological prop; encouraging one to let go of what is inessential

Star Thistle — lack of generosity; clinging to material possessions as a form of security

Trillium — greed and lust for power and possessions

Vine — wanting leadership power for selfish ends

Grief

(See also Death and Dying)

Bleeding Heart — to release a relationship which has ended, or death of a loved one

Borage — uplifting and renewing the heart with courage; heart balm for grief

Dandelion — releasing feelings of grief or emotional pain which are stuck in the body

Evening Primrose — deep soul pain, ability to encounter traumatic abuse in early infancy and childhood, especially rejection and abandonment

Fuchsia — contacting grief that may be emotionally repressed

Golden Ear Drops — releasing tears of grief that may have been held back, especially during childhood

Honeysuckle — letting go of the past, coming into the here-and-now so that life can go on after death or loss

Love-Lies-Bleeding — profound feelings of melancholia and anguish, especially when the soul suffers privately and is cut off from others

Sagebrush — accepting the pain and emptiness of any kind of loss

Star Of Bethlehem — calming and soothing after the shock of death or other tragedy

Wild Rose — not accepting the tragic events of life; withdrawal or numbing due to grief

Yerba Santa — internalized sadness due to past trauma, melancholy; deeply internalized pain stored in the heart and chest

Groundedness

(See also Centeredness, Daydreaming)

Alpine Lily — disconnected from female body; inability to integrate higher feminine spirituality with essential experience of the female body

California Wild Rose — difficulty coming into the body; lack of vitality or enthusiasm for life

Canyon Dudleya — difficulty accepting ordinary or mundane reality, desire to inflate or exaggerate reality

Clematis — being present in the here-and-now; for those who feel "floaty" or dreamy

Corn — bringing spirituality through the body and into the Earth

Fawn Lily — bringing spiritual forces more into earthly life, especially when there is a tendency to retreat or hold back

Golden Yarrow — staying embodied, especially when energy leaks from solar plexus

Hibiscus — experiencing sexuality as a positive expression of the body

Indian Paintbrush — igniting forces of physical vitality for higher, creative work

Lady's Slipper — strong spiritual forces which are not fully grounded and integrated; lacking in focus and clear connection with one's destiny

Manzanita — feeling at home in the physical body and earthly world; feeling the body as a source of emotional nourishment

Queen Anne's Lace — distortion of psychic forces due to emotional instability or sexual feelings; for balanced and grounded psychic opening

Rosemary — tending to overly discarnate states; reduced ego forces that cannot properly come into the body; forgetfulness, memory loss

Saint John's Wort — protection when feeling one's consciousness is too open and expanded

Shooting Star — feeling at home on the Earth and in human life; overcoming deep-seated alienation

Sweet Pea — finding roots in community life; developing a sense of place

Vervain — zealous or fanatic activity which overrides body awareness

Guilt

(See also Shame)

Deerbrush — mixed motives; unclear intentions; to purify and integrate the innermost feelings of the heart

Elm — feelings of guilt and misery when one can't measure up to expectations; to develop a more honest assessment of one's capabilities

Golden Ear Drops — repressed feelings of guilt associated with early childhood experiences

Mullein — listening to the voice of conscience; developing moral sense of right and wrong

Pine — self-blame; being hard on oneself; assuming guilt out of proportion to actual circumstances

Pink Monkeyflower — covering up, fear of exposure, not trusting that others will understand; profound shame

Pink Yarrow — undue guilt; emotional merging with others which results in misplaced feelings of guilt

Habit Patterns

Cayenne — breaking free of habitual behavior; fiery catalyst for change

Chestnut Bud — constant repetition of experiences without learning from them; attachment to habit patterns which are regressive and limiting

Morning Glory — to overcome destructive habits; to develop lifestyle patterns based upon healthy rhythms

Rock Water — holding overly strict and unyielding habit patterns based upon extreme ideals of discipline and control

Sagebrush — breaking free of old identities and habits which are no longer appropriate; finding what is essential or true for oneself

Walnut — letting go of habits or lifestyle patterns taken on from the influence of others

Hardness

Baby Blue Eyes — hard, numb exterior; cynical or bitter attitude toward life experience

Beech — hard, judgmental attitude toward others, demanding; unrealistic standards of perfection for others

Dandelion — extreme tension from overactivity, leading to hardness or stiffness in the body

Dogwood — hard, limiting emotions; self-abusive due to previous abuse from others; accident-prone and self-destructive

Morning Glory — harsh lifestyle; habits which are hard on the body; out of touch with gentle and subtle energy levels

Nicotiana — appearance of hard exterior or tough posture; bodily strength at the expense of the emotional life

Oak — strong, unyielding will in struggle, not knowing when to surrender

Pine — hard attitude toward oneself; extreme self-judgment and blame

Pink Monkeyflower — inability to be vulnerable due to feelings of shame or fear of rejection

Poison Oak — creating a hard exterior; inability to show vulnerability; projecting anger or other hostile emotions; fear of intimacy

Quince — integrating the softer, feminine aspect when also needing to be strong and self-directed

Rock Water — being hard on oneself by creating overly strict standards or personal regimens

Star Tulip — lack of receptivity to the inner voice or to the spiritual realm; softening of soul forces

Harmony

Angelica — to feel the harmonious weaving of soul life with higher realms, especially the angelic realm

California Poppy — feeling harmony within oneself, especially balancing the tendency to seek outside oneself for fulfillment

Chamomile — to restore emotional harmony after upset

Fuchsia — bringing repressed emotions to awareness so they can be harmonized with one's conscious awareness

Lavender — to bring emotional calming; to soothe after overly intense spiritual activity

Lotus — harmonizing and enhancing meditative experience; integrating spiritual identity with the personality

Quaking Grass — creating harmony within a group; blending of individual egos

Shasta Daisy — creating harmonious patterns in work and thinking; the harmony of integrative thinking

Star Tulip — harmony in the relationship of the soul to the spiritual world; feeling attunement to higher realms; developing inner listening

Hate

(See also Dislike)

Black Cohosh — twisted love or love-hate relationships, tending toward violence

Crab Apple — self-hate, especially with obsessive concern over impurity or contamination

Holly — hostility toward others out of a feeling of jealousy; sibling rivalry or other forms of negative competition

Oregon Grape — expecting hate from others; acting according to the lowest, rather than the highest, potential in others

Pine — undue blame and hatred of oneself; inability to accept one's mistakes

Scarlet Monkeyflower — explosive emotions, especially anger, due to feeling of powerlessness or repressed rage

Snapdragon — verbal expressions of criticism and hostility toward others; tendency to lash out verbally at others

Willow — resentment, blame of others; hatred which continues over time, turning to bitterness

Healers

Agrimony — masking one's own pain and suffering in order to appear in control; attachment to the image of healer as one who is beyond pain

Calendula — ability to listen to clients; ability to be warmly receptive as well as dynamically active in a healing practice

Centaury — false ideals of service leading to overly servile attitudes; becoming drained and depleted rather than replenished by healing work

Deerbrush — recognizing and applying true higher motives for healing work

Golden Yarrow — staying receptive and engaged in the healing process without becoming overly vulnerable

Impatiens — inability to be receptive to client's true needs; tendency to over-schedule clients, to be rushed or impatient with difficult clients

Mallow — conveying qualities of personal warmth and nurturing in healing practice

Mariposa Lily — imparting feminine forces of nurturing and care; positive mother archetype

Oak — taking on the role of healer as hero; needing to learn when to set limits

Pink Monkeyflower — fear of self-exposure or vulnerability in role as healer

Pink Yarrow — tendency toward emotional merging with others; unconscious emotional identification which results in a loss of objectivity and inner strength

Red Chestnut — excessive worry and anxiety about the well-being of one's clients; to develop the ability to project healing, comforting thoughts

Self-Heal — contacting true inner healing capacities; shifting focus from personality of healer to the healing process

Shasta Daisy — ability to think holistically about a client's condition, to integrate the many different parts of the symptom picture into a meaningful portrait

Sunflower — ability to convey warm radiance from within; compassionate presence of Self; positive father archetype

Yarrow — overabsorption of others' suffering, resulting in feelings of depletion; need for more psychic detachment

Yellow Star Tulip — intuiting client's Higher Self; acting on one's inner sense of what is needed for client's true healing; compassionate presence

Zinnia — becoming overly somber and serious when exposed to the daily suffering of others; bringing humor and light-heartedness to one's healing approach

Healing Process

Agrimony — denial of pain or of the need for healing

Angelica — protection and nurturing from spiritual guides, receiving help during difficult healing journey

Arnica — releasing armoring from parts of the body or psyche which have been deeply wounded or traumatized; to instill etheric wholeness after surgery or accidents

Black-Eyed Susan — for any form of denial during the healing process, to accept one's illness and to face the deeper or "shadow" qualities of the healing journey

Borage — upliftment when heavy-hearted or discouraged

California Wild Rose — inability to be fully committed to healing; apathy; engaging the heart in the healing process, increasing one's will to live

Canyon Dudleya — overdramatizing healing or suffering; accepting ordinary and mundane step-by-step process of healing; integrating healing changes gradually rather than dramatically

Cerato — following one's own guidance in the healing process, especially when inundated by the advice of others

Chestnut Bud — to break repeated patterns in illness; to learn lessons or messages from suffering

Crab Apple — when obsessed with healing, especially the need for cleansing and purification; overly strict expectations or dismay about imperfections

Echinacea — re-building core Self when damaged from extreme trauma, major surgery or other devastation; bringing strength when deeply shattered

Fairy Lantern — regressive tendencies in therapeutic process; stuck in childlike pattern of dependency; fixation on child rather than adult Self

Fuchsia — presentation of psychosomatic symptoms that may be masking real pain and suffering

Gentian — to restore one's faith and perseverance when setbacks occur in the healing process

Golden Ear Drops — contacting painful memories, authenticating and deepening emotional experience

Gorse — attachment to suffering, extreme melancholy or depression

Heather — obsession with one's symptoms, compulsion to talk constantly about one's problems

Impatiens — unwilling to accept the slow process of healing journey, wanting to move too quickly without absorbing the inner experience of healing

Lavender — nervous tension; allows full relaxation in order to receive benefits of healing work

Love-Lies-Bleeding — finding meaning in one's suffering; to move beyond personal to transpersonal level of understanding about one's pain; to stimulate the immune system

Manzanita — difficulty integrating bodily component into healing work, favoring mental or cognitive approach

Mariposa Lily — contacting core feelings from childhood; providing a mantle of protection when doing difficult work with childhood or mother issues

Milkweed — extreme dependency; illness which obliterates one's conscious awareness; a need for healers who act as surrogate parents

Mountain Pennyroyal — cleansing toxic thoughts; to clear states of negativity or psychic contamination which impede the healing process

Mustard — accepting the dark as well as the light; having the courage to work through painful emotions and bouts of depression

Olive — physical renewal after exhaustive illness; recuperation from major surgery or trauma

Penstemon — courage to continue improving Self despite challenges, especially physical pain or handicap

Pine — being hard on oneself in the healing process; internalizing guilt, inability to forgive oneself and move forward

Pink Monkeyflower — difficulty letting down barriers, or allowing others to help by sharing one's true feelings and suffering

Pink Yarrow — hypersensitive to the healing process, adverse reaction to medication or to the therapeutic process because feelings seem magnified and intense

Pretty Face — willingness to go through a period of ugliness or discomfort; desire for beauty and perfection which inhibits one from staying with the intensity of the healing process

Rosemary — unable to be present in physical body, to bring physical healing all the way into the body, to feel safe during body work or massage

Sagebrush — willingness to go through a stage of aloneness and emptiness as a prerequisite to change

Self-Heal — core remedy to ignite self-responsibility in the healing process, especially to encourage the belief that one can be healed; to break over-dependence on therapist or therapies

Shasta Daisy — to integrate different therapeutic approaches or information received about healing

Sunflower — balancing ego forces, between positive self-image and honest self-examination

Walnut — making major transitions in the healing process; supporting profound transformation and re-ordering of life

Wild Rose — engaging oneself in the recovery process when there has been a long, lingering illness, with a tendency toward apathy and withdrawal

Yerba Santa — releasing emotional congestion in the heart; restoring ability of the heart to breathe out deep pain and grief

Heart

Aloe Vera — replenishing the creative forces of the heart when feeling burned out or depleted

Alpine Lily — for women: integrating the deeper feelings within the heart with unconscious feelings in the lower female organs

Baby Blue Eyes — opening the heart to the loving presence of the spiritual world, ability of the soul to feel benevolent guardianship when lacking in trust and faith

Bleeding Heart — healing the broken heart, for ending relationships, separation or death of loved one; to develop more emotional self-sufficiency

Borage — feeling disheartened or discouraged, heavy-heartedness or grief; bringing cheerful and buoyant courage

California Wild Rose — strengthening and vitalizing the heart; counteracting feelings of apathy by bringing compassion for others and interest in life

Dandelion — over-achiever; bringing balance to the heart by moving from "human doing" to human being

Fawn Lily — greater flow of spiritual forces through the heart, especially when there is a tendency to contain or reserve one's spirituality for oneself

Forget-Me-Not — spiritualizing the love currents of the heart; ability of the heart to understand and accept karmic or eternal aspects within relationships

Holly — vexations of the heart: jealousy, envy, hatred; feeling lack of love; opening the heart to the universal abundance of love

Impatiens — frenetic, over-impulsive, or fast-paced lifestyle which places extreme stress on the heart

Love-Lies-Bleeding — to allow and to understand intense and deep feelings of suffering, leading the heart to greater compassion and understanding

Mariposa Lily — feeling the warmth and nurturing quality of one's heart; mothering as a heart force

Nicotiana — to counteract the use of stimulants or other physical measures to rouse the heart; energizing the heart by activating the soul life and contacting real feelings

Pink Monkeyflower — allowing feelings to flow through the heart more easily; contacting authentic feelings despite fear or shame

Pink Yarrow — to distinguish true heart forces of compassion from overly sympathetic or dysfunctional merging with others

Yerba Santa — release of constriction in the heart region, especially feelings of sadness; release of accumulated psychic toxins caused by deep-seated emotional repression

Hesitation
(See also Ambivalence, Certainty, Confidence, Decisiveness)

Cerato — uncertainty about one's own values; over-dependence on the advice of others

Fairy Lantern — waiting for others to take responsibility; helplessness

Larch — uncertainty, lacking in confidence

Mimulus — holding back due to fears of everyday life

Scleranthus — fluctuating between two possibilities when making decisions

Tansy — difficulty being decisive; tendency to lethargy, "sitting on" one's energy

Home and Lifestyle
(See also Father and Fathering, Mother and Mothering)

Beech — hypersensitivity to environment in home, compulsion to have everything in order; intolerance of others' imperfections

Buttercup — feelings of worthlessness or low self-esteem in domestic role

Canyon Dudleya — inability to identify with ordinary household tasks or daily living responsibilities; aversion to a practical routine, craves excitement or glamour in unbalanced manner

Crab Apple — compulsive cleaning or ordering of living quarters, especially an aversion to anything unclean or out of order; alternatively, for lack of hygiene in living environment, need to purify and set in order

Fairy Lantern — living with parents or in dependent situation beyond young adult stage, inability to face world or work responsibilities

Fawn Lily — treating home as a retreat; spiritual introversion leading to social isolation

Filaree — attachment to mundane aspects of household, allowing activities such as cleaning to loom out of proportion, depriving one of greater participation in social or worldly life

Honeysuckle — home filled with nostalgic items or memorabilia to an extreme degree, so that soul is not living in present time

Impatiens — performing household tasks quickly or irritably, without real interest or participation of the soul

Indian Pink — scattered or disheveled quality in living environment; quick pace of life or whirl of activities that prevent one from feeling centered or calm in one's home

Iris — dull, drab or ugly living environment; inattention to color and form, lack of creativity or soul interest in home and environment; excessive use of television or other forms of escapism which stifle creative activity in home and lifestyle

Madia — inability to complete simple household tasks, easily distracted; chaotic living quarters due to inability to focus attention

Mariposa Lily — to bring maternal warmth and nurturing presence to home

Mimulus — being housebound or shut-in; not venturing out of home due to various "everyday" fears or phobias

Morning Glory — lack of rhythm in living habits such as eating and sleeping, chaotic lifestyle or living environment due to erratic habits

Mountain Pennyroyal — to purify home or environment, especially when contaminated by psychic or astral debris such as disturbed thoughts or negative energies of others

Pink Yarrow — easily absorbing emotional environment of one's home; oversensitivity to or merging with one's surroundings without appropriate ego boundaries

Pretty Face — desire for home to appear beautiful in conformance to others' standards; being out of touch with inner sense of what pleases or satisfies the soul

Sagebrush — purifying and simplifying one's lifestyle, especially when home and surroundings are congested and disorderly; overly materialistic accumulation of objects in home

Shasta Daisy — bringing parts of living environment into greater wholeness and relatedness; bringing harmony to chaotic or disorderly home

Star Tulip — developing quiet inner presence in one's home; allowing home to become a source of soul experience

Sweet Pea — homelessness or social isolation; moving frequently, inability to feel home as connected to a place on Earth and part of larger social community

Tansy — inability to complete household tasks; unfinished projects due to lethargy and procrastination

Walnut — to move out of or change current living situation, to establish new home or lifestyle rhythms

Zinnia — finding joy and interest even in mundane tasks; childlike wonder and pleasure in daily living

Honesty

(See also True to Self)

Agrimony — acknowledging inner conflict; for those who cover up true feelings

Black-Eyed Susan — to counteract denial; to examine repressed psychological material; emotional honesty with oneself

California Poppy — looking honestly within oneself instead of trying to escape through spiritual glamour, drugs, or dream-like experiences

Canyon Dudleya — inflation of psychic experiences; compulsion to exaggerate reality in order to feel spiritual

Fuchsia — expressing basic emotions rather than false emotionality which covers up true feelings

Goldenrod — conforming to others' patterns of social behavior to win approval, not being true to oneself

Mullein — acknowledging inner guidance, conscience; tendency to lie, lack of truthfulness with oneself or others; shutting off one's inner voice

Pink Monkeyflower — showing true feelings despite fear of exposure or censure

Sagebrush — inappropriate identity or self-image which needs to be released; internal purification; to develop greater integrity and clarity

Scarlet Monkeyflower — recognition and appropriate expression of powerful emotions such as anger or rage

Snapdragon — to contact core feelings of anger and sexuality, especially when misplaced as aggression toward others

Hostility

(See also Anger, Resentment)

Baby Blue Eyes — detached hostility masquerading as cynicism

Beech — hostility expressed as criticism or condemnation of others

Holly — hostility due to feelings of separation or rivalry; actively expressing hostility to others

Oregon Grape — expectation of hostility from others; paranoia

Poison Oak — projecting hostility as a way of avoiding intimacy; hostile behavior which keeps others from making contact

Snapdragon — hostility expressed by biting words and other verbal criticism

Tiger Lily — transmuting hostile or aggressive tendencies; developing feminine balance and inclusiveness

Hysteria

(See also Emergency)

Canyon Dudleya — susceptibility to mediumism or unbalanced psychism; exaggerated emotions which prevent an objective and ordered experience of life

Chamomile — extreme emotional upset; crying and other distraught behavior

Cherry Plum — out of control, erratic or destructive behavior

Cosmos — overexcited mental activity, accompanied by rapid but inarticulate speech

Five-Flower Formula — to bring immediate calming

Fuchsia — false emotionality; powerful emotions or physical suffering which are psychosomatic expressions of deeper but unrecognized feelings

Mugwort — overemphasis on psychic life which leads to emotional imbalance

Pink Yarrow — pathological merging with others' emotions, resulting in hysteria or other extreme displays of emotion

Purple Monkeyflower — profound fear or panic, especially as a negative state of spiritual consciousness, overwrought psychic imagination or projection due to fear

Red Clover — fear and panic in group situations; easily influenced by mass media or thought-forms

Rock Rose — panic and hysteria in extreme situations, when facing death or destruction; fear of ego death

Idealism

Beech — overly perfectionist ideals; harsh standards which are imposed on others

Blackberry — bringing ideals into practical manifestation; integration of thinking and willing

California Wild Rose — activation of true ideals; ability to engage heart forces in life work

Centaury — wanting to be of service but must find inner balance between others' and own needs

Clematis — impractical ideals and visions; dreaminess

Fawn Lily — strong spiritual ideals that need to be shared with others

Larkspur — positive idealism, altruistic leadership

Mountain Pride — ability to speak out for one's ideals; active commitment

Rock Water — overly strict ideals for oneself and others; inflexible idealism

Vervain — strongly held ideals and beliefs which can lead to fanaticism; overly intense in promotion of one's ideas to others

Immobility

(See also Inertia, Resistance)

Blackberry — unproductive thought patterns which do not manifest in the world

Cayenne — lack of sufficient catalyzing, fiery forces; emotional or physical paralysis

Golden Yarrow — performance anxiety, wanting to act but too sensitive

Iris — feeling weighed down; to develop winged aspects of the soul life, to mobilize artistic and creative impulses

Larch — paralysis due to fear of failure; inability to take risks

Morning Glory — erratic habits, addictions

Rock Rose — paralyzed by fear of death or destruction

Scleranthus — inability to make a decision, thus preventing forward movement

Tansy — sluggish, lethargic, overly phlegmatic, indecisive

Wild Oat — inability to choose career or life direction; being stuck in unfulfilling work

Immune Disturbances

(See also Body, Environment, Psychosomatic Illness)

Beech — over-identification with exterior surroundings, leading to sensitive, reactive, or critical behavior and immune dysfunction

Crab Apple — oversensitivity and obsession with impurity leading to reduced ability to tolerate toxins; hyperallergic

Echinacea — maintaining the integrity and essential nature of oneself despite circumstances of degradation, abuse or environmental assault; for compromised immune system

Garlic — attraction to mediumism, opening oneself physically and psychically to parasitic entities

Lavender — hypersensitivity leading to nervous exhaustion and related stress to immune system

Love-Lies-Bleeding — to increase immune response by finding meaning in one's illness or disease; to shift from victim to participant in healing process

Morning Glory — compromised immunity due to damaged etheric body; need to rebuild rhythmic connection to Nature and etheric body

Nasturtium — lowered vitality and immunity due to overly intellectual lifestyle

Olive — extreme fatigue and exhaustion; depletion of one's defenses, both physical and psychic

Self-Heal — strengthening one's own health-creating forces; self-responsibility as a pathway to self-healing

Walnut — following one's own convictions; creating inner strength and integrity of Self

Yarrow — oversensitivity to one's social or physical environment; absorption of psychic or physical toxins, leading to fatigue and depletion

Yarrow Special Formula — vulnerability to negative energies and substances in the environment, such as radiation, electromagnetic fields, allergens, pollution

Impatience

Calendula — difficulty listening to others; need for more receptivity

Cosmos — to regulate the flow of thoughts coming from higher mental planes; too-rapid speech or thinking patterns

Impatiens — expecting others to go faster, impatience with the seemingly slow pace of life

Poison Oak — susceptible to irritation or anger; antipathetic rather than sympathetic tendencies

Inadequacy

Buttercup — feeling that one's life or vocation is not important

Elm — feeling inadequate to one's responsibilities; overanxious striving for perfection

Evening Primrose — feeling unlovable or unwanted due to childhood rejection or abuse

Fairy Lantern — feeling that one cannot cope with adult responsibilities; unfinished emotional work with inner child

Golden Yarrow — feeling that one is not capable of performing; overanxious and oversensitive to others

Goldenrod — socially insecure, trying to measure up to others' standards

Iris — feeling uncreative; feeling that one is inartistic

Larch — self-censorship; fear of failure or being judged as inadequate

Milkweed — feeling unable to cope with life or normal ego demands; extreme feelings of dependency

Pine — never feeling that one is good enough; being hard on oneself

Pink Monkeyflower — sense of shame; core feeling of unworthiness

Pretty Face — never feeling beautiful enough

Sticky Monkeyflower — feelings of sexual inadequacy or awkwardness

Sunflower — self-effacement; lack of balanced ego forces

Indecision

(See also Ambivalence, Conflict, Decisiveness, Hesitation)

Cerato — inability to trust in one's inner knowing, overly reliant on advice from others

Larch — indecision due to lack of self-confidence

Mullein — inability to connect with one's inner guidance, or to find inner values for decision-making

Scleranthus — fluctuating between two possibilities, "back and forth" deliberation

Tansy — delaying decisions, not acting when action is called for; procrastination

Wild Oat — wavering about life purpose and vocation; lack of life direction, the chronic "seeker"

Individuality

Centaury — suppression of true individuality in order to serve the needs of others

Chrysanthemum — contacting one's true spiritual Self, shift from over-identification with lower persona

Echinacea — reclaiming one's integrity and dignity despite prior abuse, trauma or devastation

Fairy Lantern — cultivating more individuality, especially as an expression of adult responsibility and initiative

Goldenrod — sense of true Self in social situations; balance between group identity and individual identity

Milkweed — poorly integrated individuality; difficulty in coping with normal demands and responsibilities of adult ego; wanting to blot out or obliterate ego

Mullein — fulfillment of one's true potential, being true to one's inner knowing of what is right

Purple Monkeyflower — developing authentic spiritual identity, especially if fear has stifled true expression

Sagebrush — ability to reflect about and observe the Self, to experience the emptiness of "not-Self;" to distinguish personality from essential spiritual identity

Self-Heal — contacting inner resources, self-reliance

Sunflower — balanced expression of ego identity; general remedy to stimulate positive individuality

Violet — to maintain self-identity in a group situation, especially when shy or nonassertive

Inertia

(See also Avoidance, Immobility, Resistance, Procrastination)

Baby Blue Eyes — cynicism which retards natural progress of soul's evolution, numbing the soul's awareness

Blackberry — inability to put ideas into action, or to ground one's vision in practical reality

Cayenne — getting stuck in old patterns of behavior; needing fiery catalyst; inability to move on to the next step in life

Chestnut Bud — unnecessarily repeating old habit patterns and life experiences; not learning one's life lessons

Morning Glory — getting stuck in destructive, addictive habit patterns

Tansy — hesitation, indecisiveness, or lethargy due to suppression of natural vitality

White Chestnut — thinking which is stuck in a mental rut, a "broken record" of repeating thoughts

Influence

Angelica — ability to receive positive influence and guidance from spiritual world

Centaury — being excessively influenced by others; weak-willed and overly subservient

Cerato — excessively influenced by the opinions and advice of others; lacking certainty of one's own convictions

Garlic — increased susceptibility to parasitic influences, both physical and psychic; weakened resistance due to fear and anxiety

Larkspur — influencing others through balanced leadership; positive charisma

Mountain Pennyroyal — clearing the mind of negative thoughts taken on from others

Pink Yarrow — absorbing or acting out thoughts and feelings of others; emotional merging

Vervain — intense and overbearing influence on others; to develop moderation and inner balance

Vine — influencing others adversely; strong-willed; limiting others' free will

Walnut — to break free from cultural or family influences or other past circumstances; freedom to follow one's own direction

Inner Child

(See also Children)

Alpine Lily — rejection of or alienation from the feminine, especially unconscious rejection of mother or mother's role in family constellation

Angelica — feeling protected and cared for by benevolent spiritual beings; feeling the presence of a Higher Power

Baby Blue Eyes — mistrust of the world, emotional insecurity due to abandonment or estrangement from father during childhood

Beech — critical judgment of others, often as displaced self-criticism; judgment of the childlike aspects of oneself

Black-Eyed Susan — recalling buried painful experiences from childhood, especially conscious recognition of repressed feelings and emotions

Bleeding Heart — accepting pain of broken relationships in family of origin, to let go and to move forward with emotional life

Buttercup — tendency to still see oneself in persona of small, vulnerable child; low self-esteem stemming from one's identity as a child

California Wild Rose — accepting the pain of childhood, especially when it may have stunted heart and will forces; moving beyond victim role to fully engaged adult role

Calla Lily — healing mixed messages about sexual identity received from one's parents in childhood; to fully reclaim one's sexual identity

Canyon Dudleya — getting attention by overinflating emotional experience; also the unconscious acting out or dramatization of childhood trauma in adult life

Centaury — compulsion to serve parents, family members or parent-like figures; dominance of the inner child by one's own adult self; neglect of inner emotional needs, lack of self-nurturing

Cerato — learning to trust one's own inner knowing which was invalidated by parents in childhood

Cherry Plum — fear of losing control, especially if deep, traumatic feelings are experienced; the ability to "let go and let God;" fear that childlike spontaneity will lead to loss of control

Chicory — behaving in childish way to get attention; neediness, inability to cope emotionally

Dogwood — feeling of awkwardness or ungainliness in the physical body, abuse or neglect during childhood which disconnects body from its innate sense of grace and beauty

Echinacea — re-patterning the core Self, rebuilding self-esteem and dignity despite profound or severe abuse or exploitation

Elm — for the "hero" who had to take responsibility to rescue the family as a child; overwhelm due to premature assuming of adult responsibilities

Evening Primrose — to accept that one may have been rejected or unwanted in utero or when born, unconscious absorption and identification of mother's or father's negativity; deep feelings of rejection and abandonment

Fairy Lantern — attachment to childlike identity as a way of pleasing elders; unconscious compulsion to repeat childhood; getting stuck in inner child therapeutic work

Fuchsia — emotional catharsis, integration of deep-seated emotions held in the body which may have never been fully experienced

Golden Ear Drops — contacting and releasing painful childhood memories, often repressed; emotional acceptance and integration of childhood experiences

Goldenrod — to individuate from family constellation, establishing one's identity apart from family structure

Holly — crippling of the heart's capacity to love unconditionally due to childhood experiences of emotional abuse, conditional love or sibling rivalry

Iris — contacting creative soul forces, especially artistic impulses which may have been suppressed in childhood

Larch — low self-esteem; expectation of failure which results in self-censoring; suppression of childlike spontaneity

Mariposa Lily — healing core relationship with one's mother, finding spiritual archetype of mother and mothering despite personal trauma or affliction

Milkweed — unconscious desire to merge with parents, inability to cope with individualized identity, compulsion to obliterate consciousness and repress ego function; over-dependence on mother or family support

Oregon Grape — overcoming childhood conditioning which expects the worst from others; mistrust and suspicion; fear of strangers, ethnic or racial prejudice learned as a child

Pine — blaming oneself for family dysfunction; feeling guilt out of proportion to real circumstances

Pink Monkeyflower — profound shame within the soul; inability of soul to express true feelings and emotions, usually due to emotional, physical or sexual abuse in childhood

Pink Yarrow — feeling psychically sensitive and overly absorbent, learned to cope as child by becoming a container for emotional refuse of family members

Pretty Face — ugly duckling or black sheep in family system, internalized feeling that one is different and unattractive

Purple Monkeyflower — overemphasis on "fearing God" in childhood religious upbringing, which has stifled childlike sense of wonder, reverence and trust

Red Clover — reacts rather than acts in family crisis, prone to emotional hysteria and group panic, unable to think or act for oneself

Rosemary — for those who learned to disembody when physically or emotionally abused; difficulty for soul to incarnate fully or warmly inhabit body

Scarlet Monkeyflower — need to contact and acknowledge feelings of anger and upset about childhood experiences; tendency to apologize for or repress powerful feelings about childhood

Self-Heal — to take responsibility for own healing, moving beyond victim role, believing that healing and recovery are possible

Shooting Star — traumatic or extremely disturbed birthing situation; when one's soul has never fully incarnated or accepted its humanity

Sunflower — healing relationship to masculine principle, especially when relationship to father has been disturbed; low self-esteem

Willow — releasing blame and bitterness for childhood pain; ability to forgive parents, other family members or teachers

Yerba Santa — unclaimed grief, especially when deep sadness or trauma from childhood is stored in the heart

Zinnia — reclaiming authentic inner child, laughter, playfulness, and light-heartedness

Insecurity

Aspen — anxiety about the unknown and the future

Baby Blue Eyes — lack of trust that the world is safe, especially due to disturbances with father or masculine principle

Calla Lily — uncertainty and confusion about sexual identity

Evening Primrose — unconscious belief that one is unwanted and unloved, due to toxic emotions absorbed in early childhood

Fairy Lantern — instability in relationships; unhealthy, immature seeking of security from others as parental substitutes

Garlic — psychic fears which drain and weaken the vitality, thus producing feelings of insecurity

Golden Yarrow — fear of performance or social contact; hypersensitivity

Goldenrod — insecurity with others expressed by false persona in a group or social situation

Mallow — social insecurities that hinder ability to make friends; developing social trust

Mimulus — feeling overly fearful, timid, fretful

Pink Monkeyflower — insecurity characterized by shame or defensiveness; emotional masking

Pretty Face — inability to radiate inner sense of beauty; social insecurity due to over-concern about personal appearance

Rosemary — not feeling safe in the physical body

Saint John's Wort — insecure sleeping alone or going to sleep (for both children and adults)

Star Thistle — lack of feeling secure in Self, with a tendency to accumulate material possessions as a way of feeling secure

Insight

(See also Awareness)

Angelica — insight into the spiritual world

Black-Eyed Susan — penetrating insight into emotions, especially when uncovering darker or "blocked" areas of consciousness

Chestnut Bud — understanding the lessons gained from life experiences

Fuchsia — awareness and understanding of emotions which are masked by false emotionality

Hound's Tongue — realizing the higher meaning of intellectual ideas or material phenomena

Mugwort — greater clarity about dream life or events outside rational consciousness

Queen Anne's Lace — blockages related to seeing, both physically and metaphysically; integration of sight with expanded sensitivity and clairvoyance

Sage — insight into the meaning of life; wisdom and acceptance

Shasta Daisy — synthesis of many ideas into one whole; seeing the pattern of the whole within the many parts

Star Tulip — inner knowing from one's own meditative attunement

Yellow Star Tulip — insight through social interaction with others, listening skills

Insomnia

Aspen — fear of the dark or the unknown; hypersensitivity to unseen forces real or imagined

Black-Eyed Susan — insomnia due to troubling thoughts which are repressed or only dimly conscious; need for the subconscious part of the Self to be relieved of toxic material

Chamomile — calming hypertension, emotional upset; releasing accumulated emotional tension held in the stomach, especially beneficial for children with difficulty relaxing at bedtime

Chaparral — intense cathartic dreams which trouble the psyche and cause fitful sleep

Dill — insomnia due to inability to assimilate one's experiences; nervous or sensory overwhelm

Lavender — overwrought nerves, especially from extreme spiritual or mental pursuits

Mugwort — disturbed sleep due to overactive dream life

Red Chestnut — insomnia due to excessive worry and concern about others

Saint John's Wort — dream disturbances, especially when connected with fear or psychic stress of any kind

White Chestnut — insomnia caused by repetitive, obsessive thoughts; unable to quiet the mind

Inspiration

(See also Intellectualism, Thinking)

Blackberry — putting ideals into practical expression; acting on one's intentions

Cosmos — ability to articulate higher inspiration in thoughts and speech

Hound's Tongue — transforming sense-bound ideas to higher imagination; tendency to materialism or earth-bound thinking

Indian Paintbrush — to ground inspired or creative activity, especially when the body is overtaxed

Iris — to spark inspired thinking and creative activity; general remedy for inspirational forces

Mugwort — to balance or integrate psychic forces with inspired thought; practical ordering of inspired thought

Shasta Daisy — synthesis of many ideas into a living whole

Star Tulip — receptivity to spiritual information; chalice-like soul qualities which serve as a container for spiritual activity

Instinctual Self

(See also Body, Lower Self, Sexuality)

Alpine Lily — alienation from feminine sexuality and sexual organs

California Pitcher Plant — integrating instinctual forces into human experience; proper use of animal or astral forces

Easter Lily — conflict about sexuality, feeling it is impure or "lower"

Hibiscus — allowing the vital power of sexuality to be integrated in one's life

Manzanita — aversion to the physical body; ignoring and rejecting basic survival instincts such as hunger and need for sleep

Pomegranate — conflicts about the feminine procreative instinct; conflicts between raising a family and having a career

Queen Anne's Lace — integration of psychic and sexual energies

Scarlet Monkeyflower — fear of instincts relating to power, survival and anger; healthy integration of these energies into one's personality

Snapdragon — contacting core emotions, especially when misplaced as verbal aggression and hostility

Sticky Monkeyflower — difficulty integrating sexual instincts with one's heart feelings; fear of intimacy which leads either to suppression of sexuality or heartless promiscuity

Tiger Lily — for those who act out aggressive, competitive instinctual drives

Trillium — transforming lower instincts of greed or lust for power

Intellectualism

(See also Inspiration, Thinking)

Cosmos — overly wordy, rapid and rambling speech which needs greater integration with the Higher Mind

Hound's Tongue — sense-bound or materialistic ideas; to develop higher imagination and perception

Nasturtium — dry intellect which suppresses vitality

Shasta Daisy — to balance analytic thinking with holistic overview; synthetic thinking

Zinnia — overly serious or intellectual; need to lighten up

Intimacy

(See also Personal Relationships, Sexuality)

Baby Blue Eyes — restoration of childlike innocence and trust; intimacy as a form of trust and openness

Basil — tendency to polarize feelings of physical intimacy and sexual desire with spiritual ideals; sexuality divorced from deeper soul feelings

Calendula — ability to express warmth, intimacy and nurturing feelings with one's words

Evening Primrose — cold or distant behavior; inability to express intimate feelings due to past rejection

Fawn Lily — to develop intimate and warm contact with others; tendency toward an aloof spirituality

Golden Yarrow — to develop social contact and rapport with others, while maintaining sensitivity

Hibiscus — fuller intimacy and soulfulness in sexual relationships, physical warmth

Mallow — greater social warmth, ability to sustain soulful relationships with others, especially friendship

Mariposa Lily — deprived of mother or parenting resulting in coldness in the soul, inability to make contact with others

Pink Monkeyflower — creating emotional distance out of profound sense of shame and guilt, inability to show others true feelings; fear of unmasking or exposing true Self to others; fear of rejection

Pink Yarrow — confusion about intimacy, between sympathetic and empathetic soul qualities; learning to establish intimacy without inappropriate merging

Poison Oak — fear of making contact with others, especially of being touched; fear of being enmeshed or engulfed, leading to hostile or offensive behavior

Shooting Star — profound alienation from human contact and human warmth; feeling that one is not fully human or fully incarnated in physical body; sense that one does not "belong" with others

Star Tulip — softness and receptivity; soul gentleness as a gateway to intimacy

Sticky Monkeyflower — fear of intimate contact, especially sexual contact; integration of feelings of sexuality with human warmth and intimacy

Violet — inability to share one's essential Self in group situations; shyness and reserve; fear of losing one's identity if too close to others

Water Violet — inability to establish intimate contact, due to a sense of disdain or social superiority

Yellow Star Tulip — to develop the ability to establish empathetic contact, to sense what another is really feeling

Involvement

(See also Apathy)

California Wild Rose — enthusiastic involvement in life; accepting life with all its pain and challenges

Evening Primrose — enhanced emotional presence; ability to make commitment in relationships by resolving childhood trauma, abuse and feelings of rejection

Fawn Lily — inability to share oneself with others due to a reclusive or overly spiritual quality within the soul

Golden Yarrow — greater involvement in life and in public affairs, despite innate sensitivity

Hornbeam — greater involvement in the tasks of life, especially when tired for no apparent reason

Mallow — involvement with others, developing warmth in friendship

Mariposa Lily — emotional connection with others; when feeling separate and unloved

Shooting Star — feeling a part of life on Earth; for those who feel alienated from Earth existence; to accept being a part of humanity

Sweet Pea — participation in community or family life; social rootedness

Trillium — involvement with others for the greater social good; overcoming lower emotions of greed

Violet — connection with others; overcoming shyness or fear that one's identity will be submerged in the group

Water Violet — sharing with others; overcoming aloofness or pride

Irritability

Beech — critical or blaming of others; often from oversensitivity to one's environment and the effect of others' behavior

Chamomile — soothing and calming for those who are easily irritated or emotionally upset

Chicory — acting overly fussy as a way of getting attention; being particularly irritable when not getting the attention demanded

Crab Apple — feeling upset by impurity and imperfection, to an obsessive degree

Dill — upset caused by overstimulation, taking in many experiences too quickly

Impatiens — irritability directed at others, especially when they are too slow or methodical; general remedy for many forms of irritation or inflammation

Indian Pink — feeling upset by frenetic activity around oneself, need for centering

Lavender — overstimulation of nerves leading to irritability and hypersensitivity

Pink Yarrow — easily upset by emotional disturbances in others; absorbing feelings of irritation from others

Poison Oak — inability to form sympathetic bond with others due to irritation and impatience; projecting hostility to keep others away

Snapdragon — extreme reactivity; easily "set off" to make verbal attacks, to "snap back" when one feels challenged or attacked

Willow — resentful lashing out at others; prone to blaming others

Yarrow — vulnerability to disturbances in the environment

Joy

Angel's Trumpet — acceptance of death as a joyous transition, deep release or liberation of the soul as an expression of joy

Baby Blue Eyes — lack of joy, paralysis of soul forces, profound cynicism

Borage — cheerful courage from within the heart; buoyancy

Holly — ability to feel happiness for others, taking joy in others' accomplishments

Hornbeam — approaching life as a dull routine; to develop joyful involvement in life's tasks

Impatiens — taking time to experience the joy of life; to experience life at an enjoyable pace

Larkspur — providing leadership with joy, charisma

Mustard — transforming depression into quiet, balanced joy

Zinnia — playfulness, childlike sense of humor

Judgment

Beech — severe criticalness, excessive judgment of others

Cerato — ability to judge for oneself, rather than relying on the opinions of others

Mullein — developing inner values and moral choices

Pine — severe self-judgment; guilt and self-blame

Queen Anne's Lace — clarity in psychic perception and judgment

Scleranthus — forming clear judgments instead of vacillating between alternatives

Leadership

Elm — overly perfectionist or overly anxious leadership

Lady's Slipper — blocked leadership potential, thwarted destiny, often accompanied by nervous exhaustion and self-doubt

Larkspur — inspiring others by example and through social service; positive charisma

Mountain Pride — warrior-like courageous leadership, ability to face adversity

Oak — never-ceasing effort in spite of poor health or reduced forces

Red Clover — leadership in crisis situations; keeping a calm center when others are in panic

Sage — calm, wise leadership; letting go of personal ambition and importance

Sunflower — radiant individuality, positive influence on others

Tiger Lily — sense of receptivity and cooperation, balancing an overly aggressive nature

Trumpet Vine — ability to speak out vigorously to the public; using the voice as a powerful instrument of leadership

Vervain — strong leadership which can become imbalanced by overintensity or fanaticism

Vine — developing leadership which respects the freedom and autonomy of others, where there is a tendency to authoritarian, despotic leadership

Learning Difficulties

(See also Awareness, Concentration and Focus, Study)

California Wild Rose — boredom or lack of interest in study material; affirming inner connection to academic or scholarly work

Chamomile — emotional hyperactivity which interferes with learning process and concentration; need for calm

Chestnut Bud — repeating errors, difficulty learning lessons

Clematis — difficulty paying attention in class, daydreaming or fantasizing

Cosmos — speech difficulties when the mind is overwhelmed by too much information

Gentian — giving up when difficulties are encountered; for the strength to persevere despite setbacks

Impatiens — difficulty paying attention; nervousness, restlessness, inability to focus; hyperactivity

Iris — lacking in creative insight or interest, inability to engage imaginative or inspirational forces; engagement of Higher Mind in mental pursuits

Madia — short attention span, flits from one activity to another

Milkweed — lack of ego strength; emotional immaturity, leading to learning difficulties; retarded development

Penstemon — physical or mental handicaps which make learning difficult; strength to persevere through long and difficult training or rehabilitation program

Peppermint — stimulating mental capacities, especially when basic temperament is dull or sluggish

Self-Heal — confidence in one's abilities when faced with learning difficulties from accident, injury or illness

Trumpet Vine — problems with speech such as stuttering

Yarrow — hypersensitivity due to environmental stress which prevents full concentration and focus; expanded psychic forces that overwhelm the mental capacities

Life Direction

Baby Blue Eyes — feeling stymied, beset by cynicism and bitterness, inability to trust in the unfolding of life events

Blackberry — manifesting intentions as concrete actions; ability to fulfill goals

Buttercup — feeling the worth of one's life work and vocation, even if not glamorous or considered important by society

California Wild Rose — accepting and responding to the challenges of life so one can move ahead with life destiny

Chrysanthemum — awareness of one's own mortality; ability to shift to true spiritual life purpose and direction

Fairy Lantern — resolving and releasing the past; to facilitate the maturation process when stuck in any developmental phase

Gentian — easily discouraged or pessimistic about one's life direction; to develop confidence and perseverance

Lady's Slipper — to integrate spiritual purpose with daily work, ground and focus spiritual destiny

Larch — confidence to follow one's creative inspiration and life destiny, especially when plagued by self-doubt

Pomegranate — for women: conflict between family and career goals

Sage — especially for advanced stages in life biography, ability to absorb life experience and impart wisdom of soul

Sagebrush — periods of inactivity or setback; ability to accept emptiness as a time of transition and inner growth

Scleranthus — vacillating between two choices; life destiny paralyzed by indecision

Shooting Star — for people who do not feel a part of humanity; enhancing the commitment to life purpose on Earth

Sweet Pea — for the constant wanderer or traveler who is unable to commit; not feeling at home in any community or place on Earth

Walnut — finding one's own direction free of the influences of others, especially family or friends

Wild Oat — confusion about vocation and life destiny; trying many kinds of work, none of which satisfy; finding an outer expression of inner purpose

Lightness

Angelica — feeling spiritual guidance and enlightenment, feeling that the soul can be uplifted; participation in higher realms of activity

Borage — upliftment of the heart, buoyancy of feeling

Cosmos — to develop mental agility; mercurial lightness in thought and speech

Hound's Tongue — feeling too weighed down, or earth-bound; overly materialistic viewpoint

Iris — ability to catalyze inspired thought, creative activity

Larkspur — joy in leadership; altruistic idealism

Mustard — uplifting heavy, depressive emotions into joyful balance

Peppermint — lightness in one's thinking; mental alertness

Pretty Face — bringing more light and radiance into the body, especially the face

Queen Anne's Lace — uplifted vision, fine-tuned perception

Saint John's Wort — feeling the strength and protection of one's inner light; particularly when consciousness is diffuse and overexpanded

Yarrow — bringing more light and strength in the aura to overcome feelings of vulnerability

Zinnia — childlike humor when overly somber or leaden

Listening

(See also Receptivity)

Calendula — hearing the deeper meaning of another's words; cultivating appreciation and respect for the speech of others

Forget-Me-Not — connection with spiritual guides and departed souls; remembering those who guide beyond the physical realm

Heather — remaining quiet so others can be heard; especially when focusing too much on one's own personal problems and needs

Impatiens — tendency to interrupt; impatience with others when they speak

Mullein — hearing inner spiritual guidance, especially in moral decision-making, values clarification

Quaking Grass — listening to the needs of others in group work

Star Tulip — hearing one's inner voice; receptivity to spiritual influences, particularly in meditation and dreaming

Yellow Star Tulip — sensing the deeper meaning or message of others, receptivity to the feelings of others; empathy

Loneliness

(See also Abandonment, Rejection)

Baby Blue Eyes — excessive detachment, numbness toward life events, lack of trust

Bleeding Heart — feeling loss and pain of a relationship which has ended; dysfunctional attachment to another, leading to extreme feelings of loneliness when emotional needs are not met

Echinacea — profound sense of devastation which makes one feel utterly alone and bereft

Elm — feeling one is alone in facing an overwhelming task; to realize that human and spiritual help is available

Evening Primrose — inability to form committed relationships, emotional distancing due to early rejection in childhood

Forget-Me-Not — feeling a connection to the Higher Self and to spiritual beings; to counteract feelings of spiritual isolation

Heather — seeking social contact by talking excessively about one's problems

Honeysuckle — loneliness expressed as nostalgia for the past; living in the "good old days" instead of connecting with others in present time

Love-Lies-Bleeding — pain and suffering which tends to isolate; to share and to learn from one's pain and suffering

Mallow — overcoming social barriers; developing trust and warmth

Mustard — loneliness and isolation which result from depression and withdrawal

Nicotiana — appearing solitary or independent but unable to express or share real feelings with others; emotional numbness

Oregon Grape — feeling cut off from others due to paranoid feelings about the intentions of others

Pink Monkeyflower — holding back from expressing intimate feelings due to fear of rejection

Sticky Monkeyflower — awkward with intimate expressions; fear of emotional or sexual intimacy due to past hurts

Sweet Chestnut — feeling cut off from spiritual source when severely tested; existential loneliness and despair

Sweet Pea — feeling cut off from community or family ties; not able to find soul feeling for "home" or one's place on Earth

Violet — feeling shy about opening to others in a group

Love

Angelica — feeling the love and care of spiritual beings

Baby Blue Eyes — opening the heart to spiritual presence, despite harsh life experiences, especially when the soul is beset by cynicism

Bleeding Heart — freedom in love; overcoming unhealthy attachments

California Wild Rose — enthusiastic involvement in life; love as an antidote to apathy

Chicory — selflessness in expressing love; letting go of possessiveness and clinging, or seeking love through negative attention

Fawn Lily — ability to translate lofty spirituality into warm, flowing impulses of love

Forget-Me-Not — understanding the deeper meaning of relationships, especially the karmic or metaphysical qualities

Holly — universal Christ-like love; compassionate understanding of others

Love-Lies-Bleeding — to come to a greater understanding of love and compassion through suffering and sacrifice

Mariposa Lily — receptivity to human love, maternal nurturing

Pink Monkeyflower — inability to express genuine feelings of love and warmth; inhibition due to fear and shame

Pink Yarrow — ability to distinguish loving and compassionate behavior from overly sympathetic merging

Yellow Star Tulip — to develop compassionate understanding for the needs of others; empathic presence

Lower Self

(See also Instinctual Self, Sexuality, Shadow Consciousness)

Alpine Lily — perception or unconscious belief that one's female body is lower or inferior

Basil — split between sexuality and spirituality; acting out sexuality as a secretive or shame-based experience

Black-Eyed Susan — insight into inner darkness or hidden aspects of oneself; conscious acknowledgment of disowned parts of the Self

California Pitcher Plant — integrating instinctual forces into one's human experience; balanced use of animal or astral forces

Chrysanthemum — over-identification with earthly life and persona; inability to contact Higher Self

Easter Lily — integrating soul purity with bodily sexuality

Fuchsia — emotional repression; inability to express genuine deep feelings

Hibiscus — integration of soul warmth and sexual passion

Lotus — spiritual pride which disowns lower energy centers

Nicotiana — excessive need to ground or armor oneself; to acquire strength at the expense of the feeling life

Pine — releasing guilt and self-blame; over-identification with negative parts of oneself

Queen Anne's Lace — to integrate emotions and sexuality with psychic life; distorted or subjective clairvoyance

Scarlet Monkeyflower — transforming anger and deep, powerful emotions; facing the shadow side of the personality

Snapdragon — to harmonize lower energy centers, especially when libido is misplaced as verbal hostility and aggression

Tiger Lily — transmuting hostility and aggressiveness

Trillium — overcoming greed or lust for power

Vine — tendency to use will to control others; developing inner obedience to higher spiritual Self

Manifestation

(See also Action, Will)

Aspen — inaction due to fear of taking risks, especially anxiety over what is unknown

Blackberry — atrophied or unexpressed will forces; putting ideals and ideas into action

Borage — developing courage and confidence, especially when feeling disheartened

Buttercup — feeling that one's contribution is not good enough, or does not count

California Wild Rose — listless and apathetic attitude; positive enthusiasm for life and life's challenges

Cayenne — igniting the will, sparking the inner drive and motivation, cutting through inhibiting habits and patterns

Centaury — overly servile mentality; empowering oneself to take responsibility and make changes

Cerato — hesitating or losing momentum; squandering resources by overreliance on others' schemes or advice

Chestnut Bud — repeating experiences rather than moving forward into real change; learning from life events

Chicory — excessive neediness which impairs one's ability to manifest; falling apart when feeling lack of support

Clematis — too floaty and dreamy; insubstantial ideas and plans, without enough commitment to the here-and-now

Crab Apple — obsessive concern with perfection which stymies ability to manifest; unable to tolerate disorder or creative chaos

Filaree — inability to manifest real life work due to enmeshment in endless details or distractions

Gentian — discouragement when there are setbacks; need to keep trying

Golden Yarrow — stepping out into the world and making changes despite inner sensitivity

Gorse — pessimistic attitude which impedes ability to see a positive outcome

Hornbeam — procrastination; feeling that one is too tired to start or continue a project

Impatiens — to consider the long view; becoming frustrated and impatient if change is not immediate

Indian Paintbrush — lacking vitality to be creative; to develop forces of will to sustain inspired projects and ideas

Iris — bringing thoughts from higher realms into creative expression

Lady's Slipper — feeling estranged from true talents and capabilities; inability to integrate higher spiritual purpose with daily work

Larch — greater self-confidence; for those who impose limits on their creative expression rather than break through barriers

Madia — staying focused on a goal, especially for those who tend to get sidetracked or lose interest

Mountain Pride — courage to take risks; to stand out or speak up, to make bold steps for change

Penstemon — persevering even when challenging or adverse situations come up; inner strength and fortitude

Pine — loss of energy and momentum by self-blame, disparaging and self-deprecating attitudes and behavior

Scleranthus — inability to make choices, vacillating; compromising one's potential through hesitation and indecision

Scotch Broom — overcoming negative or hopeless images of the world; developing the capacity for positive, selfless service

Shasta Daisy — integrating many facets of a project, bringing coherence, organization, and order

Tansy — feeling strong inertia; overly phlegmatic forces which impede true self-expression and manifestation

Trumpet Vine — healthy self-assertion, especially for speaking up and projecting oneself

Walnut — breaking old ties that hinder, setting change in motion without being hampered by past influences

Wild Oat — scattered talents and interests; lack of passion and commitment for long-term goals or career; ability to choose vocational opportunities which reflect life purpose

Martyrdom

Canyon Dudleya — seeing oneself as suffering out of proportion to real experience, overdramatizing and exaggerating one's experiences

Centaury — tendency to be a "doormat" for others, lacking inner sense of individuality

Chicory — feeling sorry for oneself; manipulating others to gain sympathy

Elm — anxiety about responsibility, feeling the weight of the world on one's shoulders

Heather — overabsorption in personal problems or trauma

Larkspur — excessive dutifulness, lack of joy; experiencing leadership as a burdensome responsibility

Love-Lies-Bleeding — tendency to internalize suffering and pain; to move beyond the weight of personal suffering to transpersonal understanding

Mustard — feeling sorry for oneself because of deep depression

Oak — balancing desire to be a hero with realistic expectations of one's strength

Penstemon — perseverance despite hardships such as a physical handicap or challenging life circumstances

Rock Water — being overly strict with oneself; self-denial

Sweet Chestnut — extreme soul anguish; feeling as if one is being punished by God

Willow — seeing oneself as the victim; blaming others for one's situation

Masculine Consciousness

(See also Father and Fathering, Sexuality)

Agrimony — false mask of how a "man should be," doesn't allow others to see real feelings; denial of emotional pain by appearing cheerful or nonchalant; often associated with drug or alcohol abuse

Aloe Vera — unbalanced work patterns which lead to burnout and exhaustion; over-identification with "fire" forces, need to evoke soothing and healing "water" aspects of Self

Baby Blue Eyes — hard and cynical attitude; loss of childlike innocence due to poor relationship to father; developing a positive masculine identity which combines strength and sensitivity

Black Cohosh — tendency to commit sexual abuse or violence, either as an unconscious urge or actual behavior

Calendula — using words to injure others; developing sensitivity to the impact of one's words on others; for healing of verbally abusive relationships or to establish a receptive mode in communication with others

Calla Lily — insecurity about male sexual identity; lack of recognition from parents who preferred a female child; finding an authentic relationship to male identity and to inner masculine-feminine balance

Dandelion — for the overachiever, strong active personality; being out of touch with real needs of the body; emotions which often manifest as extreme body tension, especially in neck and shoulders

Elm — feeling of being all alone in carrying the burden of responsibility; feeling unequal to the task; to accept the help of others and of spiritual forces

Fairy Lantern — patterns of immaturity, the *puer eterna* or eternal child; reluctance to accept adult responsibilities due to unresolved childhood problems; "Peter Pan" syndrome

Golden Ear Drops — overcoming the cultural bias that men do not cry; to contact painful feelings and wounds from the past

Hound's Tongue — developing one's inner, imaginative capacities, especially when preoccupied with work, news, computers, spectator sports; developing the soul's capacity for imagination and wonder

Impatiens — always being in a hurry, inability to be present with others; excessive fiery forces which create tension and irritability

Larch — developing true self-confidence despite shyness and low self-esteem; for blockages to self-expression that may manifest as throat afflictions, also for adolescent boys during voice change

Larkspur — positive leadership traits; charismatic enthusiasm which is able to engage and inspire others

Mountain Pride — warrior-like courage, masculine archetype of strength; confronting and transforming adversity in a positive manner

Nicotiana — tough exterior achieved through numbing of emotions; seeming not to care or appearing to be "cool;" needing to contact real feelings in the heart

Oak — provider and protector of others; balancing strength and struggle within one's limits and letting go when necessary; the Hero archetype

Oregon Grape — fear and hostility toward others which can often erupt in violence; particularly helpful for group animosities such as in adolescent gangs and ethnic conflicts

Penstemon — inner masculine strength in the face of grave challenges of life, such as injury, economic or physical adversity

Pink Monkeyflower — fear of intimacy and vulnerability, often due to shaming or abuse as child; inability to express deep emotions, or woundedness; fear of touching or being touched by other men; fear of being judged as effeminate if vulnerability is shown

Poison Oak — manifesting overly Martian qualities, inability to be vulnerable; creating barriers and showing hostility rather than real feelings; fear of being engulfed in the feminine

Rock Water — strict disciplinarian for oneself or others; stone-like qualities of the soul which need to become more organic, flexible and yielding

Sage — relating to elders or to one's own higher wisdom; reflecting and learning from life experience; the Wise Man archetype

Scarlet Monkeyflower — becoming aware of repressed rage, particularly for men who feel a sense of powerlessness or impotence

Star Tulip — softening overly masculine qualities, bringing forth the anima, or inner feminine aspect of the man; deepening the ability to feel emotions; enhancing dreams, contemplative life, poetry and art

Sticky Monkeyflower — fear of intimacy in sexuality; excessive or repressed sexuality as a way of avoiding true intimacy

Sunflower — helping to express one's own unique sun-like radiant individuality; for low self-esteem manifesting either as puffed up egotism or a self-effacing attitude

Tiger Lily — tendency to overly masculine traits, especially aggression; bringing more feminine balance

Trillium — for overly ambitious men who desire power and wealth at any cost; forsaking relationships in pursuit of soulless materialism

Vine — showing excessive masculine power and control; seeing masculine as dominant and feminine as submissive

Wild Oat — difficulty in finding a vocation, or avoiding a career choice by doing many odd jobs; finding the inner calling to a line of work

Zinnia — burying oneself in work, being out of touch with childlike or joyful parts of oneself; allowing time for play and adventure

Massage

Arnica — easing shock or trauma, especially when injury or trauma may still be stored in the body

Calendula — bringing overall warmth and healing through one's touch; massage as a form of "listening" between two people; use in tandem with herbal oil of Calendula

Chamomile — soothing and relaxing, especially to stomach and solar-plexus region; often given before a massage

Crab Apple — cleansing, particularly when applied topically or when combined with Self-Heal in a creme; for those who feel upset about physical impurity or imperfection

Dandelion — releasing emotional tension stored throughout the body, especially in the musculature; use with Dandelion Massage Oil

Dogwood — releasing hardened emotions stored in the body, especially when there may have been physical or sexual abuse

Lavender — relaxing to head, neck, and shoulders; releasing blocked spiritual energy

Manzanita — embodiment; greater awareness brought to the massage and the part of the body being massaged; good for both the practitioner and the massage client

Mugwort — to stimulate warmth and circulation, especially female flows such as menstruation, birthing, or nursing; use with Mugwort herbal oil

Nasturtium — rejuvenating and refreshing, awakening and vitalizing

Olive — bringing renewal when there is extreme fatigue

Pink Monkeyflower — direct application on the body for those who feel bodily shame, especially about sexuality

Pink Yarrow — emotional oversensitivity and merging by the client or massage practitioner

Rosemary — fully engaging the physical body, bringing healing all the way into physical body to warm and enliven physical presence

Saint John's Wort — psychic oversensitivity, and oversensitivity to light; use with herbal oil of Saint John's Wort

Self-Heal — bringing new life forces; promoting overall health

Star Tulip — opening and sensitizing both client and practitioner to the massage

Yarrow — for body workers who merge with or absorb too much psychic tension from their clients; for clients who are oversensitive to their environment

Yerba Santa — release of emotional tension stored in chest region, often experienced as respiratory symptoms

Materialism and Money

(See also Greed)

Aloe Vera — workaholism, depletion of life forces through overwork; inability to enjoy simple pleasures of life

Angelica — restoring spiritual connection; to instill awareness that there is more to life than the material world

California Poppy — compulsion to buy many new things, attraction to anything alluring, filling life with things outside oneself rather than from within

Chrysanthemum — to confront mortality; for those who accumulate wealth and power in an attempt to make earthly life permanent

Crab Apple — obsession with perfection, desire to have perfect home or environment, over-dependent on external environment for inner well-being

Filaree — obsession with money, especially with detailed accounting; losing perspective of importance of money in relationship to other parts of life

Hound's Tongue — seeing the world in materialistic or merely physical ways, dulled and deadened in inner life by an over-worldly viewpoint

Iris — restoring a sense of soul beauty and artistry, for those who calculate and value only what is utilitarian, efficient, or income-producing

Larkspur — awakening feelings of altruism and balanced leadership; for those who may use leadership skills only for business or profit

Poison Oak — wanting to conquer the world; aggressive Mars-like qualities which overcompensate for a fear of intimacy

Sage — bringing deeper forces of wisdom and consideration; for those who tend to think in terms of short-term profit and private gain

Sagebrush — learning to live more sparingly, to discern what is essential and to let go of excess

Star Thistle — for those who find it hard to be generous, who count their possessions and regard personal security in terms of material wealth

Sunflower — ego aggrandizement, for those who pursue fame and fortune as exterior forms of recognition

Tiger Lily — overly competitive business drive; learning cooperation and trust

Trillium — greed for material power and status; desire to accumulate possessions, often leading to emotional and physical congestion; purifying the root or survival chakra

Vine — for those who use money and power as a way of exerting control over others

Yellow Star Tulip — sensitivity to the sufferings of others and the Earth, balancing business life with social and moral awareness

Zinnia — ability to lighten up, especially for workaholics who take money and business affairs too seriously and need to enjoy life

Meditation

(See also Spiritual Emergency or Opening)

Angel's Trumpet — ability to penetrate to spiritual threshold, especially when dying; conscious dying process

Angelica — awareness of benevolent spiritual forces, protection and guidance from higher realms

California Poppy — extreme fascination or involvement with psychic powers or techniques; confusing spiritual glamour with authentic spiritual experience

Fawn Lily — prefers quiet and meditative experience, out of balance with worldly involvement

Forget-Me-Not — enhancing awareness of spiritual guidance or communication with those outside the physical world

Hound's Tongue — tendency to overly materialistic or sense-bound consciousness, preventing meditative experience

Impatiens — resistance to taking the time to cultivate the inner life; feeling too hurried to meditate

Lavender — overstriving in meditative work, often leading to nervous exhaustion; nervous conditions resulting from unbalanced meditative life

Lotus — enhancing spiritual awareness; deepening meditative experience

Milkweed — use of meditation techniques to blot out or stupefy consciousness; inappropriate suppression of healthy ego forces

Mugwort — awareness of dreams; conscious control of psychic life

Purple Monkeyflower — inability to sustain meditative or spiritual practices due to fear of spiritual world

Queen Anne's Lace — balanced opening of third eye; integration of psychic life with emotional life

Star Tulip — overcoming blockages to spiritual receptivity; inner listening ability

White Chestnut — quieting repetitive or obsessive thoughts; stilling the mind

Menopause

(See also Mid-Life Crisis)

Aloe Vera — feelings of burnout and exhaustion; need for a "pause" to rejuvenate body and redirect creative forces

Alpine Lily — resistance to bodily changes and fluctuations during menopause, not wanting to stay in body; need for body and soul to harmonize

Beech — moody, hypersensitive or critical due to feelings of extreme vulnerability or instability

Black Cohosh — extreme tension in reproductive organs or pelvic region; dark, clotted or obstructed menstrual flow, often accompanied by anger, rage or other emotional tension

Black-Eyed Susan — avoidance or denial of menopausal symptoms; inability to accept menopause as a natural transition in life

Borage — profound grief at cessation of menses, especially if unable to conceive child or find mate

Buttercup — feeling dried up or worthless; low self-esteem around image of oneself as an older woman

Canyon Dudleya — tendency toward hysteria or emotional exaggeration; unleashed psychic forces due to menopause, which need to be harmonized and grounded

Crab Apple — experience of physical toxicity or congestion due to cessation of menstrual flow; need for body to purify and re-align

Easter Lily — pronounced reproductive disturbances or toxicity in reproductive organs around menopause; resolving tensions around polarities of sexuality and spirituality

Echinacea — feeling physically overwhelmed, disturbed immune function; menopause experienced as shattering and disruptive, loss of female identity

Fairy Lantern — inability to release reproductive function, unresolved feelings from childhood or from motherhood; desire to dress or look much younger than one really is

Fuchsia — strong emotional reactions and bodily symptoms such as flushing, or headaches; integration of emotional and bodily awareness, moving energy down and through the body

Hibiscus — reduced sexual response; physical or emotional dryness, lack of warmth or sensation in sexual experience; to redefine sexuality in a new context not related to procreation

Iris — enabling the soul to become more creative, transfer of creative forces from womb to higher chakras

Lavender — frayed nerves or insomnia, excessive or erratic energetic patterns associated with menopause, needing calming

Mariposa Lily — to resolve issues around conception and mothering; to transform identification with mother role; to examine own mother's attitude toward menopause

Olive — extreme physical exhaustion and fatigue due to difficult menopausal transition

Pink Yarrow — excessive emotions during menopause; erratic or profuse bleeding patterns; hypersensitivity

Pomegranate — feeling that time is running out on the "biological clock;" desire for conception near time of menopause; to resolve issues regarding conception and career goals

Pretty Face — feelings of physical ugliness or low self-esteem due to cultural emphasis on youthful beauty; to find inner beauty and appropriate grooming and cosmetic measures which enhance rather than mask the true Self

Rosemary — to balance heat regulation in body; alternately hot or cold; ability to incarnate fully into the body and integrate bodily warmth with soul warmth

Sage — Wise Woman archetype, to move to new aspects of the Self; ability to bless and value life experience

Sagebrush — feelings of emptiness or loss due to cessation of menses; ability of psyche to let go of old identity

Scarlet Monkeyflower — intense feelings and emotions, especially anger, sometimes producing bodily symptoms such as rashes or flushes

Self-Heal — viewing menopause as a healthy transition; taking inner responsibility for wellness; to transform negative medical model of menopause as illness or misfortune

Sticky Monkeyflower — developing new patterns of intimacy; transforming sexual identity as part of menopausal transition

Tiger Lily — eruption of strong animus forces, need for "soul estrogen" to balance and re-align feminine and masculine parts of the Self and develop a positive relationship to one's masculine side

Zinnia — viewing menopause as positive and freeing, celebrating and experiencing soul joy as part of menopausal transition; integration of Inner Child and Wise Woman archetypes

Mental Clarity

(See also Awakeness, Concentration and Focus, Thinking)

Cosmos — overly active mental state, need for greater clarity and integration with higher spiritual thought

Hound's Tongue — raising sense-bound thinking into higher spiritual understanding

Madia — focus and concentration

Milkweed — mental impairment, reduced ego forces, need to re-awaken core identity

Mountain Pennyroyal — insight into negative thoughts and thinking patterns taken on from others

Peppermint — overcoming mental lethargy, increasing alertness

Rabbitbrush — ability to stay aware of many different details simultaneously; mental flexibility

Rosemary — feeling foggy or forgetful, when spiritual consciousness cannot penetrate through body

Shasta Daisy — synthesizing ideas into a meaningful whole; archetypal thinking

Mid-Life Crisis

(See also Menopause)

Agrimony — addressing hidden or stifled parts of oneself which need honest examination; especially if using drugs or alcohol to hide real feelings

Aloe Vera — feelings of burnout and exhaustion from pushing oneself to achieve career goals or social status

Black-Eyed Susan — bringing to light parts of the Self which are submerged, which operate largely as shadow forces in mid-life crisis

Borage — deep and unexplained feelings of grief and loss over that which has not been fulfilled or achieved

Buttercup — accepting one's destiny, especially when feeling that one has not achieved outer importance or social prominence

California Wild Rose — feelings of resignation or apathy; going through the outer motions of daily responsibilities without inner connection

Chrysanthemum — over-identification with fleeting material or worldly goals; need for the soul to establish deeper values, to face death and other forms of impermanence

Dandelion — for the over-achiever, with major stress or toxic accumulation in the body; allowing the body to relax and become more soulful

Elm — overwhelmed due to life's responsibilities, to revitalize and re-align with true aims of Higher Self

Fairy Lantern — desire to relive youth, unbalanced psychological need to date younger persons, or appear younger than one actually is; irresponsibility toward family, friends or work

Honeysuckle — extreme feelings of nostalgia, reliving past experiences, excessive longing for old relationships; believing the past is better than present circumstances

Iris — feeling weighed down by the ordinariness or dullness of the world, inability to see one's Self or potential with fresh creative vision; lack of artistic or soulful activity

Manzanita — reclaiming connection with body, especially if body is overweight or devitalized

Oak — learning to surrender and accept limits, especially for one who has strongly identified with the role of provider or hero

Pretty Face — imbalanced or obsessive concern about one's physical aging; contacting inner beauty within the soul rather than simply through physical artifice

Sage — reviewing or reassessing one's life direction; to gain a higher perspective or to glimpse the right direction for one's destiny

Sagebrush — letting go of outer attachments or material possessions, to empty and purify in order to experience clarity; especially when the soul feels encumbered or entangled in present circumstances

Self-Heal — physical or psychological healing crisis; awakening the Self to its own responsibility and purpose for living

Sweet Chestnut — profound periods of suffering during mid-life; especially when the soul feels cut off from spiritual guidance; feelings of anguish or existential loneliness

Trillium — excessive drive for power or possessions, which has left the soul congested or burdened; transforming personal desires into higher social values

Walnut — for individuals in mid-life crisis who must make a clear and definite break with current circumstances in order to continue to evolve; courage to follow one's destiny

Moderation

Aloe Vera — moderation in the use of creative and vital forces; for the tendency to overwork

Canyon Dudleya — slower pace for spiritual and psychic development; letting go of desire for psychic or emotional drama

Dill — assimilating many sensory impressions with consciousness

Impatiens — moderation of overly impulsive actions

Lavender — overstimulated; to moderate excessive or extreme spiritual or meditative practices which deplete the nerves

Morning Glory — erratic lifestyle and habits which deplete vital energy

Vervain — following the middle way, moderation in feelings and actions; counterbalancing overenthusiasm or fanaticism

Morality

Basil — secrecy and deception in sexual behavior; integrating sexuality and spirituality

California Poppy — to distinguish and develop inner moral forces as a counterbalance to psychic techniques or other forms of spiritual glamour

Cerato — over-dependence on others for moral values; uncertainty about one's own thoughts and feelings

Chestnut Bud — learning moral lessons from one's experience; for the tendency to repeat past errors

Crab Apple — obsessive sense of morality; preoccupied with impurity and imperfection

Deerbrush — mixed or hidden motives which undermine one's moral stance; for sincerity and openness

Easter Lily — conflicts about sexual morality; alternating between promiscuity and prudishness

Holly — developing compassion and understanding for others; overcoming jealousy and hatred

Mountain Pride — becoming a spiritual warrior to combat evil or injustice in the world; to act upon one's convictions

Mullein — developing a sense of conscience; overcoming deceitfulness toward oneself and others

Pine — extreme moral standards applied to oneself in a punishing way; regret over past actions which paralyzes the soul

Purple Monkeyflower — fear-based moral values; courage to develop one's own sense of truth

Rock Water — overly rigid sense of morality; confusing strict ascetic rules with moral behavior

Scleranthus — inner knowingness to distinguish right from wrong; making ethical decisions; to overcome hesitation and indecisive wavering

Star Thistle — generosity and sharing; overcoming stinginess born of fear of lack

Trillium — altruistic sacrifice of personal ambition or desire for the common good; overcoming greed and lust for power and possessions

Vine — tyrannical domination of others; to encourage respect for the individuality of others

Yellow Star Tulip — moral sense born of an awareness of the consequences of one's actions; sensitivity to the suffering of others

Mother and Mothering

(See also Children, Feminine Consciousness, Home and Lifestyle, Pregnancy)

Alpine Lily — embodied presence, able to experience motherhood as a physically nurturing and rewarding experience

Beech — overly critical of one's child, extreme demands for perfection projected onto the child due to one's own hypersensitivity

Buttercup — feeling low self-esteem about identity as mother, compared to other social roles

Canyon Dudleya — hysterical tendencies in mothering role; creating trauma-drama situations for oneself, child or family system; finding an ordered and simple approach to mothering and homemaking roles

Centaury — confusing mothering with servitude; lack of strength in mothering role; excessive compliance with children's demands

Cherry Plum — feeling that one is beyond the limits of coping or out of control due to extreme stress, such as caring for a sick child

Chicory — emotional neediness in mother or child: tendency to manipulate child in order to receive love and attention for oneself; or to help a child who is overly dependent on mother

Corn — contacting the archetype of the Earth Mother; nurturing abilities through physical connection to Earth

Elm — assumes responsibilities of motherhood, but later feels despondent and overwhelmed; overanxious striving for perfection as a mother

Evening Primrose — rejection of child in utero, extreme disturbance in mother-child bond, absorption of toxic emotions by child from mother

Fairy Lantern — tendency to over-mother, need to keep child in overly dependent relationship; emotional immaturity which prevents one from assuming full responsibilities of adult motherhood

Fawn Lily — integration of high spiritual ideals with mundane demands of mothering role; to create spiritual presence in home environment; using spiritual forces to protect and nurture others; compassionate sensitivity

Forget-Me-Not — making a decision to have a child; to stimulate awareness of karmic connection with the incarnating soul

Impatiens — does things for the child, rather than allowing child to learn or experience; wants things done quickly

Indian Pink — handling simultaneous demands from children and household responsibilities; intense activity which robs one of feeling centered or truly present

Iris — home and mothering role feels dull or dowdy; for channeling inspired forces of creativity into mothering and homemaking role

Mariposa Lily — bonding in childhood with mother; building rapport between mother and child; general remedy for instilling positive mother archetype

Milkweed — unconscious regression and merging with mother or mother figure beyond normal developmental stage

Pomegranate — conflict about use of feminine creative forces, sometimes absorbed from the mother; conflict between personal mother role and "world mother" role

Quince — conflicts between power and love in feminine forces; need to integrate power with feminine softness; vacillating between being overly strict or overly permissive as a mother; often used for single and/or working mothers

Red Chestnut — over-fretful concern about child; over-identification with child instead of being in touch with one's own self

Scarlet Monkeyflower — episodes of uncontrolled rage or power plays with child; facing one's own feelings of repressed anger

Star Thistle — disturbances in the bond to the mother which predispose the child to seek excessive material rewards as a form of security

Star Tulip — developing receptivity as a mother, trusting one's own guidance and intuition in mothering role; ability to contact the spiritual identity and true needs of the child

Yellow Star Tulip — compassionate attunement to one's child; ability of mother to sense real feelings and needs of child

Zinnia — seeing motherhood as a grim responsibility; lack of joy or spontaneity in mothering; to play with and enjoy child's world; to contact one's own inner child

Motivation

Blackberry — putting ideas into action

California Wild Rose — enthusiasm and positive involvement in life

Cayenne — stagnant forces of will which need to be fired into action

Deerbrush — purity of intention; for those with unconscious or mixed motives

Gorse — counteracting feelings of hopelessness, especially about personal affairs

Larch — stronger confidence to carry out one's creative inspiration and intention

Mountain Pride — warrior-like stamina in the face of adversity and challenge

Scotch Broom — seeing opportunity for service in spite of difficulties; maintaining motivation to serve

Tansy — low motivation, lethargy, procrastination; to develop true self-interest and motivation for work and other tasks

Negativity

Beech — seeing others critically; harsh judgment

Black Cohosh — for those with powerful magnetic energy which often attracts the negativity of others

Holly — inability to open heart to love for others

Mountain Pennyroyal — purging the mind of negative thoughts or entities which are already within the psyche; clearing out negativity taken on from others

Oregon Grape — projection of negativity onto others, imagining hostile intentions of others; paranoia

Pink Yarrow — sensitivity to negative emotional influences; "psychic sponge" type

Poison Oak — tendency to be angry or hostile to others as a way of warding off intimacy

Scarlet Monkeyflower — strong anger or power plays, often unacknowledged

Snapdragon — verbal negativity and hostility directed toward others

Willow — bitter and resentful, unable to forgive

Yarrow — vulnerability to negative influences, especially of mental or psychic nature; needing a protective psychic shield

Yarrow Special Formula — negativity in environment due to chaos, geopathic or technological imbalance; sensitivity to environmental toxicity such as pollution and radiation

Nervousness

Aspen — acute sensitivity to influences which are not consciously seen or understood

Canyon Dudleya — nervous depletion or excessive excitability from psychic or mediumistic experiences

Chamomile — emotional tension, particularly in stomach and solar plexus region

Cherry Plum — nervousness stemming from fear of losing control

Cosmos — nervous speech patterns which are too rapid, speaking which cannot keep pace with or adequately access higher thought

Garlic — emotional fears that drain or plague the psyche, producing nervousness

Golden Yarrow — acute sensitivity, desire of soul to be more visible but feeling too vulnerable

Indian Pink — maintaining centered attitude amidst confusion

Lady's Slipper — prone to nervous idiosyncrasies, inability to focus and harness spiritual forces and express them in one's body and work

Lavender — oversensitivity to spiritual and mental activity; tendency to be high-strung; frayed nerves

Mimulus — nervousness due to everyday fears and worries

Morning Glory — nervous problems from overstimulation or chaotic lifestyle; drug and alcohol abuse

Nicotiana — using smoking or similar addictive substances to calm or numb the nervous system; to develop greater awareness of underlying feelings which contribute to nervousness

Pink Yarrow — oversensitivity due to emotional absorption; feeling and internalizing disturbances from the environment and from others

Purple Monkeyflower — extreme fear or apprehension related to spiritual or occult phenomena

Rosemary — feeling ill at ease in physical body, cold extremities

Vervain — overly enthusiastic; frayed nerves from overstriving

Non-Attachment

Angel's Trumpet — acceptance of death and dying process as appropriate transition for the soul

Bleeding Heart — developing healthy non-attachment in personal relationships

Calendula — listening to the other, non-interference and receptivity

Chrysanthemum — accepting transitory nature of earthly life without morbidity or despair

Filaree — letting go of common worries or obsessive fastidiousness with trivial things; need for a larger perspective

Goldenrod — detachment from what others think, from false persona as a social prop

Love-Lies-Bleeding — intense attachment to one's personal pain and suffering, thus excluding involvement of others; to move to a higher level of understanding about one's suffering

Rock Rose — shifting identification from the physical body and ego to the Higher Self, particularly when facing threat of death

Sage — non-attachment to achievement or recognition, ability to contact inner wisdom, equanimity and peace

Sagebrush — letting go of the inessential aspects of the Self; experiencing emptiness as a positive state

Trillium — non-attachment to power and wealth; social altruism

Nostalgia

Chrysanthemum — desire for youthfulness and attractiveness, especially when associated with a past phase of life; to accept the aging process

Fairy Lantern — inability to accept maturity; longing to return to childhood, often because of unresolved emotional issues

Forget-Me-Not — strong attachment to the memory of one who has died; to shift consciousness to awareness of the departed soul in spiritual world

Honeysuckle — dwelling in past thoughts and memories which are romanticized as "better times"

Obsession

Crab Apple — obsession with impurities, diet, hygiene or personal faults

Filaree — preoccupation with inessentials; compulsive worry

Heather — preoccupation with one's own problems, excessive need to discuss them with others

Pink Monkeyflower — obsessive-compulsive behaviors stemming from sexual abuse or shaming

Purple Monkeyflower — obsessive-compulsive behavior due to ritual or occult abuse; extreme superstition or ritual behavior conducted out of fear

Red Chestnut — fixation on fears for others; fantasized worries about what might happen to loved ones

Rock Water — obsession with strict standards for oneself; extreme asceticism

Sticky Monkeyflower — compulsive or obsessive sexuality due to fear of real intimacy

Vervain — strong attachment to one's point of view; overzealous need to convert others

White Chestnut — recurring thoughts and worries; mind stuck in a rut

Overview

Filaree — involvement with too many details; too-narrow interest; obsessive worry

Quaking Grass — seeing the working of the whole group and all individuals within a group

Rabbitbrush — mastery of many details, consciousness which effectively embraces the big picture

Sage — ability to perceive life events with greater perspective and detachment

Shasta Daisy — bringing diverse ideas into wholeness; archetypal insight

Trillium — working for the greater whole, collective consciousness which overrides personal gain

Overwhelm

(See also Stress, Tension)

Canyon Dudleya — emotions easily agitated; overstimulated by life events; tendency toward hysteria

Chamomile — overwhelming emotional tension, especially in the stomach or solar plexus

Cherry Plum — fear that overwhelm will lead to breakdown and loss of control

Corn — overwhelmed by crowded city life, inability to feel connection to physical body or Earth

Cosmos — confusion from too many thoughts, especially when speaking

Dill — inundated by too many sense impressions and experiences; overwhelmed when beginning a large task

Elm — feeling one's responsibility is too much; feeling overextended and isolated

Hornbeam — intimidated by the tasks of everyday life; feeling a lack of energy to go on

Indian Pink — overwhelmed by the intensity of surrounding activity; need to get centered

Lavender — overloaded by the influx of too much spiritual energy; nervous overwhelm

Oak — going beyond one's natural limits; innate strength which is pushed too far

Pink Yarrow — taking on too much emotional intensity from others

Rabbitbrush — confusion by too many details; inability to hold many aspects in simultaneous awareness

Red Clover — influenced by group emotions; crowd hysteria or panic

Paranoia

(See also Fear)

Aspen — feeling threatening forces or entities, but unable to bring them into consciousness; fear of the unknown

Black Cohosh — suspicious of others, often based on current or past experiences of violence and abuse

Holly — tendency to see others as unloving or unaccepting

Oregon Grape — expecting hostility from others; profound paranoia

Pink Yarrow — tendency to absorb emotions of others; uneasiness in crowds

Purple Monkeyflower — unbalanced religious beliefs or spiritual practices that lead to fear and paranoia; inability to experience spiritual phenomena in a calm and objective manner

Perfectionism

Agrimony — desire to appear emotionally perfect and acceptable; the "pleaser"

Alpine Lily — attached to spiritual pole of femininity; viewing bodily organs or female sexuality as lower or imperfect

Beech — tending to blame and criticize others due to high standards of perfection

Buttercup — never feeling one's contributions are good enough; inferiority complex, need to accept oneself

Centaury — being a slave to the perfectionist standards of others; not developing one's own viewpoint

Cerato — relying on the advice of others instead of learning from one's own mistakes

Chamomile — becoming easily upset; difficulty dealing with challenging emotions or strife

Crab Apple — needing body and environment to be perfect; upset if even small details are out of place or if there is any impurity or flaw

Dandelion — over-planning one's life; enslaving the body to impossible standards of performance

Elm — wanting to be the hero; high standards for performance leading to frustration and overwhelm

Fawn Lily — retreating from daily strife; feeling secure in a reclusive setting which is more spiritually perfect

Filaree — obsession with details out of proportion to their real importance; draining energy through worry and over-concern

Gentian — feeling that lack of success means ultimate failure; inability to keep trying

Impatiens — wanting everything to proceed rapidly, easily irritated or upset by blundering of others

Larch — so sure of failure that an effort to try is often curtailed; paralysis due to impossibility of achieving perfection; fear of mistakes

Lavender — high standards and intense spirituality which lead to oversensitivity and nervous affliction

Lotus — viewing oneself as spiritually advanced; difficulty in recognizing the pitfall of spiritual pride

Manzanita — feeling disgusted by one's physical body; seeing perfection only in what is spiritual

Pine — inability to forgive oneself for errors; self-deprecation when one's performance is less than perfect

Pretty Face — impossibly high standards of beauty; never feeling beautiful enough

Red Chestnut — wanting no harm to befall others; over-concerned and over-protective of others

Rock Water — harsh ascetic standards which deny the soul pleasurable involvement in life

Scarlet Monkeyflower — stuffing core levels of anger and rage in order to appear "nice"

Vervain — fanatical, overstriving; wanting others to become perfect by adopting one's standards and beliefs

Vine — expecting perfection from others; using one's will to enforce obedience from others

Water Violet — drawing back from involvement with others; feeling disdain for others

Willow — blaming others for adverse situations; inability to accept and let go

Perseverance

Baby Blue Eyes — ability to regain trust and faith in spiritual destiny despite harsh experiences

Gentian — perseverance despite setbacks; especially when discouraged or depressed

Larch — continuing even after mistakes; seeing mistakes as learning lessons

Mountain Pride — strength and perseverance to fight worldly ills; spiritual warrior

Oak — strong forces of perseverance; Mars-like fortitude, but with a need to know when to let go

Penstemon — ability to catalyze inner strength, despite obvious handicaps and obstacles

Scotch Broom — maintaining faith despite obstacles and difficulties in the outer world, especially with a tendency to depression

Personal Relationships

(See also Brokenheartedness, Intimacy)

Basil — ability to integrate sexuality and spirituality in relationships; to heal relationships based on secrecy or hidden sexual liaisons

Bleeding Heart — clinging possessiveness and emotional co-dependence; to develop more freedom and objectivity in relationships

Buttercup — to develop one's sense of self-worth and self-esteem

Calendula — communication, receptive listening with others; warmth in verbal intercourse; to heal argumentative tendencies

California Wild Rose — overcoming apathy and lack of concern about others

Chamomile — calming emotional trauma or hypersensitivity in relationships

Chicory — using negative behavior to get attention; emotional neediness

Evening Primrose — inability to form committed relationships; afflicted relationships due to feelings of abandonment and rejection in childhood

Fairy Lantern — relating to others as parental figures, feigning helplessness or dependency

Forget-Me-Not — perceiving deeper karmic bonds within relationships, ability to acknowledge spiritual destiny and intent of relationship

Goldenrod — assuming false persona in effort to please others or to annoy others for negative attention; to retain individual integrity in relationships and social situations

Heather — seeking social contact by talking about one's problems; excessive preoccupation with oneself

Holly — letting go of jealousy and envy in relationships

Mallow — ease in developing friendships; warmth and trust; overcoming rejection complex and other social barriers

Mariposa Lily — healing mother-child bonding; developing nurturing aspect of all relationships

Oregon Grape — acknowledging the good will of others; ability to perceive that others are loving and caring; to counteract paranoid tendencies

Penstemon — strength and perseverance despite difficulties in relationships

Pink Monkeyflower — shame and emotional masking, inability to express true feelings or make emotional contact

Pink Yarrow — oversensitivity to others, lack of appropriate emotional boundaries

Poison Oak — difficulty in yielding or showing a soft side; fear of vulnerability; creating barriers, displaying hostility

Quaking Grass — cooperation with others in group work

Scarlet Monkeyflower — power and anger issues in relationships

Shooting Star — feeling alien; profound sense of not fitting into human society, of being a stranger to Earth

Snapdragon — improper expression of emotions through verbal aggression and hostility

Star Thistle — sharing and generosity, giving of oneself; tendency to be miserly or stingy

Sticky Monkeyflower — dealing with issues of intimacy and sexuality; overcoming fear of intimacy; integrating sexuality with heart feelings

Sunflower — healing father relationship; afflicted masculine aspect or animus, which distorts relationships

Sweet Pea — relating with others, finding community and social bonding; developing a sense of belonging to a community

Tiger Lily — cooperation with others; to balance aggressive or egotistic tendencies

Trillium — working for the common good; transforming personal survival impulses to social values

Violet — shyness, holding back in a group out of fear of being absorbed by others

Water Violet — overcoming aloofness with others, especially the feeling of disdain or pride

Yellow Star Tulip — empathy for the feelings of others; compassionate presence and insight

Perspective

Angel's Trumpet — viewing death as a transition rather than an ending

Angelica — awareness of the profound influence of spiritual beings on one's life

Canyon Dudleya — shifting perspective to include ordinary events and calm flowing of life, when prone to over-dramatizing one's experiences

Filaree — seeing petty concerns in the larger context of life destiny

Forget-Me-Not — ability to include spiritual world and beings in perception of daily events

Hound's Tongue — transforming overly materialistic perspective; ability to contemplate matters in spiritual terms

Queen Anne's Lace — objective clairvoyance, ability to receive psychic impressions without emotional distortion

Rabbitbrush — gaining an overview of many details; to see the big picture

Sage — widened perspective based on life wisdom, ability to rise above daily affairs and concerns; detachment and reflection

Scotch Broom — seeing difficulties as opportunities for service in a challenging world

Shasta Daisy — understanding how diverse ideas form a meaningful whole; ability to see patterns and relationships in mental and emotional life

Pessimism

Baby Blue Eyes — profound cynicism and paralysis of soul forces; loss of innocence

California Wild Rose — cynicism and apathy; lacking a sense of destiny or meaning in life

Gentian — feeling doubt and discouragement, particularly after a setback

Gorse — pessimism with regard to one's personal affairs; doubt and discouragement

Larch — expectation of failure; lack of belief in one's own talents and capacities

Oregon Grape — misperceiving the intentions of others as hostile; having a "chip on the shoulder"

Penstemon — counteracting pessimism by actively facing adversity and setbacks with fortitude and courage

Scotch Broom — pessimism in the face of obstacles imposed by world situation; rallying one's positive forces for higher service

Possessiveness

Bleeding Heart — possessiveness in relationships, out of an excessive dependence on the other for self-validation; holding on to a relationship from a need to live vicariously through the other person

Chicory — needy or demanding; feeling one never has enough attention from others

Star Thistle — stinginess, inability to share oneself or possessions

Trillium — greed and lust for power and possessions; possessiveness due to personal ambition

Power

Black Cohosh — transforming darker psychic energy, to wrestle with inner demons or shadow energies

Blackberry — lack of strong forces of will; inability to manifest in the world

California Pitcher Plant — weakness or excessive strength of instinctual forces; integration of one's instinctual aspects

Centaury — being controlled by others' expectations; ability to serve in freedom and to resist exploitative relationships

Chicory — being manipulative in relationships, especially due to emotional insecurity and neediness

Chrysanthemum — attachment to power and position; fear of death

Fairy Lantern — giving away personal power, feigning helplessness or over-dependence

Lady's Slipper — integration of spiritual power into root chakra; spiritualized sexuality and grounded spirituality

Larkspur — exercising the power of leadership through charisma; providing an inspirational example

Mountain Pride — inner power to fight for what one knows to be true in one's heart

Nicotiana — appearance of being powerful and in control which is achieved through numbing or suppressing one's more sensitive and subtle feelings

Pink Yarrow — giving personal power away by "bleeding" into others' energy fields

Quince — conflicts about power, especially for women; need to integrate power with love

Scarlet Monkeyflower — fear and conflict about owning one's emotional power, especially anger or rage

Snapdragon — strong vital power and magnetism which can turn to verbal abuse when misdirected

Sunflower — balanced power and ego strength; radiant individuality

Tiger Lily — aggression and overstriving; need to bring feminine balance

Trillium — greed for power; drive to accumulate material wealth

Vine — domination of others; personal power achieved through control of others

Pregnancy

(See also Children, Mother and Mothering)

Alpine Lily — experiencing one's reproductive organs in a positive way during conception and pregnancy; ability to conceive and to sustain pregnancy

Angelica — spiritual protection for the incoming child

Bleeding Heart — letting go of a child which has been miscarried or aborted

Borage — to soothe heart pain and grief after a miscarriage or abortion

California Wild Rose — ability to anchor the new life on Earth; for difficult pregnancies

Calla Lily — mixed messages about sexual identity when in utero, strong parental preference for male or female child which confuses incarnating soul

Cerato — developing trust in one's inner knowing; relying on the strength of one's inner guidance when choosing prenatal and natal care

Chamomile — balancing the emotional ups and downs of pregnancy; calming and soothing, especially when there is nausea and stomach upset

Cherry Plum — extremely stressful pregnancy or labor, when one feels "I can't take any more"

Corn — grounding and centering in the body; contacting Earth Mother qualities

Easter Lily — cleansing of sexual organs, especially when conception is blocked

Evening Primrose — unconscious or conscious destructive intent to fetus during pregnancy, unwanted child; absorption by child of toxic emotions during pregnancy

Five-Flower Formula — trauma or accident during pregnancy or birth; for stressful or extremely challenging birth

Forget-Me-Not — contacting the incarnating spirit, remembering one's karmic connections in the spiritual world

Gorse — postpartum depression

Lavender — nervous stress and oversensitivity

Manzanita — acceptance of physical body during pregnancy, offsetting feeling of ugliness or awkwardness in the body; experiencing the body as the spiritual temple of the incarnating soul

Mariposa Lily — bonding with the incoming child; confidence about mothering; general remedy for positive mothering forces during pregnancy and birth

Mugwort — overdue pregnancy, to release "moon" or "flowing" forces; to assist in drawing child out of mother's body during labor

Mullein — deciding whether to carry a child, getting in touch with one's moral values, listening to guidance from Higher Self

Olive — fatigue from missed sleep; exhaustion from long labor

Penstemon — strength to persevere during challenging and difficult pregnancies, especially when there is much physical stress

Pink Yarrow — oversensitivity to the emotions of others; cries easily; emotional vulnerability to influences in the home or workplace when pregnant

Pomegranate — conflicts between career and home life; positive direction of feminine creative forces

Quince — for women who must balance strength and nurturing, who must be competent and strong in the world and receptive and nurturing at home

Red Chestnut — worry and concern about pregnancy or for new child; over-anxious

Scleranthus — doubts and indecision during the many life changes brought about by pregnancy; bringing inner equanimity

Shooting Star — helping the soul come rightly into Earth; for possible miscarriage, premature birth or traumatic labor

Star Tulip — to build trust in one's own mother instincts; to encourage inner receptivity and listening forces

Walnut — transition in each stage of pregnancy, especially in releasing the child at birth; to accept new role as mother

Yarrow — "holding in" the forces of pregnancy, overcoming tendency to premature birth, bleeding or spotting; for oversensitivity to the environment which may develop during pregnancy

Yarrow Special Formula — added protection against radiation, pollution or other harmful environmental toxins

Yellow Star Tulip — developing telepathic communication with child; sensitive awareness of child's needs

Prejudice

(See also Community Life and Group Experiences)

Angelica — ability to see the spiritual core of each person rather than outer physical characteristics; harmonization of individual guardian angel with larger cultural folk soul

Beech — negative image of others, critical; projecting faults onto others due to prejudicial standards

Black-Eyed Susan — perceiving others as evil or bad due to repression of negative material in one's own psyche; to honestly examine shadow forces which manifest as racism and other prejudice

Buttercup — internalizing racial, sexual or other stereotypes projected from others; low self-esteem through absorption of negative images from others

Calendula — inability to listen to what others are really saying; argumentativeness; resolving differences by establishing respectful dialogue

Canyon Dudleya — inciting mass hysteria or derogatory stereotypes; creating exaggerated pictures of others based on emotional demagoguery rather than objective truth

Centaury — internalizing master-slave relationship; acting to please others due to social conditioning; ability to learn one's own strength as a true basis for service

Deerbrush — out of touch with real feelings, acting in culturally accepted or conventional ways while harboring opposing feelings inside; ability to act from the inside out

Goldenrod — lack of true individuality or inner strength; following cultural conventions or stereotypes even when wrong or harmful, in order to be accepted by others

Holly — generally indicated for prejudice of any kind; opening heart to true human compassion; feeling connected to others in human family, inclusive rather than exclusive behavior

Honeysuckle — inability to accept current social reality; belief that there were better times in the past; wanting to return to an old way of living based on racial, sexual or other social stereotypes

Mountain Pride — taking a stand for truth or social justice, despite opposition; warrior-like courage in the face of prejudice

Mullein — developing own internal sense of right and wrong; independent moral conscience able to make judgments and develop values apart from social prejudice

Oregon Grape — seeing other groups of people or communities as violent or undesirable, expecting the worst from such groups; primary feelings of hostility and mistrust which fuel prejudice

Penstemon — ability to persevere, to believe in oneself despite social challenges or prejudice; transforming feelings of persecution through inner strength and determination

Pine — self-blame, feeling that one is bad or unworthy; counteracting paralysis and dysfunction due to self-deprecation and stereotypes of inferiority

Pretty Face — inability to see unique racial or other physical characteristics as inherently beautiful; internalized image of ugliness due to social stereotypes; finding one's own inner radiance

Quaking Grass — ability for neighborhoods, communities and other groups to work in harmony; resolution of individual differences or prejudices for the greater wholeness of the group

Red Clover — susceptibility to mass hysteria or other forms of group thought; developing calm, self-aware behavior

Saguaro — to examine beliefs and traditions imparted from ancestral family; to cultivate positive connection with cultural roots and overcome prejudicial beliefs or superstitions

Vervain — fanatical belief in one's one ideology or political program; inability to recognize the beliefs of others

Vine — to transform the belief that social relationships are based on dominance and submission, or that one group should be submissive to other

Walnut — breaking from unhealthy family ties or cultural traditions which are prejudicial; the strength to find one's own path

Water Violet — belief that one is better or superior by virtue of culture, class or race; staying aloof and not wanting to be contaminated

Pride

(See also Egotism, Self-Aggrandizement, Self-Esteem)

Buttercup — healthy pride in one's accomplishments even if not considered great by societal standards

Larch — pride and confidence in one's creativity, especially when doubting one's abilities

Lotus — spiritual pride, ungrounded spirituality; crown chakra overdeveloped in relationship to other energy centers

Pretty Face — healthy pride in one's appearance; inner beauty which illumines physical features

Sunflower — egotistical sense of self-importance; overbearing individuality

Water Violet — excessive pride; keeping one's distance from others; feeling better than others

Procrastination

(See also Avoidance, Inertia, Resistance)

Blackberry — putting ideas into action; awakening the will to manifest one's vision

Cayenne — strong catalyst to mobilize the will when feeling stuck

Clematis — avoidance of tasks at hand; dreamy disposition

Hornbeam — feeling lack of energy due to emotional resistance to one's work

Larch — putting off action out of fear of failure or lack of self-confidence

Tansy — acting on what one knows needs to be done; overcoming lethargy and deep emotional blockages to one's true energy

Protection

Angelica — ability to contact spiritual realms on the soul level; to feel help from higher, beneficent forces

Garlic — protection from psychic parasites which drain one's vitality

Golden Yarrow — protection when the soul desires more social involvement despite innate sensitivity

Lavender — soothing when exposed to too much nervous stimulation

Mariposa Lily — protection of child from harmful influences; mothering mantle of warmth and sensitivity

Mountain Pennyroyal — to expel negative psychic entities or forces that have become attached to the aura

Pink Yarrow — emotional vulnerability; promoting emotional centering and strength

Poison Oak — overly defensive and self-protective; for those who guard vulnerable feelings by showing a hard exterior

Purple Monkeyflower — feeling more protection and trust regarding one's spiritual experience, especially if characterized by fear

Red Clover — insulation from group panic and hysteria; ability to think for oneself

Saint John's Wort — protection during dreaming and from adverse astral influences; trust in divine protection

Walnut — freedom from outside ideas and influences that stymie or subvert one's direction in life

Yarrow — protection from negative thoughts or environmental influences through the strengthening of one's inner light

Yarrow Special Formula — energetic protection from radiation and other noxious environmental influences

Psychosomatic Illness

(See also Body, Immune Disturbances)

Arnica — to release the effects of past trauma; often masking or preventing insight into current illness

Canyon Dudleya — conditions that come and go rapidly, often appearing worse than they actually are; unconscious need to receive attention through the drama of illness

Fawn Lily — tendency toward weakness and fatigue, fragile and delicate temperament, overly spiritual

Fuchsia — emotional repression of authentic feelings, often manifesting as acute illnesses such as headaches

Lavender — tendency to headaches and nervous problems due to overstimulation of spiritual forces

Pink Monkeyflower — sexual or other bodily dysfunction brought about by profound sense of soul shame, or violation of core self

Pomegranate — PMS and other women's complaints from unresolved feelings about female creativity and reproduction

Queen Anne's Lace — distortions in vision, especially when masking emergent clairvoyance

Scleranthus — shifting symptoms, constant energetic changes; difficulty determining true illness

Self-Heal — contacting the true source of healing in any illness; self-responsibility

Star Of Bethlehem — clearing the effects of past trauma; soothing and reorienting the body to its soul-spiritual Self

Wild Rose — sickness which lingers or lasts longer than expected; loss of interest in life

Yerba Santa — tendency toward respiratory illness from deep-seated melancholy

Purification

(See also Catharsis, Cleansing, Release)

Chaparral — cleansing of subconscious emotions or psychic toxins from drug use or other traumatic experiences driven into the subconscious

Crab Apple — over-concern with physical toxins; clearing of toxins whether real or imagined

Deerbrush — clarity in the heart with regard to inner intentions, especially when there are mixed motives

Easter Lily — purification of sexual organs, or of emotions centered in the sexual organs; conflict between purity and sexuality, or a sense of uncleanness in the sexual organs

Evening Primrose — cleansing of toxic psychic emotions absorbed by child in utero or early infancy, especially abuse and rejection

Golden Ear Drops — release of toxic childhood memories stored in the heart, often expressed in deep crying

Mountain Pennyroyal — to cleanse psychic infestation; to revitalize the auric field

Sagebrush — shedding of false identity; releasing what is no longer essential to one's destiny

Star Tulip — spiritual purification; becoming more open and receptive in meditation and dream life

Quiet

Angelica — feeling comfort and protection of higher realms

Chamomile — emotional quietude and calm

Indian Pink — inner stillness despite intense activity

Madia — inner silence and concentration; letting go of scattered thoughts and inner chatter; focus

Sage — inner peace and equanimity, especially as a result of life experience and reflection

Sagebrush — deep emptiness, pregnant silence as a way of stilling the soul

Star Tulip — inner peace and receptivity; inner listening

White Chestnut — mental repose; ability to empty and still the mind when agitated

Receptivity

(See also Listening, Sensitivity, Vulnerability)

Angelica — receptivity to guidance and guardianship from angelic realms

Calendula — hearing the message and intent of another, especially in verbal communication

Forget-Me-Not — openness to spiritual guides or karmic connections beyond earthly dimension

Lotus — openness to higher spiritual awareness

Mallow — receiving the warmth and love of others

Mariposa Lily — receptivity to human love; mother-child bonding

Mugwort — keeping psychic balance as intuitive faculties are opening

Mullein — hearing the voice of conscience

Sagebrush — experiencing emptiness as a precondition to change and transformation

Star Tulip — receptivity to spiritual worlds; especially listening to one's inner voice

Violet — openness to the warmth of others in a group

Yellow Star Tulip — emotional receptivity, empathy; ability to listen and feel the experience of others

Rejection

(See also Abandonment, Failure, Loneliness)

Angelica — feeling that one is taken care of by higher spiritual forces, regardless of rejection by others

Baby Blue Eyes — early rejection and lack of support hardened into cynical, mistrustful attitude

Black Cohosh — addiction to relationships despite rejection or abuse, difficulty letting go

Bleeding Heart — feeling spurned by lover or other partner, unable to release emotional attachment

Buttercup — feeling insignificant compared to others; low self-esteem

Chicory — feeling overly needy, sorry for oneself; never feeling there is enough love or support

Crab Apple — feeling dirty or unclean, not good enough or pure enough

Dogwood — feeling and often being awkward and accident-prone; feeling unlovable and often a victim

Echinacea — feeling utterly devastated and shattered in soul and body by abuse and trauma; loss of essential dignity

Evening Primrose — rejection or abandonment in utero and in infancy leading to feeling of coldness and emotional distance in the soul; sexual and emotional repression due to profound fear of rejection

Gentian — discouragement due to rejection or failure, inability to recoup and move on

Goldenrod — fear of social censure, developing false persona in order to be accepted by others

Holly — belief that there is not enough love; feeling unloved, jealous or envious of others who appear to have more

Honeysuckle — dealing with rejection by dwelling in past when times were better, unable to face pain of actual circumstances

Larch — so afraid of failure that creativity is stunted or curtailed; self-censoring; expecting rejection or failure

Mallow — difficulty in initiating and sustaining friendships, inability to generate soul warmth

Mariposa Lily — estrangement from mother or other early childhood trauma which leads to patterns of feeling unwanted and unloved

Oregon Grape — projection of hostility and assumption of negative judgments from others, leading to rejection both real and imagined

Pine — being hard on oneself, self-deprecation; being one's own worst enemy

Pink Monkeyflower — holding deep feelings inside; not feeling that others will accept or understand; profound shame

Pretty Face — feeling ugly, feeling judged by outer standards of beauty; needing to let own soul radiance shine forth

Scarlet Monkeyflower — belief that one will be rejected if strong feelings are expressed, especially anger; trying to be the "nice" person

Shooting Star — feeling rejected by human community; feeling alien, as though not fitting in

Sticky Monkeyflower — fear of intimacy and rejection, especially in sexual relationships

Sweet Chestnut — feeling abandoned, even by God; feeling hopeless and alone

Sweet Pea — not feeling one fits into community, or geographic location; feeling homeless

Willow — dwelling in feelings of rejection, letting them turn into bitterness and blame; lacking forgiveness

Rejuvenation

(See also Devitalization, Vitality)

Aloe Vera — reviving exhausted creative forces

Baby Blue Eyes — restoration of childlike innocence and trust within the soul

California Wild Rose — awakening to life; enthusiasm and involvement in life

Hibiscus — rejuvenation when sexuality is depleted; to bring warmth and vitality in sexual response

Indian Paintbrush — to revive creative expression, especially earthy vitality

Iris — re-awakening of artistic abilities, especially higher inspiration

Morning Glory — awakening of fresh "morning" forces when depleted by erratic sleep patterns or drug use

Nasturtium — to awaken body and revive feelings, when dry or depleted from too much intellectual work

Olive — re-invigoration of strength and energy after a long struggle or physical exhaustion

Self-Heal — to catalyze inner recuperative powers in all healing situations

Relaxation

(See also Energetic Patterns, Tension)

Canyon Dudleya — to calm overexcited or hysterical tendencies

Chamomile — letting go of nervousness and ` emotional tension; difficulty in sleeping, insomnia; especially good for children

Dandelion — release of tension and stress held in the body, especially the musculature

Dill — difficulty relaxing due to over-stimulation of nerve-sense system from too many impressions and experiences

Elm — trusting one has the help needed; letting go of undue worry

Five-Flower Formula — immediate relaxation before more specific therapy can be initiated

Lavender — calming overstimulated nerves; helping to ground one's energy

Morning Glory — nervousness due to erratic life patterns or addictions

Red Chestnut — tension due to excessive anxiety and worry about others

Vervain — moderation, de-stressing; letting go of overstriving and excessive zeal

White Chestnut — letting go of obsessive, repetitive thoughts and worries directed inward

Release

(See also Catharsis, Purification)

Angel's Trumpet — letting go of physical body in dying process, or for any profound soul transition

Bleeding Heart — releasing unhealthy attachment in relationships; for death of loved one, to end a relationship, or to continue a relationship based on emotional freedom

Chamomile — releasing nervousness and emotional tension; for difficulty in sleeping, insomnia; especially good for children

Cherry Plum — overcoming fear of losing control; trusting intuition, inner guidance

Chestnut Bud — releasing old habit patterns; learning the lessons of life

Chicory — to let go of emotional neediness, or excessive demand for attention

Chrysanthemum — acceptance of one's mortality, ability to accept the impermanent nature of earthly affairs

Dandelion — letting go of emotional tension held in the muscles

Dogwood — release of hardened emotions from past trauma

Evening Primrose — releasing toxic emotions absorbed unconsciously in infancy

Filaree — letting go of trivial or petty worries that drain or misdirect the true intentions of the Higher Self

Fuchsia — releasing false or hyper-emotionality which blocks contact with real feelings

Golden Ear Drops — release of childhood emotional pain, especially through tears

Honeysuckle — releasing nostalgia for the past; coming into present time

Love-Lies-Bleeding — to understand and release intense pain and suffering which may be overly personalized; transcendence

Mountain Pennyroyal — expulsion of negative thoughts, particularly those taken on from others

Oak — knowing when to let go of struggle; ability to yield

Pink Monkeyflower — release of emotional fears and shame, especially rejection from others

Sagebrush — to shed false identity, old lifestyle or personal identity that is no longer appropriate; to release excess baggage in body or psyche

White Chestnut — to quiet and release obsessive, repetitive thoughts and worries

Yerba Santa — release of past emotional traumas stored within the psyche, felt especially in the chest region and in the breathing; ability to breathe out emotional tension

Repression

Agrimony — repressing real feelings due to politeness or superficial social standards

Black-Eyed Susan — lack of awareness of one's "shadow" side or unaccepted parts of the Self

Centaury — repressing one's own need for expression in order to please others

Chaparral — traumatic or psychically overwhelming material which works as a toxic poison in the subconscious

Dandelion — holding tense emotions in the body

Evening Primrose — repression of core emotions and sexual feelings, due to emotional and sexual abuse in childhood

Fuchsia — suppression of true emotions, often covered by false emotionality

Golden Ear Drops — repression of painful childhood memories; hidden traumatic experiences

Hibiscus — inhibition of sexuality, especially difficulty integrating soul warmth with sexual function

Larch — blockage of creative expression

Nicotiana — repression of feeling life in the heart, especially when accompanied by addiction to tobacco or other substances

Pink Monkeyflower — holding back true feelings of intimacy and love out of fear of exposure, shame

Purple Monkeyflower — unconscious fear of the occult; especially if brought about by intense and unbalanced involvement in spiritual or cultic group

Rock Water — self-repression through over-strictness

Scarlet Monkeyflower — holding back or denying anger and strong emotions out of fear; over-control of one's emotions to appear "nice"

Snapdragon — repressed metabolic and libido energy, often misdirected as verbal anger toward others

Sticky Monkeyflower — inhibition of sexual feelings due to fear of intimacy

Tansy — suppression of one's energy and feelings in order to keep the peace, or to deal with emotional overwhelm

Vine — trying to repress the free will of others

Yerba Santa — constriction of emotions, especially sadness and grief held in the chest and lungs

Resentment

(See also Anger, Blame)

Baby Blue Eyes — cynical and detached feelings which prevent one from feeling the goodness of others

Holly — resentment due to misperceived favoritism; jealousy and envy

Oregon Grape — resentment of others; seeing other people's actions in negative light; expecting the worst from others

Willow — blaming others or one's situation, bitterness

Resistance

(See also Avoidance, Denial, Inertia, Procrastination)

Agrimony — denial of emotional pain as a way to resist doing inner work, covering feelings with a mask of cheerfulness

Angel's Trumpet — fear of death; resistance to letting go of life or to crossing the spiritual threshold

Black-Eyed Susan — difficulty penetrating into the dark, "shadow" aspects of the personality

Blackberry — putting thoughts into action; overcoming resistance to manifestation

California Wild Rose — holding back from full involvement in life; resisting the experience of life's pain by disengaging from life

Cayenne — breaking through resistance; catalyzing the will

Cerato — not following inner guidance; resisting doing what one knows needs to be done; self-doubt and invalidation

Chestnut Bud — not learning lessons of experience; repeating mistakes

Chrysanthemum — difficulty accepting the aging process; attachment to outer image, youth or materialistic values

Clematis — resistance to being in the present by daydreaming or fantasizing about the future

Dandelion — emotional holding expressed as muscular tension, armoring

Fairy Lantern — not wanting to accept adult responsibilities; stuck in an immature stage of development

Fuchsia — resistance to one's true feelings, often expressed as false emotionality or psychosomatic complaints

Golden Ear Drops — difficulty contacting childhood emotions; brings awareness of painful experiences from the past

Honeysuckle — resistance to being in the present by nostalgia for the past

Hornbeam — inner resistance to facing the daily responsibilities of life, expressed as fatigue and lack of involvement

Impatiens — not accepting the seemingly slow pace of life or of others; irritation, annoyance at circumstances; not able to flow with life events

Manzanita — difficulty being in the body; resistance to healing processes because of deep aversion to physical incarnation

Morning Glory — difficulty facing the day due to depletion of vitality; need for fresh, etheric forces to greet the morning

Pink Monkeyflower — fear of exposing feelings when opening up to inner work

Poison Oak — fear of having one's boundaries violated, thus resisting social and intimate contact

Quaking Grass — difficulty working with group process; need to yield to or consider the needs of others

Rock Water — rigidity, inflexibility; difficulty opening up to feelings

Saguaro — resistance to authority; alienation and conflict with authority figures

Scarlet Monkeyflower — difficulty accepting and working with strong emotions such as anger or power issues

Self-Heal — inner resistance to taking responsibility for one's own healing process; over-dependence on outside help, not helping oneself

Star Thistle — holding on to material possessions out of fear of lack; resistance to sharing with others

Star Tulip — lack of spiritual receptivity; resistance to inner work, meditation; blockage of awareness of dreams, spiritual guidance

Tansy — inertia, difficulty getting moving, lethargy; resistance to true expression of one's energy

Water Violet — aversion to social involvement, difficulty getting socially involved

Responsibility

Centaury — taking care of others, but not of oneself; feeling overly responsible for others

Chicory — feeling responsible for others in a possessive, clinging way; manipulates care of others to receive attention for oneself

Elm — feeling overburdened or overwhelmed with responsibility; tendency to be overly perfectionist, or heroic

Fairy Lantern — inability to accept adult responsibility, inappropriate clinging to childlike role

Larkspur — balanced leadership in the world; counteracts tendency to be either over-dutiful and grim, or "puffed up" with self-importance

Mountain Pride — spiritual warriorship in adverse times; social responsibility

Oak — easily accepting responsibility due to strong abilities, but overextending and pushing beyond real limits

Red Chestnut — feeling responsible for the problems of others; worry and anxiety on their behalf

Willow — taking responsibility for life experiences rather than blaming others; counteracts bitterness

Restlessness

(See also Nervousness)

California Poppy — constant fascination and experimentation with psychic techniques or religious cults

Canyon Dudleya — dissatisfaction with quiet or ordinary pace of life, often creating melodramatic situations to excite oneself and others

Dill — too many experiences taken in by the senses and nerves; overstimulated

Impatiens — restlessness due to impatient, quick temperament

Lady's Slipper — restlessness when accompanied by nervous exhaustion and sexual depletion

Lavender — highly nervous and sensitive, tendency toward insomnia; highstrung

Morning Glory — nervous problems due to erratic lifestyle and chaotic living habits

Scleranthus — indecisiveness, constant alternation between one choice and another

White Chestnut — mental restlessness; constant chatter of thoughts

Wild Oat — for the "jack of all trades," trying many vocations but unable to find true life purpose

Scatteredness

(See also Attention, Concentration and Focus)

Clematis — tendency to daydream; avoiding the here-and-now with fantasies of the future

Five-Flower Formula — immediate centering when thrown out of balance by stress or traumatic circumstances

Indian Pink — taking on many activities at once; frazzled or frenetic energy; need center oneself

Madia — inability to focus on one thing, tendency to be distracted by inessentials

Rabbitbrush — bringing awareness to several simultaneous activities

Scleranthus — switching from one idea to another; scattered due to indecision

Shasta Daisy — scattered thinking; need for integration and meaning

Sweet Pea — for the wanderer unable to establish roots, homeless or vagabond

Wild Oat — inability to find life direction, wandering from one job or activity to another

Seeking

California Poppy — imbalanced fascination for psychic and spiritual experiences; to develop inner awareness and integrity

Cerato — seeking the advice of others; overly dependent on outside validation

Goldenrod — desiring others' approval in social situations, or negative attention through social disapproval

Self-Heal — continual seeking of various healing regimens without inner willingness to be healed

Sweet Pea — lack of social connectedness and roots; perpetual seeker

Wild Oat — searching for true vocation in life, with a tendency to try many different jobs

Self-Acceptance

Alpine Lily — acceptance of female self, as expressed in the physical body; often relating to lack of acceptance by mother

Baby Blue Eyes — feeling at ease with oneself; trusting in the goodness of the world, thus able to let down one's defensive guard

Buttercup — accepting the worth of one's life, vocation, or lifestyle

Crab Apple — acceptance of oneself instead of focusing on impurities and imperfections

Echinacea — reclaiming positive spiritual identity, even when violated, shattered or assaulted

Larch — confidence in one's inner strength and abilities

Mariposa Lily — warm and loving acceptance of oneself; ability to feel maternal nurturing

Penstemon — accepting handicaps or afflictions; making the best of difficult situations

Pine — release of guilt and self-blame; ability to forgive oneself for not being perfect

Pretty Face — acceptance of one's physical features with their imperfections

Self-Heal — knowing the inner power of self-healing; accepting that the Self is capable of transformation

Sunflower — ability to shine, to emanate true Self, to believe in oneself

Self-Actualization

Baby Blue Eyes — moving forward in life despite harsh experience, to regain spiritual trust as condition of soul evolution

Blackberry — putting ideas into action; overcoming inertia

Buttercup — knowing one's true worth despite worldly standards

Centaury — developing strong sense of Self, for those overly dominated by others

Chrysanthemum — shifting from ego-identification with personality to higher spiritual identity

Cosmos — developing capacity for higher thought; integration of mental faculties with spiritual essence

Echinacea — ability to experience a sense of wholeness, despite extreme threats to the inner Self

Golden Yarrow — ability to take soul forces or artistic impulses into the world, despite sensitivity

Iris — catalyzing soulful, more artistic aspects of the Self

Lady's Slipper — acceptance of one's inner spiritual authority and life destiny, ability to integrate and ground spirituality

Milkweed — profound estrangement from core Self, difficulty in coping with normal demands and responsibilities of adult ego

Mullein — fulfillment of one's true potential, especially when there is a moral conflict about values and goals

Quince — balancing love forces with power and strength

Self-Heal — taking responsibility for one's own well-being, facing one's karma

Sunflower — radiant expression of individuality; positive selfhood

Tansy — contacting true source of one's energy; moving beyond procrastination and lethargy

Wild Oat — finding one's true vocation, especially for those who have tried many different kinds of work and are still dissatisfied

Self-Aggrandizement

(See also Egotism, Pride)

Canyon Dudleya — inflating psychic and emotional experiences in order to appear spiritually and psychically extraordinary to others or oneself

Larkspur — leadership with selfish motivations; lack of altruism

Lotus — exaggerated sense of one's spirituality; inflated belief that one is especially spiritually evolved

Snapdragon — use of personal power to intimidate others, especially through verbal abuse

Sunflower — unbalanced egotism; feeling need to receive adulation from others

Trillium — lust for power and greed for material wealth

Vine — tendency to control others; desire for power over others

Self-Concern

Chicory — demanding emotional energy and attention out of proportion to real needs

Crab Apple — obsessive concern with one's faults, imperfections and impurities

Fawn Lily — overemphasis on spiritual activity which insulates Self from involvement and challenge in the world

Filaree — compulsive concern about trivial or inconsequential aspects of life; "picky"

Heather — excessive preoccupation with one's problems; needing to talk about them with others

Love-Lies-Bleeding — intense physical suffering or other psychic pain which overwhelms the consciousness and isolates the soul from involvement with others

Mimulus — personal fears and worries about everyday problems; fretful nature

Self-Effacement

Buttercup — belittling oneself; not feeling own self-worth; shyness about sharing one's gifts with others

Centaury — being a "doormat" for others; unhealthy need to be the servant

Fairy Lantern — feigning helplessness or dependency, playing childlike role to please others

Larch — lack of belief in one's talents or capabilities; lack of confidence; holding back, hesitation due to expectation of failure

Mimulus — fretful and fearful, seeing oneself as weak and vulnerable

Pine — hard on oneself, dwelling on past mistakes; extreme feelings of guilt

Pink Monkeyflower — emotional masking, unable to express true feelings due to shame

Pretty Face — feeling physically ugly, ashamed of appearance; excessive concern with cosmetic grooming

Sunflower — suppression of individuality; not feeling strong sense of Self

Violet — holding back in groups out of fear of losing identity; shyness

Self-Esteem

Black-Eyed Susan — integrating "shadow" aspects into one's sense of Self; emotional honesty to examine disowned aspects of Self

Buttercup — knowing one's true worth with others

Calla Lily — inability to integrate sexual identity with sense of Self; confusion or regret about core sexuality

Centaury — ability to serve others out of a feeling of self-worth, rather than servitude

Cerato — strength to follow one's inner guidance

Cosmos — inability to express complex thoughts or to verbalize one's deeper aspects to others

Echinacea — core sense of Self which is severely abused or assaulted; regaining integrity and dignity of core Self

Evening Primrose — feeling that one is unloved and unwanted due to actual trauma, abuse or neglect in early childhood

Fairy Lantern — inability to see oneself as full-fledged adult, conflicted feelings about oneself as child

Goldenrod — feeling one's own individuality and strength, especially under strong pressure for social conformity

Heather — tendency to see Self in terms of one's problems; preoccupation with personal suffering

Larch — confidence in one's expressive and creative abilities

Lotus — ability to feel Self as an expression of spirituality; contact with Higher Self; for spiritual pride if spirituality is unbalanced

Mallow — confidence in social situations

Pretty Face — poor personal grooming or excessive grooming and cosmetic masking due to internal image of oneself as ugly; ability to bring forward inner beauty from the soul

Purple Monkeyflower — inability to contact core spiritual identity due to ritual abuse or other fear-based religious experience

Sage — taking a more detached view of life and life experiences; ability to view the Self within a larger panorama of events

Sagebrush — lack or loss of fame and fortune, considered as a blow to the Self; accepting personal loss; shedding parts of the Self which are no longer appropriate for true destiny

Sunflower — sun-like, radiant individuality; owning the "I" or Self

Trumpet Vine — strong, vital speaking and self-expression, out of inner self-confidence

Self-Expression

(See also Communication, Speaking)

Beech — tendency to make critical comments; need to learn to be more praising and supportive in communications

Buttercup — increased sense of inner confidence and self-worth when speaking to others

Calendula — generating warmth and healing forces in one's words; ability to balance speaking and listening

Cosmos — speech which is too rapid or overly intellectual, not integrated with higher thought, lacking deeper concepts

Heather — overly talkative tendencies, especially concerning one's problems

Iris — soul-imbued forces; artistic impulses in speaking, poetry and drama

Larch — confidence in expression; when there is a tendency to doubt one's abilities

Mountain Pride — taking risks in communication, including healthy confrontation, speaking one's truth

Snapdragon — overly aggressive energy which manifests as verbal abuse or biting comments

Sunflower — boastful, drawing attention to oneself and accomplishments

Trumpet Vine — vitality in speaking and other forms of expression, especially when blocked or lacking in force

Violet — to share warmth with others, especially when there is a tendency to retreat or hold back

Selfishness

(See also Egotism, Greed, Pride)

Bleeding Heart — emotional attachment to others; co-dependent behavior

Chicory — emotionally possessive, needing undue attention

Chrysanthemum — overly attached to position and power, especially as a result of deep fears about one's own death and mortality

Fawn Lily — spiritual selfishness, need to share spiritual forces with others

Heather — preoccupation with one's own problems

Holly — inability to feel love or admiration for others

Star Thistle — stinginess, feeling of lack, holding on to what one has rather than sharing

Trillium — seeking personal gain and power

Water Violet — seeing oneself as better or higher; holding back out of disdain for others

Yellow Star Tulip — lack of awareness of what others are feeling; empathetic attunement

Sensitivity

(See also Receptivity, Vulnerability)

Angelica — feeling protected and guided; awareness of spiritual guardianship at times of stress

Aspen — hypersensitive to things unseen or unknown; need for psychic balance

Beech — oversensitivity to others and to the environment, leading to a hypercritical nature; blaming others for one's suffering

Calendula — true perception and sensitivity in listening to another; allowing warm, nurturing communication with others

Chamomile — subject to emotional tension; overactive solar plexus; moody or tearful

Chaparral — absorbing disturbing or violent images, either from direct experience or mass media; psychic toxicity

Golden Yarrow — seeking more active involvement in life despite acute sensitivity; vulnerable but needing to be visible

Lavender — oversensitivity to spiritual energy; high-strung

Love-Lies-Bleeding — tendency toward melancholia or intense personal suffering due to extreme sensitivity; to enable the soul to expand its sensitivity to compassionate awareness of others

Mountain Pennyroyal — absorbing or receiving negative thoughts from others; psychic and mental toxicity

Mugwort — sensitivity to threshold experiences, especially dreaming

Nicotiana — inability to cope with sensitivity, compulsion to numb or deaden the soul's experience

Pink Monkeyflower — extreme sensitivity, characterized by shame and emotional masking; inability to show real feelings

Pink Yarrow — oversensitivity to the emotions of others; internalizing others' problems as one's own

Poison Oak — fear of one's feelings, inward sensitivity; coping by projecting a hostile or aggressive exterior, avoiding intimacy

Purple Monkeyflower — extreme sensitivity characterized by fear of spiritual phenomena in particular; hypersensitivity and fear leading to unbalanced psychic experiences

Queen Anne's Lace — distorted psychic impressions due to disturbances in emotional life; to promote balanced clairvoyance

Red Chestnut — over-concern about the problems of others; fear and worry

Saint John's Wort — overexpanded psyche; vulnerability to harmful influences

Star Of Bethlehem — soothing acute sensitivity and trauma

Star Tulip — openness to spiritual realms; inner receptivity

Walnut — overcoming susceptibility to old ideas and influences, especially when ready to break with the past

Yarrow — sensitivity to negative influences in physical or psychic environment

Yarrow Special Formula — vulnerability to environmental toxins; susceptible to allergies, environmental sensitivity

Yellow Star Tulip — understanding and intuiting deeper feelings and spiritual essence of others; compassionate sensitivity

Seriousness

Canyon Dudleya — allowing small episodes of life to appear overly dramatic; overinflating psychic experiences; taking spiritual-psychic phenomena too seriously

Fairy Lantern — to develop more depth and seriousness; to move from child identity to adult consciousness

Hornbeam — approaching life as a dull routine; lack of joy

Nasturtium — overintellectualization, lacking vitality

Rock Water — being overly strict with oneself

Vervain — being overly fanatical about one's ideas; political or social agenda which overwhelms social relationships

Wild Oat — becoming more serious and directed about life and vocation

Zinnia — overly serious, lacking humor; somber and severe approach to life

Service

(See also Altruism)

Centaury — sacrificial service which drains or depletes rather than inspires

Fawn Lily — protecting and nurturing others; reclusive spiritual impulses transformed into compassionate service to the world

Larkspur — positive, balanced leadership; joyous service

Mariposa Lily — developing mothering forces, serving children; also to develop the positive mother archetype in any kind of service

Mountain Pride — strength to speak out, to make changes despite societal inertia or opposition

Scotch Broom — seeing world difficulties as opportunities for service

Tiger Lily — feminine impulses balancing masculine assertiveness in business life

Trillium — developing cooperation with others for mutual support

Vine — transforming tyrannical tendencies to positive service for others

Water Violet — increasing interaction with others; overcoming aloofness or haughtiness

Yellow Star Tulip — empathetic consciousness; understanding the needs of others

Sexuality

(See also Desire, Feminine Consciousness, Intimacy, Masculine Consciousness)

Alpine Lily — full engagement of female energies in sexual expression; integration of sexuality with spiritual feminine Self

Basil — to integrate sexuality and spirituality in a love relationship, especially when viewed as opposing polarities; sexuality often expressed in secretive ways, such as sexual addiction, pornography or shame-based sexuality

Black Cohosh — sexually abusive or destructive relationships; feeling that one is entangled or caught in a negative relationship

California Pitcher Plant — transforming instinctual qualities of sexuality into what is truly human

Calla Lily — confusion about sexual orientation; balance of one's male and female sexual forces

Crab Apple — feeling of shame, that sexuality is unclean

Dogwood — hardening of sexual forces, especially as a result of trauma or abuse; restoring grace and innocence

Easter Lily — conflicts between promiscuity and prudishness, between inner purity and expressions of sexuality

Evening Primrose — repression of sexual feelings, emotional distance in sexual relationships due to profound trauma, rejection or abuse in early childhood

Fairy Lantern — tendency in either men or women to stay in prepubescent sexuality

Fuchsia — genuine sexual feelings often sublimated into other psychosomatic emotions

Hibiscus — responsiveness in male and female sexuality, especially integration of soul warmth with physical passion; ability to experience love and warmth in sexual relationship with partner

Lady's Slipper — depletion of sexual forces often accompanied by nervous exhaustion; energy imbalance between crown and lower chakras

Larch — generally indicated for men; feeling that one is inadequate, or cannot measure up to expectations of sexual performance; impotence; to balance creative and procreative forces

Manzanita — accepting the body, feeling good about one's physical nature

Mariposa Lily — healing sexual abuse from childhood; healing premature exposure to adult sexuality which destroys innocence and wonder of childhood

Pink Monkeyflower — ability to express feelings of love and intimacy, fear of exposure; shame of sexual organs, often due to past violation or abuse

Pomegranate — expression of feminine forces through procreation and through creativity in the world; the integration of these polarities

Purple Monkeyflower — ritual sexual abuse involving cultic beliefs which distorts the soul's experience of sexuality

Queen Anne's Lace — integration of sexuality with psychic forces; balance between lower chakras and third eye function

Snapdragon — lack of integration of libido, misplaced as aggression and verbal hostility toward others

Sticky Monkeyflower — fear of intimacy, of dealing with sexual energy; unbalanced sexual expression manifesting either as repressed or overactive sexuality

Shadow Consciousness

(See also Lower Self)

Baby Blue Eyes — feeling pulled down by cynicism, inability to make spiritual contact

Black Cohosh — actively confronting or wrestling with shadow Self or the shadow aspects of another person

Black-Eyed Susan — clearer insight into covered-up or darkened emotions; ability of Higher Self to recognize and own its shadow side

California Pitcher Plant — proper harnessing of raw instincts or animal power

Scarlet Monkeyflower — awareness and transformation of "darker" emotions, especially anger and power

Snapdragon — inability to recognize authentic feelings of libido, masked as anger and aggression toward others

Vine — darkened forces of will which control others; to spiritualize the will by making a conscious connection with the Higher Self

Shame

(See also Guilt)

Agrimony — covering shame with a mask of cheerfulness; a carefree demeanor which hides inner torment

Alpine Lily — deep alienation from the female body; shame based on distorted cultural images of female sexuality, or on beliefs absorbed from one's family, particularly the mother

Basil — splitting of sexuality from spirituality, leading to shame-producing or aberrant sexual behavior, often deceptive and secretive

Buttercup — sense of worthlessness, feeling unimportant

Calla Lily — confusion about sexual orientation or same-sex attraction; shame about sexual feelings

Crab Apple — feeling that one is contaminated, impure or flawed in some fundamental way

Easter Lily — feeling that sexuality is impure, unspiritual, "lower"

Golden Ear Drops — repressed childhood memories associated with shame-producing experiences; cathartic release of painful emotions from the past

Larch — fear of making a mistake, feeling exposed to the ridicule of others; paralyzed by fear of being shamed, self-censoring

Pine — self-blame and criticism; feeling that one's life is a failure

Pink Monkeyflower — fear of exposure, that others will discover something terrible about oneself; profound shame

Pretty Face — feelings of shame associated with one's appearance; feeling ugly and unlovable

Purple Monkeyflower — shame stemming from occult or ritual abuse, leading to fear and submission to the power of others

Scarlet Monkeyflower — nonacceptance of powerful emotions such as anger; feeling that one's emotional shadow must be hidden and repressed, that it is "lower," shameful and dangerous

Sharing

Calendula — communicating warmly with others

Centaury — knowing one's limits in sharing with others; ability to say "No" when appropriate

Chicory — giving love without the need to get something in return

Fawn Lily — sharing spiritual gifts with others; overcoming tendency to hold back or stay uninvolved

Holly — opening heart to receive and give love

Mallow — developing friendship and social warmth

Pink Monkeyflower — feeling safe exposing oneself to others, opening up to others despite fear

Star Thistle — giving of oneself to others, especially when there is a tendency to stinginess

Trillium — overcoming "survival" instincts which prevent true sharing and cooperation with others

Violet — keeping a sense of individuality when sharing with a group, especially when there is fear that one will be submerged in the group

Water Violet — opening to others; overcoming aloofness; sharing oneself through social service to others

Shock

Arnica — maintaining the connection with Higher Self or ego forces during trauma; healing past shock or trauma

Echinacea — pronounced assaults to the inner Self; deeply shattering or destructive experiences

Five-Flower Formula — overall recovery from shock and trauma, especially for immediate use

Lavender — shock to the nerves from too many spiritual forces coming through the body

Pink Monkeyflower — violation or abuse which leads to emotional closure and profound soul shame

Saint John's Wort — out-of-body or other psychic experiences, especially leading to nerve depletion

Self-Heal — recuperative healing from shock

Star Of Bethlehem — soothing, maintaining inner peace after trauma; healing effects of past trauma, often repressed at the time

Shyness

Buttercup — lacking sense of self-worth, of having something of value to share with others

Larch — confidence in one's inner strength and abilities; suppression due to fear of making mistakes

Mallow — social insecurity; tendency to create barriers to friendships due to lack of trust

Mimulus — various fears in social situations; specific phobias which lead to withdrawal or introversion

Violet — fear of losing oneself in a group; genuinely shy

Water Violet — aloofness, social reserve; holding back from social contact

Sluggishness

Blackberry — difficulty taking action on one's intentions

Cayenne — catalyzing the will with a fiery stimulus to overcome inertia and resistance

Hornbeam — mental resistance to work or daily affairs

Morning Glory — inability to incarnate into the body in the morning; difficulty arising from bed

Peppermint — mental lethargy; inability to catalyze mental faculties

Tansy — physical lethargy due to indecisiveness or procrastination; paralysis of energies

Softness

Baby Blue Eyes — restoration of childlike innocence and trust

Calendula — listening to others; healing warmth; gentle receptivity

Deerbrush — fostering innocence and purity of the heart; gentle cleanser and softener

Dogwood — restoring gentleness, grace, innocence and openness; transforming hardened physical or emotional aspects of Self

Golden Yarrow — remaining in contact with others, softening without merging

Mariposa Lily — opening to the maternal, nurturing part of the Self; ability to impart soft, comforting qualities

Pine — overly hard attitude toward oneself, unable to forgive oneself

Pink Monkeyflower — showing one's softer, more vulnerable emotions without fear of rejection or shame

Poison Oak — fear of one's soft or feminine side, projecting overly Mars-like exterior

Quince — conflict about softness or femininity in relation to power

Star Tulip — spiritual openness; listening and receptivity through the feminine forces

Yellow Star Tulip — empathy and compassion for others; enveloping and nurturing sensitivity

Soothing

Calendula — the healing power of listening; warmth in communication

Chamomile — calming emotional tension or upset

Lavender — bringing inner peace, calming nervousness

Mariposa Lily — bringing mother forces of protection and comfort

Star Of Bethlehem — soothing when suffering from shock or trauma; restores inner peace

Soulfulness

Alpine Lily — greater inner space for the feminine self, especially the tendency to squeeze out or limit the full-bodied physical expression of the feminine

Angelica — perceiving and receiving help from higher worlds; sensing the soul within a larger matrix of spiritual life; attunement with spiritual beings who guide and guard

Deerbrush — purity and openness of heart; ability of the soul to become a container for higher worlds by healing personal distortion

Forget-Me-Not — awareness of spiritual and karmic factors in relationships; soul-based relationships which recognize eternal as well as temporal factors

Holly — ability to feel one's soul connection with others; soul communion

Iris — creating a chalice or inner vessel for receiving higher inspiration; active expression of the soul life through creativity

Sagebrush — experiencing inner space within the soul, apparent emptiness as a precondition for self-awareness

Star Tulip — receptive awareness; contacting higher worlds of thought

Yellow Star Tulip — perceiving the inner soul life of others; deep feeling for others

Yerba Santa — sense of internal space which feels toxic and congested; restoring sanctity of the heart center

Speaking

(See also Communication, Self-Expression)

Calendula — contacting the healing power of the word; using words as a positive healing force; overcoming argumentativeness; adding warmth to one's voice and speech

Canyon Dudleya — to calm and harmonize speech which excites or whips up the emotions of others; political or religious demagoguery

Cosmos — speaking with clarity and depth when speech tends to be too rapid or inarticulate; integration of ideas into coherent self-expression; translating higher thought into mental concepts

Garlic — fear when speaking, often associated with stage fright and a ghostly pale look; feeling drained or paralyzed

Golden Yarrow — providing an emotional buffer, especially for the solar plexus; ability to project one's voice despite anxiety

Heather — self-absorption; talking about one's problems, drawing excessive attention to oneself when speaking

Larch — confidence in self-expression, especially for low self-esteem

Madia — scattered, unfocused talking

Mimulus — shyness, timidity; swallowing words, nervousness when speaking

Red Clover — speech which is full of fear and anxiety absorbed from others

Snapdragon — lashing out, using cutting or biting words

Sunflower — projecting positive self-image when speaking

Trumpet Vine — clarity and vitality in verbal expression; dramatic stage presence

Vervain — forceful or compelling speech which does not recognize others' free will; intense beliefs which are imposed on others

White Chestnut — repetitive chattering; going over and over the same thoughts

Spiritual Emergency or Opening

(See also Emergency, Meditation)

Angel's Trumpet — experiencing death as genuine spiritual experience, spiritual initiation; overcoming resistance of the soul to impending death, or any significant soul transition

Angelica — protection when opening to spiritual experience; ability to sense benevolent higher forces at work in one's life, and the guidance and guardianship of higher realms

Arnica — bringing Higher Self in renewed relationship to the body; helping soul to keep connected with physical body after injury, shock, or spiritual opening

Aspen — fear of the unknown when crossing a spiritual threshold

Baby Blue Eyes — to counterbalance cynicism; when the soul feels estranged from the spiritual world, thus retarding its spiritual development

California Poppy — fascination or glamour in spiritual experiences; over-emphasis on psychic phenomena or techniques rather than true spiritual and moral development

Canyon Dudleya — tendency to unbalanced or hysterical states of psychism or mediumism; overemphasis on spiritual experiences in proportion to ordinary life events

Corn — grounding spiritual energy through the body, experiencing the body as a microcosm of the Earth

Fawn Lily — craving spiritual and meditation experience as a retreat from daily life

Forget-Me-Not — connection with spiritual guides; remembering those who guide beyond the physical realm

Garlic — tendency to be drained by lower entities due to fear of the spiritual world; psychic infestation

Indian Paintbrush — polarizing spiritual energy currents in the body between Heaven and Earth, especially while doing highly creative work

Iris — bringing more soulful aspects to spiritual identity; integration of artistic expression with spiritual process

Lady's Slipper — integration of inner spiritual authority with real life tasks, harmonization of crown and root chakras

Lavender — harsh or overly strenuous spiritual practices leading to nervous overload

Lotus — enhancing and opening spiritual consciousness; balancing overdeveloped spirituality which is not integrated with other aspects of Self

Love-Lies-Bleeding — seeing larger spiritual purpose or meaning when suffering intense physical pain or mental anguish

Milkweed — unbalanced spiritual practices which blot out or obliterate healthy ego structure; over-dependence on spiritual leaders or dogma

Mountain Pennyroyal — invaded or taken over by other entities; psychic toxicity, often due to harmful occult or meditative techniques

Mugwort — sensitivity to threshold experiences, especially dreaming; ability to integrate psychic life with ordinary consciousness

Purple Monkeyflower — profound fear of spiritual opening, often due to fear-based religious beliefs or occult ritual abuse; to develop calm and objective relationship to spiritual phenomena

Queen Anne's Lace — integration of sexuality with psychic awareness, especially when distorted or unbalanced in either direction; developing objective clairvoyance

Rock Rose — identification with the Higher Self when facing threat of death or death-like initiation experience

Rock Water — overly strict approach to spiritual life; asceticism or other forms of rigidity which deny the joy of true spiritual experience

Rosemary — inability to integrate spiritual experiences with body; body becomes cold and stiff while in meditation or prayer

Saint John's Wort — protection while outside the body, especially during dreams, or from overly expanded or psychic states of mind; generally indicated for all stages of spiritual opening

Star Tulip — softening any resistance to the spiritual realm; ability to feel soul communion with higher spiritual forces

Sweet Chestnut — faith when facing the "dark night of the soul;" meeting a severe spiritual test that stretches the soul to the limit

Yarrow — overexpansion of spiritual Self leading to acute sensitivity; need for protection; overly porous auric field

Spontaneity

(See also Flexibility)

Cayenne — fiery catalyst to break through stagnant situations

Iris — artistic creativity; inspired approach to the commonplace in life

Larch — flowing creative expression; not censoring oneself

Rock Water — flowing attitude toward life; letting go of perfectionist and overly rigid behavior

Zinnia — childlike laughter and delight; ability to break free from overly planned schedules and routines

Strength

Black Cohosh — confronting and transforming negative power aspects in relationships

California Pitcher Plant — meeting the world with courage and strength through harnessing instinctive forces; indicated for weak digestion; inability to assimilate astral elements into the psyche or body

Centaury — courage and strength to say "No" to others; overly servile mentality

Echinacea — strengthening one's core integrity, ability to contact and realize deepest aspects of Self

Fairy Lantern — strength to become fully adult, to move developmental process forward

Golden Yarrow — strength and centeredness; to be more active in the world despite anxiety or sensitivity

Indian Pink — maintaining one's inner center of gravity despite intense activity and demands on oneself

Milkweed — ego strength to cope with one's core identity; to develop the individuated Self, especially when tendency is to blot out or annihilate Self

Mountain Pennyroyal — strength and clarity of thought; distinguishing and clarifying own thoughts from other influences

Mountain Pride — warrior-like strength in the face of obstacles and adversity; courage to confront evil or wrongdoing

Nicotiana — false persona of strength or toughness; to integrate emotional awareness and sensitivity with real strength

Oak — fortitude during long struggle; endurance; realizing the limits of one's endurance

Penstemon — inner strength in the face of adversity; the ability to meet extreme challenges

Pink Yarrow — emotional strength; for those who compromise their vitality by absorbing the emotional toxicity of others

Quince — developing the strength of love, especially to balance the need for power with feminine receptivity

Scotch Broom — tenacity of purpose in spite of obstacles, especially with tendency to despair about the world

Snapdragon — for those with strong personal power, often misdirected as aggression

Sunflower — healthy ego strength; strong, radiant individuality

Walnut — courage to follow one's own path despite outer influences

Yarrow — integrity of the aura, especially when too open to environmental or psychic influences

Yarrow Special Formula — strengthening the body and mind when physically assaulted by environmental toxins, chaos or radiation

Yerba Santa — wasting away of strength; tendency to melancholia and introversion

Stress

(See also Challenge, Overwhelm, Shock, Tension)

Aloe Vera — overwork, burnout; misuse of fiery creative forces

Chamomile — calming and soothing; especially after crying and other intense emotions

Cherry Plum — fear that extreme stress will lead to breakdown and loss of control

Dill — feeling overwhelmed by impressions, too much stimulation, such as in travel; helpful when starting a large project

Elm — feeling overwhelmed by responsibility; taking on too much

Five-Flower Formula — bringing balance after extreme stress; especially for temporary situations or as a first step

Impatiens — impatience, frustration, irritation; trying to go too fast

Indian Pink — remaining calm and centered in the midst of intense activity

Lavender — nervous overwhelm; soothing and calming

Pink Yarrow — picking up emotional and psychic negativity from others; psychic "sponge" qualities which lead to nervous overwhelm

Rosemary — inability to incarnate properly into body; feeling cold and depleted when under stress

Star Of Bethlehem — soothing trauma after severe stress

Vervain — overenthusiasm and extremism, leading to nervous breakdown or depletion

Yarrow — stress due to negative thoughts and intentions of others

Yarrow Special Formula — allergic or oversensitive responses to the environment; stress due to frequent exposure to computer terminals, low level radiation, or electromagnetic fields

Study

(See also Concentration and Focus, Learning Difficulties, Thinking)

Chestnut Bud — to learn from past mistakes; difficulty in learning, repeating mistakes, lacking insight

Cosmos — organizing and harmonizing thought processes into coherent communication

Dandelion — extreme tension in neck and shoulders from excessive desk work

Hound's Tongue — to spiritualize thinking; overly analytical, materialistic thinking which is devoid of imagination, wonder and reverence for life

Iris — bringing artistic and soulful impulses into study; integration of creativity with learning and study

Lavender — nerves which are depleted from too much study

Madia — developing concentration and focus; overcoming distractions

Nasturtium — devitalization due to mental activity; stimulating depleted life forces

Peppermint — increasing mental alertness

Rabbitbrush — mastering many details at one time

Shasta Daisy — integrating information into a whole; able to see overall meaning in details; analysis balanced by archetypal thinking

Yarrow Special Formula — depletion due to spending many hours working in front of a video display terminal (computer screen)

Zinnia — too much study; overly serious and somber personality

Surrender

Angel's Trumpet — soul surrender at time of death, joyful liberation and transition

Aspen — trust in spiritual guidance when facing the unknown

Centaury — unhealthy surrender to the will of another, being a "doormat"

Cherry Plum — surrender to the wisdom of the Higher Self or a Higher Power when feeling desperate or out of control; ability to "let go and let God"

Love-Lies-Bleeding — ability to accept and endure physical or emotional pain; to find meaning and purpose in one's suffering

Oak — struggling beyond limits, not knowing when to surrender

Rock Rose — surrender and trust when facing threat of death or initiation experience

Sweet Chestnut — extreme anguish and despair when severely tested, requiring the soul to surrender to a Higher Power

Wild Rose — giving up too easily in illness; overly resigned to illness

Synthesis

Chestnut Bud — understanding of experiences so they need not be repeated

Cosmos — integration of speech with thinking

Lotus — integration of all soul forces into a harmonious spirituality

Rabbitbrush — overview of many details of a situation, assimilating simultaneous realities

Shasta Daisy — gathering together of many ideas into a living picture; to see the overall meaning; archetypal insight

Tension

(See also Overwhelm, Relaxation, Stress)

Chamomile — releasing emotional tension held in the stomach region

Dandelion — emotional tension stored throughout body, especially in musculature; also for a tendency to cramping

Garlic — paralysis in solar plexus due to fear; stage fright

Golden Yarrow — tension when performing or speaking, due to oversensitivity

Impatiens — mental tension and impatience

Iris — tension especially in the neck region; unable to feel inner freedom of the soul

Lavender — high-strung; nervous tension

Nicotiana — coping with tension by using addictive substances, especially tobacco

Purple Monkeyflower — extreme tension or fear, especially of spiritual experiences

Snapdragon — holding tension in jaw and mouth, grinding teeth; tense and terse manner of speaking

Vervain — fanatical straining for a cause or ideal; extreme intensity leading to physical tension

Yerba Santa — releasing emotional tension held in the chest region

Thinking

(See also Inspiration, Intellectualism, Mental Clarity, Study)

Angelica — to spiritualize thinking forces, to make thinking activity more meditative and spiritually active

Blackberry — creative power of thought; especially channeling thinking into the will

Cosmos — integration of thinking and speech, conveying higher thought in an articulate manner

Hound's Tongue — receptivity to spiritual thought; interpreting sense-impressions in the light of spiritual reality; to awaken dull and overly materialistic thinking

Impatiens — finishing others' thoughts for them; to modulate and harmonize impatient and overhasty thinking

Mountain Pennyroyal — strength and clarity of thought, clearing the mind of negativity

Nasturtium — overuse of thinking forces; need to be more in touch with life experience

Peppermint — awake thinking, overcoming mental sluggishness

Rabbitbrush — ability to master many details at one time; alert attention and presence of mind

Shasta Daisy — archetypal, holistic thinking; able to synthesize many ideas into whole thoughts and concepts

White Chestnut — repetitive and obsessive thoughts; need for mental quietude

Time Relationship

(See also Nostalgia)

Aloe Vera — overly intense pace of life preventing one from living in the moment, too burned out to enjoy life

Arnica — deep shock and trauma from past which cripples and hinders full availability of life forces

Black-Eyed Susan — inability to confront and acknowledge past experience; denial which keeps one from living fully in the present

Blackberry — using forces of will to shape and mold future; feeling stagnant; inability to create future possibilities

Bleeding Heart — powerful emotional attachment to past, inability to face present pain and loss

California Poppy — always living for anticipated future experience, seeking more stimulation rather than allowing present moment to be integrated

California Wild Rose — holding back from present moment, not wanting involvement

Cayenne — stagnating, needing catharsis and breakthrough to take next step; stuck in old patterns

Chestnut Bud — repeating past mistakes, inability to learn the lessons of experience

Clematis — awareness which is not connected with the here-and-now; dreamy, lacking full bodily presence

Dandelion — pushing oneself, over-planning and over-scheduling; trying to compress too much experience into too little time

Elm — feeling overwhelmed by present events, inability to step back and get perspective

Gorse — melancholic attachment to past problems which creates pessimistic outlook for future

Honeysuckle — dwelling on nostalgic memories of "good old times" as a way of sedating the soul; inability to accept present reality

Hornbeam — aversion to present time and tasks, causing depletion of energy

Impatiens — always wanting things to go faster; irritable and impatient, feeling there is never enough time; inability to be in the present time

Indian Pink — feeling overwhelmed by present moment, inability to center or breathe properly due to intensity of life

Lavender — experiencing present moment too intensely, needing to relax and ground

Madia — inability to focus on present moment's tasks; getting easily sidetracked, dispersing energy

Mimulus — fear there will not be enough time for daily tasks of life

Morning Glory — inability to live rhythmically in time, erratic eating and sleeping patterns which rob one's body of vitality

Pine — difficulty letting go of past events; dwelling on one's past mistakes and failures; extreme feelings of guilt and remorse

Sage — seeing large sweeps of time, making sense of life biography and destiny

Sagebrush — releasing past identifications and identities which are no longer appropriate; ability to accept the naked possibility of the present moment

Tansy — avoidance of living in present by overly slow and phlegmatic response, inertia

Zinnia — feeling burdened and pressured by time; needing to restore spontaneity and humor

Tolerance

(See also Acceptance, Flexibility)

Beech — seeing the value of differences in others; tending to judge or hold unrealistic expectations of others

Calendula — tolerance for what others are saying, receptivity

Impatiens — accepting the different (slower) rhythms and pace of others

Quaking Grass — ability to work with the ideas of others in a group

Rock Water — overly rigid standards of perfection in diet or lifestyle which inhibit the true flow of life; needing more tolerance and inner flexibility

Vervain — allowing others to have their own beliefs, even if different than one's own strongly held beliefs

Vine — respecting the free will of others; letting others express themselves freely

Willow — releasing blame and resentment toward others; forgiveness

Toner

Angelica — to spiritualize the consciousness; to help the soul feel supported and protected

Borage — uplifting the heart; bringing a sense of buoyancy and ability to radiate courage

California Wild Rose — rousing the heart to engage the soul fully in life

Lotus — general spiritual enhancer for many combinations

Morning Glory — smoothing erratic habit patterns which affect the life energy

Mugwort — balancing overall psychic life

Pink Monkeyflower — to keep the heart open in all therapeutic work, to allow the inmost Self to be seen and heard by others

Self-Heal — balancing other powerful essences and therapies; bringing self-confidence in one's own healing ability

Shasta Daisy — synthesizing and integrating other therapies; helping all issues and illnesses to be seen within the larger wholeness

Star Tulip — softening and sensitizing the soul; creating greater receptivity

Yarrow — providing overall strength, to make the Self more whole and vital; knitting together the aura

Yerba Santa — heart balancing for emotionally cathartic essences; providing a gentle release

Transcendence

Angel's Trumpet — transcendence of soul from physical plane, conscious dying

Baby Blue Eyes — ability of the soul to go beyond harsh or unfair life experience; rebuilding innocence and trust within the soul

Echinacea — reconstellating the Self; affirming core identity in spite of extreme assaults to dignity, identity or health

Hound's Tongue — spiritualizing overly materialistic thinking

Iris — rising above the mundane routine to heightened levels of creativity

Love-Lies-Bleeding — profound pain and suffering which moves soul beyond its personal limits; transpersonal awareness

Rock Rose — going beyond individual identity; great courage when facing life-threatening or other extreme challenges

Sagebrush — cultivating inner emptiness as a catalyst for change, to go through the soul's experience of the abyss

Sunflower — raising the lower ego to the "Sun Self"

Sweet Chestnut — transcendence of Self when stretched beyond all limits; intense anguish which leads to spiritual breakthrough

Transition

(See also Breakthrough)

Angel's Trumpet — moving from earthly life to spiritual existence; death and dying process

Forget-Me-Not — ability to transform relationship with one who has died by following his/her transition to spiritual world

Morning Glory — gaining a fresh perspective; breaking destructive habit patterns

Sagebrush — letting go of inessentials that no longer serve a purpose; inner purification

Walnut — breaking free of old ties and habits; inner strengthener

True to Self

(See also Denial, False Persona, Honesty)

Agrimony — acknowledging one's inner conflict

Centaury — serving others while remaining true to oneself

Chrysanthemum — commitment to true spiritual identity rather than lower persona

Cosmos — accessing and communicating deepest thoughts of Self to others

Echinacea — maintaining one's core identity when threatened or assaulted

Fairy Lantern — accepting genuine adult Self, rather than childish persona

Golden Yarrow — helping oneself stay connected and receptive to others, despite sensitivity

Goldenrod — remaining true to individual identity in group situations, especially when tending to please or seek approval from others

Milkweed — developing one's core ego identity, especially when there is an unconscious desire to regress or obliterate ego

Mullein — following voice of conscience; ability to identify Self with higher truth, to activate moral life

Pink Yarrow — inability to distinguish one's true feelings from others' emotions

Queen Anne's Lace — ability to separate personal emotions or projections from objective psychic information

Sagebrush — shedding past identity which is no longer appropriate

Walnut — remaining true to one's unique life destiny, rather than being influenced by the ideas or beliefs of others; breaking unhealthy links

Yarrow — protecting integrity of Self when it is too porous or too easily penetrated by the environment

Trust

(See also Faith)

Angelica — deep trust in the divine guidance in our lives, especially when facing the unknown or crossing the threshold of death

Aspen — ability to penetrate to the unknown, to trust that the Self can encounter subtle planes; to overcome fears of the unknown

Baby Blue Eyes — when the soul no longer trusts due to harsh life experience; feeling abandoned by spiritual world; restoration of childlike innocence and trust, renewed spirituality

Basil — building trust through communication and openness in relationships, especially when there is a tendency toward secrecy or deception

Cerato — relying on one's own inner guidance, especially when uncertain and hesitant

Cherry Plum — surrender to the intuitive guidance of life; "letting go and letting God"

Forget-Me-Not — trusting one's intuition and inner knowing; knowing that one is supported by allies in the spiritual world

Mallow — learning to trust as the basis of friendship; difficulty making friends due to lack of trust

Mariposa Lily — trusting the bonding relationship between mother and child; feeling the nurturing aspect of all relationships

Oregon Grape — trusting the good will of others, especially when tending to misperceive others' intentions

Purple Monkeyflower — developing deep trust in one's own spiritual identity and experience, especially when fearful or paranoid

Saint John's Wort — trust in divine protection in the world and in all that surrounds us; to integrate spiritual forces with bodily awareness

Self-Heal — trust in one's own self-healing powers, in the ability to be well

Vitality

(See also Devitalization, Rejuvenation)

Aloe Vera — to restore life forces and replenish the heart center; especially for the feeling of being burned out from too much "fire" or creative force

Alpine Lily — bringing more vital female energy when feminine is too abstractly spiritual or ungrounded

Arnica — repairing life energy after shock or trauma

California Wild Rose — enthusiasm for life, overcoming apathy

Fawn Lily — vitality which is depleted from overemphasis on spiritual life; tendency to become frail or fragile

Hibiscus — sexual vitality and responsiveness

Indian Paintbrush — stimulating vitality in creativity; when creative forces are not properly integrated with life forces

Lady's Slipper — nervous exhaustion and sexual depletion

Morning Glory — reawakening life energy, and sparkle of life

Mountain Pennyroyal — clear, vital thinking, especially when threatened by thoughts and energies absorbed from others

Nasturtium — overly dry intellectualism; needing more earthy vitality

Peppermint — developing awake and alert thinking

Self-Heal — awakening the inner self-healing power; integration of etheric vitality with spiritual consciousness

Trumpet Vine — lively creative expression, ability to energetically project one's voice and actions

Wild Rose — rallying life forces to fight a long illness; overcoming a tendency to apathy and resignation

Vulnerability

(See also Receptivity, Sensitivity)

Centaury — overly subject to the will of others; servant mentality which depletes one's true strength

Golden Yarrow — coping with extreme sensitivity and vulnerability, especially when in public; ability to remain open to others while still feeling inner protection

Love-Lies-Bleeding — easily wounded, or suffering greatly; to find meaning in one's suffering within a larger human context

Nicotiana — becoming more vulnerable, more in touch with real feelings of the heart

Pink Monkeyflower — becoming more vulnerable and open to others, when hiding essential parts of the Self

Pink Yarrow — susceptibility to emotional influences; excessive personal identification with the emotions of others

Poison Oak — fear of vulnerability, coping by projecting a hard exterior

Red Clover — susceptibility to group panic and hysteria

Saint John's Wort — extreme vulnerability to psychic influences or fear-producing experiences, especially in dreams

Yarrow — being easily affected by the negative attitudes and intentions of others

Yarrow Special Formula — susceptibility to negative or harmful influences in the physical environment

Warmth

Calendula — healing warmth of one's words in communication with others

California Wild Rose — igniting the heart; rousing the soul with warm feelings of love for life and for others

Cayenne — fiery warmth in the will forces

Fawn Lily — unthawing spiritual forces, aligning spiritual forces with the heart

Hibiscus — integration of soul warmth and physical warmth in sexual expression

Mallow — creating warmth in contact with others; fostering friendship

Mariposa Lily — maternal, nurturing qualities; feeling surrounded by a mantle of warmth and love

Nasturtium — greater connection with life; when the thinking forces are too cool and detached from life experience

Rosemary — inability to fully contact or experience soul warmth, often with poor circulation or coldness in the physical body

Sticky Monkeyflower — creating warmth and intimacy in relationships; overcoming fear of being vulnerable or rejected

Yellow Star Tulip — warm and compassionate attention for others; empathic concern

Will

(See also Manifestation)

Blackberry — bringing balanced forces of will to abstract or visionary thoughts; putting ideas into action

California Wild Rose — rousing the will to become involved in life; enthusiasm

Cayenne — igniting the will when moving too slowly, or stuck

Centaury — strength of will to say "No" to others when appropriate

Indian Paintbrush — bringing greater metabolic forces of will into creative process; earthy vitality

Mountain Pride — will to confront and challenge despite opposition; ability to take risks

Oak — will forces which may be too strong; tendency to overdo; hero complex

Penstemon — healthy use of will forces to confront obstacles and impediments

Saguaro — willful rebellion against authority

Snapdragon — misplaced forces of will, aggression and verbal abuse

Tansy — will forces which are too sluggish, procrastination; need to bring conscious awareness to dysfunctional will qualities

Trillium — greed or striving for power; will forces devoted to survival or materialistic goals

Vervain — using personal will to convert others to one's view; pushing with the will beyond reasonable limits; overzealousness to the point of fanaticism

Vine — imposing one's will on others

Wild Rose — rallying the will to face a health crisis, overcoming a tendency to apathy and resignation

Wisdom

(See also Awareness, Insight)

California Poppy — knowing that spiritual wisdom is within, rather than seeking it in gurus or experiences of spiritual "highs"

Cerato — trusting in one's inner knowing

Chestnut Bud — learning the lessons of life experience

Cosmos — expressing wisdom in speech; able to gather higher thoughts and express them clearly

Hound's Tongue — spiritualizing the thinking process; ability to see the deeper essence within material reality

Lotus — spiritual wisdom from opening of the crown chakra; balancing spiritual knowledge with feeling from the heart

Sage — discovering the inner wisdom of life experiences; inner contentment and peace about the meaning of one's life

Saguaro — openness to ancient wisdom, the knowledge of elders

Shasta Daisy — synthesis in thinking life; able to integrate many ideas into a coherent philosophy and world view

Star Tulip — receptivity to spiritual wisdom through meditation and dreams

Work and Career Goals

Blackberry — inability to manifest goals, paralyzed will forces

Buttercup — unwarranted feelings of low self-esteem or shame about one's job or lifestyle

California Poppy — inability to settle or commit to a career, being continuously fascinated by allure of more fame, fortune or glamorous experience

California Wild Rose — lack of enthusiasm for one's work; apathy or indifference, "filling in time"

Canyon Dudleya — inability to accept ordinary routine or everyday responsibilities, desire for glamour or excitement

Cayenne — being stuck in unhealthy work habits; catalyst for change

Centaury — overly servile attitude to work; not meeting real capacities of Self

Dandelion — tendency to overwork, resulting in bodily tension and stress

Elm — taking on too many responsibilities, resulting in feeling overwhelmed

Fairy Lantern — irresponsible work patterns; inability to accept work as a part of adult maturation

Fawn Lily — highly sensitive and spiritually attuned, but often feeling fatigued or drained by work; feeling one's work is chaotic or stressful, preferring retreat or isolation

Hornbeam — "Monday morning blues;" often feeling tired when at work; to identify and tap an authentic source of energy and commitment to work

Impatiens — feeling impatient when working with others, preferring to work alone in order to get goals accomplished quickly

Iris — feeling bored with work or career, to develop more creative forces; work experienced as dull and lackluster without creative interest

Lady's Slipper — depletion and exhaustion due to inability of soul to contact true life purpose; work which does not reflect real destiny

Larch — poor job performance or lack of promotion despite real abilities; lack of confidence or expectation of failure

Larkspur — exercising leadership skills in work; joyful service

Oak — pressing to the limits of endurance in work and responsibilities; learning how to receive help from others

Pomegranate — conflict between work and home, especially for women who are mothers; uncertainty about one's creative priorities

Quaking Grass — finding right relationship to work group, especially when in conflict about personal feelings and group values or responsibilities; difficulty working in groups; harmonizing individual personalities to accomplish group tasks

Rabbitbrush — stress or overwhelm due to demanding nature of job, especially when many details require simultaneous attention and awareness

Tansy — procrastination or lethargy with regard to work and responsibilities; unconscious repression of real energy source for work

Trillium — desire to work motivated largely by survival, or by need to accumulate material security; finding higher ideals in work

Vine — compulsion to be in control or dominant when working with others; learning receptivity and social leadership skills

Wild Oat — lack of life direction, many different work experiences without cohesive meaning or purpose; general remedy for finding sense of vocation and meaning in one's work

Zinnia — workaholism, inability to play or relax, overwork which leads to a dulling of the soul life

Part III

Flower Essence
Qualities and
Portraits

Table of Flower Essence Profiles

Agrimony *Agrimonia eupatoria* (yellow) English Kit

Positive qualities: Emotional honesty, acknowledging and working with emotional pain, obtaining true inner peace
Patterns of imbalance: Anxiety hidden by a mask of cheerfulness; denial and avoidance of emotional pain, addictive behavior to anesthetize feelings

Cross-references: Acceptance Addiction Avoidance Calm Cheerfulness
Co-Dependence Community Life and Group Experience Conflict Denial
Eating Disorders Escapism False Persona Healers Healing Process Honesty
Masculine Consciousness Mid-Life Crisis Perfectionism Repression Resistance Shame
True to Self

The Agrimony personality appears happy, enthusiastic, popular, and seemingly at peace with the world. However, if one is able to know such a person on a deeper level, it becomes clear that something is deeply troubling the soul. At the heart of such suffering is a secret torment that is hidden, not only from others, but most importantly from the Self. There may be a strong attraction to drugs, particularly alcohol, in order to maintain the mask of cheerfulness. Such persons have often been raised with strict social conventions of politeness or repression, and find it difficult to show or admit vulnerability or pain. This conditioning is particularly strong in men who have been taught that it is unmanly to show feelings. Another variation of this attitude appears among those on a spiritual path who try to emulate a state of bliss by denying or repressing troubling emotions. The Agrimony person needs to find peace as an inner soul reality, rather than an outer state of behavior which others validate. It is their lesson that true inner peace comes from honestly acknowledging pain and transforming it, rather than masking it with a superficial veneer of good cheer or polite tolerance.

Aloe Vera *Aloe vera* (yellow)   Professional Kit

Positive qualities: Creative activity balanced and centered in vital life-energy
Patterns of imbalance: Overuse or misuse of fiery, creative forces; "burned-out" feeling

Cross-references: Action Ambition Body Creativity Devitalization Dryness Energetic Patterns Exhaustion and Fatigue Heart Masculine Consciousness Materialism and Money Menopause Mid-Life Crisis Moderation Rejuvenation Stress Time Relationship Vitality

Those needing Aloe Vera "burn the candle at both ends." They have an innate abundance of fiery forces, but tend to overuse these forces and literally "burn out." Typical of the Aloe Vera type are "workaholics" whose drive is so intense that they neglect their emotional and physical needs, often sacrificing rest, food, and social contact in order to accomplish their goals. Such an attitude cripples the ability to experience life in a heart-felt way, impoverishing the feeling life, and draining the body of vital energy. While will-power can carry such persons quite far, eventually they reach a point of exhaustion, burnout, or breakdown. Aloe Vera helps the soul and body aspects to come into greater harmony, by bringing the nourishment which comes from the *water* polarity of life — the *flowing* qualities of renewal and rejuvenation. When the soul learns to balance the fiery forces of the will with the fountain of feeling from the heart, a tremendous outpouring of positive creativity and spirituality can be realized.

Alpine Lily *Lilium parvum* (red-orange)   Research Kit

Positive qualities: For women, acceptance of one's femininity grounded in a deepened experience of the female body
Patterns of imbalance: Overly abstract sense of femininity; disembodied, alienation from or rejection of female organs as "lower"

Cross-references: Acceptance Adolescence Alienation Ambivalence Body Conflict Feminine Consciousness Groundedness Heart Inner Child Instinctual Self Lower Self Menopause Mother and Mothering Perfectionism Pregnancy Self-Acceptance Sexuality Shame Soulfulness Vitality

Alpine Lily helps the feminine soul experience a more vibrant relationship to the female body. While this remedy can sometimes be indicated for men who are addressing inner feminine aspects of themselves, it is primarily beneficial for women who harbor a psychological split in their relationship to the feminine principle. These women tend to favor that which is more cosmic and virginal, and find it difficult to identify with the earthly aspect of the feminine. They have many spiritual attributes and actively use higher feminine forces, but do not integrate this consciousness with the physical body. Negative impressions of the female body are often unconsciously absorbed from the mother or from the larger culture. Because the soul does not fully identify with or inhabit its female body, physical stress and disharmony can result in the reproductive organs, in the sexual function, or in the biological experience of pregnancy and nursing. Alpine Lily stimulates the integration of the feminine and female selves, promoting circulation between the higher and lower energy centers. The soul learns that its full energy and potential depends on the utilization of the bodily female as well as the spiritual feminine.

Angel's Trumpet *Datura candida* (white) Research Kit

Positive qualities: Spiritual surrender at death or at times of deep transformation; opening the heart to the spiritual world
Patterns of imbalance: Fear of death, resistance to letting go of life or to crossing the spiritual threshold; denial of the reality of the spiritual world

Cross-references: Aging Attachment Calm Death and Dying Denial Emergency Grace Joy Meditation Non-Attachment Perspective Release Resistance Spiritual Emergency or Opening Surrender Transcendence Transition

Angel's Trumpet is used especially for the soul's capacity to experience death, or any profound transformation, in a way which is conscious and free. A key word in understanding Angel's Trumpet is *surrender* — for situations when it is no longer appropriate to fight death, or for ego surrender, when the soul must utterly submit itself to a process of spiritualization. With Angel's Trumpet, the soul can experience these processes as joyous transitions rather than as fearsome ordeals. The soul realizes that death is a form of birth when seen from the spiritual world, and comes to recognize those spiritual beings who wait on the other side. This remedy is helpful in hospice work, in wartime, during natural disasters and for all occasions when we are called to minister to loved ones who are departing from physical form. It is also helpful for therapists who must guide the soul through deeply transformative, "rebirthing" processes. Angel's Trumpet facilitates profound soul opening, transforming the fear of death into the conscious awareness of spiritual life.

Angelica *Angelica archangelica* (white)   Research Kit

Positive qualities: Feeling protection and guidance from spiritual beings, especially at threshold experiences such as birth and death

Patterns of imbalance: Feeling cut off, bereft of spiritual guidance and protection

Cross-references: Abandonment Addiction Adolescence Aging Awareness Brokenheartedness Centeredness Certainty Children Death and Dying Denial Dreams and Sleep Egotism Emergency Environment Faith Fear Grace Harmony Healing Process Influence Inner Child Insight Lightness Love Materialism and Money Meditation Perspective Pregnancy Prejudice Protection Quiet Receptivity Rejection Sensitivity Soulfulness Spiritual Emergency or Opening Thinking Toner Trust

The modern human soul suffers in a way which is unique and tragic, for it must face profound spiritual isolation and separation through living in a materialistically dense and technologically abstract world culture. The Angelica flower essence addresses the soul's experience of compression and restriction by quickening the thinking and perception processes. The soul becomes more able to perceive and discriminate its connection to the subtle sheaths surrounding the physical world. Angelica especially encourages the individual to develop a relationship with the spiritual world, transforming an overly abstract or intellectual viewpoint into a genuine feeling for spiritual presence and spiritual beings. This awareness is particularly enhanced for that group of spiritual beings who immediately border the human kingdom: the angels. Through a living relationship with the angelic realm, the human soul receives guardianship and guidance in daily affairs, and protection at times of crisis or during threshold experiences. This feeling of being protected and cared for is of enormous importance to the inner life, giving the soul great strength and courage for its work in transforming and healing the world. Angelica is broadly indicated for many flower essence formulas and is particularly important at threshold times such as birth, death, festival celebrations, or other major life passages.

Arnica *Arnica mollis* (yellow)   Professional Kit

Positive qualities: Conscious embodiment, especially during shock or trauma; recovery from deep-seated shock or trauma
Patterns of imbalance: Disconnection of Higher Self from body during shock or trauma; disassociation, unconsciousness

Cross-references: Addiction   Animals and Animal Care   Body   Emergency
Energetic Patterns   Healing Process   Massage   Psychosomatic Illness   Shock   Spiritual
Emergency or Opening   Time Relationship   Vitality

Arnica helps to heal deep-seated shock or trauma which may become locked into the body and prevent full healing recovery. Especially during accidents or violent experiences, the Higher Self or soul disassociates from its physical vehicle, and may never properly re-enter certain parts of the body despite seeming recovery. This remedy can be especially helpful for unlocking many puzzling or psychosomatic illnesses, which do not respond to obvious treatment. When Arnica is used for such cases, the soul will often relive or re-experience the emotional trauma which accompanied the original experience. In this way the soul is finally able to integrate the experience and to fully inhabit the part of the body which suffers. Arnica can also be used on a short-term first-aid basis to allow rapid recovery from trauma. It especially helps the soul attain greater awareness of the parts of the psyche or body which may be under-utilized in the individual's full expression of Self.

Aspen *Populus tremula* (green/gray) English Kit

Positive qualities: Trust and confidence to meet the unknown, drawing inner strength from the spiritual world
Patterns of imbalance: Fear of the unknown, vague anxiety and apprehension, hidden fears, nightmares

Cross-references: Addiction   Animals and Animal Care   Anxiety   Children   Courage
Faith   Fear   Insecurity   Insomnia   Manifestation   Nervousness   Paranoia   Sensitivity
Spiritual Emergency or Opening   Surrender   Trust

The Aspen personality has a disproportionately developed astral body, especially in relationship to the ego, or conscious awareness. Such persons readily receive impressions from other planes of reality; however, these intimations are perceived on the subconscious level, and often produce feelings of fear and foreboding. Aspen flower essence quiets and subdues the astral body so that the spiritual ego can gain greater strength and awareness. This flower is very helpful for children who are oversensitive to unseen and unknown influences, and can also be indicated for those who may have prematurely opened their astral sheaths through drug use or occult ritual. Aspen essence calms and harmonizes the innate psychic capacities of such individuals, by allowing the conscious mind to receive and process more information. In this way, Aspen brings greater strength and confidence, and balanced use of soul forces.

Baby Blue Eyes *Nemophila menziesii* (light blue) Research Kit

Positive qualities: Childlike innocence and trust; feeling at home in the world, at ease with oneself, supported and loved; connected with the spiritual world
Patterns of imbalance: Defensiveness, insecurity, mistrust of others; estrangement from the spiritual world; lack of support from the father in childhood

Cross-references: Abandonment   Acceptance   Addiction   Adolescence   Aging
Alienation   Aloofness   Blame   Children   Cynicism   Depression and Despair   Dullness
Faith   Father and Fathering   Feminine Consciousness   Forgiveness   Gloom   Hardness
Heart   Hostility   Inertia   Inner Child   Insecurity   Intimacy   Joy   Life Direction
Loneliness   Love   Masculine Consciousness   Perseverance   Pessimism   Rejection
Rejuvenation   Resentment   Self-Acceptance   Self-Actualization   Shadow Consciousness
Softness   Spiritual Emergency or Opening   Transcendence   Trust

Those who need Baby Blue Eyes feel unsure of themselves and are unable to trust in the goodness of others and of the world. Such individuals did not receive proper emotional support during childhood, and in particular may have lacked a healthy connection with the father or father-figure as a positive force of protection and guidance. If the father is absent, emotionally or physically, or if he is erratic and threatening (as with alcoholic violence), then the child is deprived of a basic sense of security and protection, and will grow up with a core belief that the world is an unsafe place in which to be. Such souls find it difficult to "let down their guard;" they tend to develop a protective shell of defensiveness, or intellectual cynicism. They especially find it difficult to be engaged in spiritual causes or pursuits, because they feel a lack of trust and support from the spiritual world. In extreme cases, this soul posture can lead not only to emotional isolation but also to antisocial or criminal tendencies, as the individual negates or reverses its positive spiritual connection. Baby Blue Eyes helps to restore the soul's original innocence and childlike trust. The soul is helped in its healing by learning to recognize goodness in others and in the world, and thus to become more accepting, positive and open in its expressions and actions.

Basil *Ocimum basilicum* (white)   Professional Kit

Positive qualities: Integration of sexuality and spirituality into a sacred wholeness
Patterns of imbalance: Polarization of sexuality and spirituality, often leading to clandestine behavior or marital stress

Cross-references: Addiction Adolescence Conflict Desire Escapism Intimacy
Lower Self Morality Personal Relationships Sexuality Shame Trust

The soul in need of Basil tends to polarize and separate the experience of spirituality and sexuality, believing that these cannot be integrated. This affliction is most evident in relationships where there is a compulsive need to seek sexual liaisons outside the main partnership. Quite often sexual activity is associated with that which is secret or sinful. There is also a very strong attraction to pornography and other forms of illicit or illegal sexuality. The soul feels great tension between the polarities of spiritual purity and physical sexuality. In the unconscious struggle to reconcile these forces, the soul often capitulates to or becomes enmeshed in debasing and dehumanizing sexual activity. Once these polarities are brought together as a conscious unity, the soul no longer feels compelled to separate them into opposing and destructive activities. Basil flower essence helps the soul to experience the world and the Self as truly sacred and whole.

Beech *Fagus sylvatica* (red) English Kit

Positive qualities: Tolerance, acceptance of others' differences and imperfections, seeing the good within each person and situation

Patterns of imbalance: Criticalness, judgmental attitudes, intolerance; perfectionist expectations of others; oversensitivity to one's social and physical environment

Cross-references: Acceptance Aging Blame Children Community Life and Group Experience Criticism Destructiveness Detail Dislike Environment Forgiveness Hardness Home and Lifestyle Hostility Idealism Immune Disturbances Inner Child Irritability Judgment Menopause Mother and Mothering Negativity Perfectionism Prejudice Self-Expression Sensitivity Tolerance

The Beech remedy helps transform the tendency to be critical due to an inner sense of inferiority and hypersensitivity which is projected onto others. Very often such persons grew up in an environment of criticism and harsh expectation, and so they inwardly feel very vulnerable and insecure. However, they learn to cope by condemning others instead of healing themselves. Another characteristic of this type is hypersensitivity to personal environments, both physical and social. Their permeability to the influences around them leads to intolerance of imperfection in others. Beech softens the soul pain such persons feel; as they re-establish connection with their Higher Self, they sense the love and unconditional acceptance that radiates from the spiritual world. Through this warmth of soul, they are able to let go of their harsh and blaming ways, to accept others in the same way that they are accepted by the spiritual world.

Black Cohosh *Cimicifuga racemosa* (white)   Seven Herbs Kit

Positive qualities: Courage to confront rather than retreat from abusive or threatening situations

Patterns of imbalance: Being caught in relationships or lifestyle which are abusive, addictive, violent; dark, brooding emotions

Cross-references: Abuse Addiction Catharsis Children Co-Dependence Courage Darkness Death and Dying Destructiveness Fear Feminine Consciousness Gloom Hate Masculine Consciousness Menopause Negativity Paranoia Power Rejection Sexuality Shadow Consciousness Strength

The Black Cohosh personality has the task of learning to wrestle with shadow parts in the Self and in others. These souls have positive gifts of powerful magnetism and charisma, with especially strong activity in their lower energy centers. Therefore, they naturally attract to themselves many challenging people and situations, which they must learn to confront. They often experience quite tangible feelings of threat or fear, which are well-warranted due to actual circumstances. Their personal life, or the lives of those around them, usually contain themes of violence, abuse, or addiction. Such souls can easily get caught in a vicious cycle of destructive energy. The quality of the inner life is often disturbed, tending toward brooding, vengeful, or even morbid thoughts. These imbalances can be reflected in physical illnesses, especially toxic or congested disturbances in the reproductive organs or general metabolism. Black Cohosh flower essence imparts the ability to confront and actively transform negative, destructive, or threatening circumstances. In this way such souls gain enormous power, and learn to balance and harness their innate strength and physical prowess.

Black-Eyed Susan *Rudbeckia hirta* (yellow/black center)

Professional Kit

Positive qualities: Awake consciousness capable of acknowledging all aspects of the Self; penetrating insight

Patterns of imbalance: Avoidance or repression of traumatic or painful aspects of the personality

Cross-references: Abuse Anger Avoidance Awareness Breakthrough Catalyst Catharsis Courage Darkness Death and Dying Denial Dreams and Sleep Eating Disorders Escapism Fear Healing Process Honesty Inner Child Insight Insomnia Lower Self Menopause Mid-Life Crisis Prejudice Repression Resistance Self-Esteem Shadow Consciousness Time Relationship

Black-Eyed Susan is a powerful catalyst for confronting parts of the personality or traumatic episodes from the past that have been kept locked away in the recesses of the psyche. Often these unclaimed parts of the psyche operate as shadow parts of the personality; for example, a person who was raped or abused may begin to exhibit the same behavior toward others later in life. In other instances this enormous repression does not manifest outwardly, but inwardly, in self-destructive tendencies or as mental or physical illness. In many cases Black-Eyed Susan is indicated for individuals who suffer from emotional amnesia and paralysis, and are totally unaware of the healing issues they must confront. What is needed in these circumstances is an increase of awareness; the ability to shine the light of consciousness into the shadows of the psyche. A great release of energy is felt in the soul once such buried parts of the psyche are consciously encountered and addressed in an appropriate therapeutic environment. Black-Eyed Susan restores great light and conscious awareness, helping the soul to integrate and transform unclaimed parts of the psyche.

Blackberry *Rubus ursinus* (white-pink) Professional Kit

Positive qualities: Exuberant manifestation in the world; clearly directed forces of will, decisive action

Patterns of imbalance: Inability to translate goals and ideals into concrete action or viable activities

Cross-references: Action Breakthrough Catalyst Challenge Children Community Life and Group Experience Creativity Decisiveness Desire Energetic Patterns Enthusiasm Escapism Frustration Idealism Immobility Inertia Inspiration Life Direction Manifestation Motivation Power Procrastination Resistance Self-Actualization Sluggishness Thinking Time Relationship Will Work and Career Goals

The Blackberry remedy helps the person who cannot make a viable connection with the will. The soul has many lofty visions and desires but is unable to translate these into concrete manifestation. Such people are often quite perplexed about the gap between their aims and what they actually accomplish. They give much consideration to their intentions, but lack the ability to organize these thoughts into specific priorities, or to manifest and execute such goals. Such persons often have a great deal of light around the head, which does not radiate and circulate properly throughout the body. The blood is often sluggish, as is the entire lower metabolism. As the light comes more into the limbs, the soul feels greater inner power to take real action in the world and to translate what is spiritual into actual change in the world. Blackberry flower essence bestows this radiant, awakened light to the will-life of the human soul.

Bleeding Heart *Dicentra formosa* (pink)   Professional Kit

Positive qualities: Loving others unconditionally, with an open heart; emotional freedom

Patterns of imbalance: Forming relationships based on fear or possessiveness; emotional co-dependence

Cross-references: Abandonment Acceptance Adolescence Aging
Animals and Animal Care Attachment Brokenheartedness Co-Dependence
Compassion Death and Dying Desire Destructiveness Feminine Consciousness
Freedom Grief Heart Inner Child Loneliness Love Non-Attachment
Personal Relationships Possessiveness Pregnancy Rejection Release Selfishness
Time Relationship

Bleeding Heart flower essence is a very powerful heart cleanser and strengthener for those who must learn the deeper spiritual lessons of love and freedom. Those needing this remedy suffer enormous pain and brokenheartedness because their feelings have been poured out so completely into another soul who is no longer present. Perhaps this happens because a loved one has died, or a cherished friend or family member has moved away. Most frequently, such anguish arises in personal relationships which have dissolved, or in relationships that are greatly afflicted. Although love for another may have many genuine aspects, very often the Bleeding Heart type has made the error of living too extensively outside the boundaries of its own Self. This intense desire for connection is often felt by the partner as emotional dependence, causing the partner to feel a need for distance. Such a co-dependent relationship is devoid of real freedom and a balanced exchange of heart energies. The loss and pain which are consequently felt by those in need of Bleeding Heart are therefore necessary experiences, when viewed from a larger perspective. Through Bleeding Heart flower essence, the soul learns to fill itself from within with strong spiritual forces, so that the capacity to love another is based on the ability to honor and nourish the Self.

Borage *Borago officinalis* (blue)   Professional Kit

Positive qualities: Ebullient heart forces, buoyant courage and optimism
Patterns of imbalance: Heavy-heartedness, lack of confidence in facing difficult circumstances

Cross-references: Animals and Animal Care Body Brokenheartedness Cheerfulness
Courage Death and Dying Depression and Despair Discouragement Faith Grief
Healing Process Heart Joy Lightness Manifestation Menopause Mid-Life Crisis
Pregnancy Toner

Borage is an excellent heart remedy, especially for the feeling of heaviness in the heart, and perhaps throughout the body. The "Borago" plant was originally called "Corago," referring to a state of courage associated with it. The word *courage* implies a soul quality intimately related to the heart (*cor* is Latin for heart); for it is through this energy center that one's essence is radiated outward to others. At times when the soul experiences too much grief, sadness, or other adversity, the heart can become contracted and heavy. We call this feeling "discouraged" or "disheartened." The soul needs to learn that it can counterbalance this fettered feeling in the heart by contacting that which is "light," or uplifting. Thus, the soul quality of courage is not so much connected to grit or strength, but to a condition of *buoyancy in the soul* which helps it to rise above, rather than sink into the weight of discouragement or depression. Borage flower essence helps the heart to experience this ebullience and lightness, filling the soul with fresh forces of optimism and enthusiasm. It is an excellent all-purpose balm and toner in many formulas when the soul needs upliftment and encouragement.

Buttercup *Ranunculus occidentalis* (yellow)   Professional Kit

Positive qualities: Radiant inner light, unattached to outer recognition or fame
Patterns of imbalance: Feelings of low self-worth, inability to acknowledge or experience one's inner light and uniqueness

Cross-references: Acceptance Aging Alienation Appreciation Children Co-Dependence Confidence Creativity Dislike Doubt Envy Failure Feminine Consciousness Home and Lifestyle Inadequacy Inner Child Life Direction Manifestation Menopause Mid-Life Crisis Mother and Mothering Perfectionism Personal Relationships Prejudice Pride Rejection Self-Acceptance Self-Actualization Self-Effacement Self-Esteem Self-Expression Shame Shyness Work and Career Goals

In the natural evolution of the soul there are phases of life, if not entire lifetimes, which require that one's essential light be contained in a quiet, simple way. Although such humble expressions may not appear remarkable by outer standards, they are enormously important times in which the soul gathers inward strength and consolidates its essence. It is important that such souls not judge themselves by conventional standards of achievement and success, becoming afflicted with feelings of self-doubt and diminished self-worth. Rather they need to recognize and honor the inner value and worth of who they truly are. In this way, they are able to shine forth with a radiant inner light that blesses and sanctifies even the most simple tasks and obligations. This remedy is very helpful for children, for those who may be physically handicapped or impaired, and for numerous phases and situations in the life cycle which require inner containment and simplicity. Buttercup flower essence helps the soul to realize and sustain its beautiful inner light, which becomes a source of great healing and peace for all whom it contacts.

Calendula *Calendula officinalis* (orange)   Professional Kit

Positive qualities: Healing warmth and receptivity, especially in the use of the spoken word and in dialogue with others
Patterns of imbalance: Using cutting or sharp words; argumentative, lack of receptivity in communication with others

Cross-references: Acceptance Appreciation Awareness Communication Community Life and Group Experience Compassion Conflict Destructiveness Grace Healers Impatience Intimacy Listening Masculine Consciousness Massage Non-Attachment Personal Relationships Prejudice Receptivity Self-Expression Sensitivity Sharing Softness Soothing Speaking Tolerance Warmth

The Calendula flower imparts a warm, golden light of healing for those souls who must learn to use "the Word" as a truly creative spiritual force. The Word (or Logos) is the source of all creation, ever renewing itself through the womb of Nature. Thus Calendula is also known as "Mary's Gold;" for the golden sun-radiance of the Word must be birthed through the receptive feminine matrix. In every human communication there is always this masculine and feminine polarity, of that which is spoken and that which is heard, or received. Calendula flower essence helps those whose innate creative potential to use the spoken word often deteriorates into argument and misunderstanding. It is especially indicated for personal relationship work, and for all healing and teaching work when the art of communication must be intensively developed as a soul force. Calendula gives great forces of warmth and benign compassion to the human soul, especially helping to balance the active and receptive modes of communication.

California Pitcher Plant *Darlingtonia californica* (green/purple)
Professional Kit

Positive qualities: Earthy vitality, especially integration of the more instinctual and bodily aspects of oneself
Patterns of imbalance: Feeling listless, anemic; disassociated from or even fearful of the instinctual aspects of the Self

Cross-references: Body Desire Eating Disorders Fear Instinctual Self Lower Self Power Sexuality Shadow Consciousness Strength

It is important for the human soul to learn to distinguish, yet not extinguish, its relationship to the animal world. As human beings we have the capacity for self-awareness and self-reflection, but through these very gifts we can also alienate ourselves from what appears to be "lower" or more instinctual. California Pitcher Plant, which is carnivorous (insect eating) and grows in boggy areas, is indicated for people who are unable to integrate their animal-like instinctual desires with their sense of human individuality. This results in a splitting off of their desire-nature, or astrality, from the physical-etheric vehicle. Such a condition can manifest as a weakness in physical vigor and strength, and especially as an inability to digest food (assimilate physical matter). At other times these same, unintegrated astral forces can work too independently through the unconscious as a shadow force, especially distorting or dehumanizing the soul's experience of sexuality. California Pitcher Plant helps the soul to harness and balance the immense forces of astrality and instinctual desire so that these energies can strengthen physical vitality, and serve human spirituality.

California Poppy *Eschscholzia californica* (gold) Professional Kit

Positive qualities: Finding spirituality within one's heart; balancing light and love; developing an inner center of knowing

Patterns of imbalance: Seeking outside oneself for false forms of light or higher consciousness, especially through escapism or addiction

Cross-references: Addiction Adolescence Balance Community Life and Group Experience Denial Desire Escapism Fanaticism Harmony Honesty Materialism and Money Meditation Morality Restlessness Seeking Spiritual Emergency or Opening Time Relationship Wisdom Work and Career Goals

The saying "all that glitters is not gold" is an apt one to describe the lesson of the California Poppy. Many times when the soul first opens to an expanded vista of spirituality, it is pulled in the direction of Luciferic light. Such light appears to be beneficial, but it actually stuns and dazes the soul, robbing it of its own inner power. Those who need the California Poppy seek spiritual glamour or enticing psychic experiences outside themselves, rather than engaging in a balanced process of spiritual and moral development. They can be attracted to a vast spectrum of dazzling phenomena, including drug use (especially psychedelic drugs), occult ritual, religious cults, or charismatic teachers. The soul can also be mesmerized by social glamour and fame, and become easily immersed in the life of media stars, and many other fleeting fads or causes. Such souls have the "wide-eyed" expectation that the spiritual gold which they seek can be found somewhere outside themselves. Because they do not strengthen and develop a solid inner life, they are often susceptible to techniques or influences which open the psychic faculties too rapidly, especially before these energies are balanced with the heart and thinking forces. California Poppy stabilizes the golden light of the heart, encouraging more self-responsibility and quiet inner development. In this way the soul finds the true treasure it seeks — the radiant sun force of the awakened human heart.

California Wild Rose *Rosa californica* (pink)   Professional Kit

Positive qualities: Love for the Earth and for human life, enthusiasm for doing and serving

Patterns of imbalance: Apathy or resignation, inability to catalyze will forces through the heart

Cross-references: Adolescence Aging Alienation Aloofness Altruism Ambivalence Apathy Appreciation Body Brokenheartedness Challenge Cheerfulness Children Choice Community Life and Group Experience Cynicism Depression and Despair Dullness Earth Healing and Nature Awareness Eating Disorders Energetic Patterns Enthusiasm Escapism Exhaustion and Fatigue Faith Groundedness Healing Process Heart Idealism Inner Child Involvement Learning Difficulties Life Direction Love Manifestation Mid-Life Crisis Motivation Personal Relationships Pessimism Pregnancy Rejuvenation Resistance Time Relationship Toner Vitality Warmth Will Work and Career Goals

California Wild Rose is among the most beautiful and fundamental of flower remedies, for it helps the soul to incarnate and really take hold of its responsibilities and tasks on Earth. It is often said that hate is not the opposite of love, only a distortion of it. Rather, it is apathy which is the true polarity of love. The ability to really care and to give oneself to life, to others, and to the Earth characterizes a truly loving soul. Many souls hold back or hesitate, not wanting to experience the pain or challenge of life on Earth. They find it hard to take emotional risks in relationships with others, preferring instead to anesthetize themselves from pain or suffering. Such souls can also suffer from deep-seated social alienation, being unable to rouse the inner fire of the heart toward compassionate caring and activity in the world. California Wild Rose is a very beneficial remedy for all stages of the life biography, and can be particularly helpful for adolescent and young adult life when the soul most especially longs to find its positive ideals, and seeks to serve the world through its life calling or vocation. California Wild Rose stimulates the love forces of the heart, so that the soul finds enthusiasm for earthly life, worldly tasks and human relationships.

Calla Lily *Zantedeschia aethiopica* (white/yellow) Research Kit

Positive qualities: Clarity about sexual identity, sexual self-acceptance; balance of masculine and feminine qualities

Patterns of imbalance: Confusion, ambivalence about sexual identity or gender

Cross-references: Acceptance Adolescence Alienation Ambivalence Balance Children Envy False Persona Feminine Consciousness Inner Child Insecurity Masculine Consciousness Pregnancy Self-Esteem Sexuality Shame

The beautiful Calla Lily helps those souls who are deeply troubled by their sexual gender. Many times such people have a strong, though usually unconscious, memory of dwelling in the spiritual world where sexual gender is not divided between male and female, but is a perfectly balanced androgynous state. It is therefore very difficult for such individuals to feel at home on Earth. In some instances requiring Calla Lily, the soul may have favored one gender over the other in a series of lifetimes, which now must be balanced for further evolution. At other times, individuals may have been born into a karmic situation in which the parents strongly preferred a particular gender, or where the person does not fit into social conventions about sexuality. These mixed messages about sexual identity cause great confusion and anguish. Calla Lily helps the soul to bring about its right orientation to sexuality, and at a higher level, to integrate the qualities of male and female in a harmonious expression. Calla Lily teaches that masculine and feminine are soul qualities which can be united within the individual, rather than simply external, physical or biological traits. In this way the personality evolves toward greater balance and harmonious soul expression.

Canyon Dudleya *Dudleya cymosa* (orange)   Research Kit

Positive qualities: Healthy spiritual opening, balanced psychic and physical energies; grounded presence in everyday life; positive charisma

Patterns of imbalance: Distorted psychic experiences; preoccupied with mediumism; overinflated involvement in psychic or charismatic experiences

Cross-references: Addiction Attachment Avoidance Calm Centeredness Community Life and Group Experience Egotism Emergency Energetic Patterns Escapism False Persona Fanaticism Feminine Consciousness Groundedness Healing Process Home and Lifestyle Honesty Hysteria Inner Child Martyrdom Menopause Moderation Mother and Mothering Nervousness Overwhelm Perspective Prejudice Psychosomatic Illness Relaxation Restlessness Self-Aggrandizement Seriousness Speaking Spiritual Emergency or Opening Work and Career Goals

Although the soul needs to experience emotional depth, it must guard against the temptation to inflate the emotional and psychic life, or to confuse it with true spiritual experience. Canyon Dudleya is indicated for those who need to bring more order, especially in the sense of "ordinariness," to the soul life. These souls have a great wealth of physical and emotional vitality which needs to be properly harnessed and harmonized by the spiritual ego. The temptation of such persons is to evade quiet, sustained development of the spiritual life in favor of intense, overly dramatic psychic-emotional experiences, which appear to be more real or more important than they truly are. Such persons can be easily attracted to mediumism, channeling, occult experimentation, or charismatic experiences which whip up the emotions or psychic fantasies. They are prone to neglect basic responsibilities, or the practical, simple ordering of their daily activities. Canyon Dudleya essence helps such a person to feel the quiet soul nourishment which is gained by appreciating the value of daily life experiences and relationships. Through realizing inner contentment, the soul does not need to stimulate itself excessively with psychic experience. Canyon Dudleya guides the soul towards more balanced spiritual opening and contained emotional presence.

Cayenne *Capsicum annuum* (white) — Professional Kit

Positive qualities: Fiery and energetic, inwardly mobile, capable of change and transformation
Patterns of imbalance: Stagnation, inability to move forward toward change

Cross-references: Action Breakthrough Catalyst Catharsis Decisiveness Energetic Patterns Enthusiasm Habit Patterns Immobility Inertia Manifestation Motivation Procrastination Resistance Sluggishness Spontaneity Time Relationship Warmth Will Work and Career Goals

Cayenne flower essence provides a catalytic spark to the soul who may be stagnating in its growth cycle. Such individuals become overly phlegmatic and complacent, not really challenging themselves with new experiences or stimulus. At other times, there may be a quality of simply feeling stuck or immobilized, unable to make real progress or change, or being caught in a pattern of procrastination and resistance. Cayenne is an important general remedy for many life circumstances, as well as in many therapeutic processes. It stimulates an energetic response in the body and soul, helping to overcome apparent blocks to progress and transformation. Cayenne ignites and sparks the soul with its fiery essence. The individual becomes more awake, and more capable of initiating and sustaining spiritual and emotional development.

Centaury *Centaurium erythaea* (pink) — English Kit
also known as *Centaurium umbellatum*

Positive qualities: Serving others from inner strength, with a healthy recognition of one's own needs; acting from strength of inner purpose, saying "No" when appropriate
Patterns of imbalance: Weak-willed, dominated by others, servile, acting to please; difficulty saying "No," neglecting one's own needs

Cross-references: Abuse Aging Authority Children Co-Dependence Compassion Desire Dutifulness Freedom Healers Idealism Individuality Influence Inner Child Manifestation Martyrdom Mother and Mothering Perfectionism Power Prejudice Repression Responsibility Self-Actualization Self-Effacement Self-Esteem Service Sharing Strength Surrender True to Self Vulnerability Will Work and Career Goals

The healthy soul needs to learn to balance its ego forces between the polarities of servitude and selfishness. Those who require Centaury lack sufficient ego strength, not realizing that the ability to give to and serve others requires a strong and radiant inner sense of Self. Such souls are easily depleted and devitalized; and more importantly, they lack a vibrant individuality which is so necessary for soul evolution. These persons are often under the illusion that they are being loving and helpful, but in reality they are not strong enough in their will forces to say "No," or to resist exploitation by others. Their vulnerability lies in their reliance on pleasing others to receive self-validation. Thus the compulsion to serve others is misplaced, for such a person neglects his or her own needs and cannot perceive the true, objective needs of others. In this way the Centaury type retards not only its own soul growth, but also the progress of those who need to learn from him or her. Centaury gives beneficial strength and integrity to such personalities, helping them to assume greater self-awareness and self-responsibility.

Cerato *Ceratostigma willmottiana* (blue) English Kit

Positive qualities: Trusting one's inner knowing, intuition; self-confidence, certainty

Patterns of imbalance: Uncertainty or doubt of oneself; invalidating what one knows, over-dependent on advice from others

Cross-references: Anxiety Authority Certainty Choice Co-Dependence Confidence Decisiveness Doubt Eating Disorders Healing Process Hesitation Indecision Influence Inner Child Judgment Manifestation Morality Perfectionism Pregnancy Resistance Seeking Self-Esteem Trust Wisdom

There are times when the soul feels cut off from its own inner truth and therefore does not develop enough self-reliance. Cerato flower essence helps such persons to translate their already considerable spiritual abilities into active decision-making. This process requires that other spiritual beings have less influence, prompting the soul to develop independent judgment. At first this comes as a shock and such persons do not feel confident enough to make their own decisions, turning instead to others for advice and counsel. While seeking advice can be beneficial in many instances, it is regressive for those who need to develop a stronger sense of their own spirituality and wisdom. Cerato develops the ability to trust one's inner knowing, facilitating innate spiritual wisdom and strength. In this way, the soul becomes more confident and certain of its true Self.

Chamomile

(white/yellow center)   Professional Kit

German Chamomile *Matricaria chamomilla*
Wild Chamomile *Anthemis cotula*

Positive qualities: Serene, sun-like disposition, emotional balance
Patterns of imbalance: Easily upset, moody and irritable, inability to release emotional tension

Cross-references: Addiction Adolescence Anger Animals and Animal Care Anxiety Brokenheartedness Calm Children Depression and Despair Eating Disorders Emergency Harmony Hysteria Insomnia Irritability Learning Difficulties Massage Nervousness Overwhelm Perfectionism Personal Relationships Pregnancy Quiet Relaxation Release Sensitivity Soothing Stress Tension

When we say that someone has a sunny disposition, we inherently recognize that such a soul has a harmonious emotional life. Like the sun which shines with constancy for all to see, so the soul must learn to regulate and harmonize its emotional life. Those needing Chamomile flower essence are subject to very changeable moods and ever-fluctuating emotions. Their "inner weather" is stormy and easily "clouded" until they shift their consciousness to remember that the sun is always shining serenely behind all the outer phenomena. People needing Chamomile tend to accumulate psychic tension throughout the day, particularly in the stomach region. They will often have difficulty letting go of their emotional stress at night, and thus suffer from insomnia. This is particularly true of children, whose myriad stomach complaints are often emotionally based. Chamomile helps such souls to release tension from the stomach and solar plexus areas, and to harmonize their inner solar forces for greater emotional peace and stability. It subdues the many small emotions which vex the soul life, helping to consolidate these into a more fundamental soul essence of serenity and equanimity.

Chaparral *Larrea tridentata* (yellow)   Professional Kit
also known as Creosote Bush

Positive qualities: Balanced psychic awareness, deep penetration and understanding of the transpersonal aspects of oneself
Patterns of imbalance: Psychic and physical toxicity, disturbed dreams; chaotic inner life, drug addiction

Cross-references: Addiction Awareness Catharsis City Life Cleansing Dreams and Sleep Insomnia Purification Repression Sensitivity

The psyche is very impressionable and absorbent — it takes in far more than the conscious mind can assimilate. The dream life acts as an important filter for the soul, digesting disturbing or chaotic experiences which may be too powerful to contact consciously. Chaparral is an important psychic and physical cleanser which is indicated when the soul has been overexposed to actual violence or disturbing images in the media. It is also a very beneficial remedy for drug detoxification, including heavy use of medical or psychiatric drugs. Drug use expands the psychic boundaries but diminishes and distorts the awake consciousness. Therefore the individual is plagued with enormous astral-emotional debris which lodges in the subconscious mind, and which must be cleansed for complete recovery. Chaparral is a very beneficial remedy for modern civilization when the soul is subject in so many ways to chaotic, violent and degrading images and experiences. It is broadly applicable, but works especially through the dream life to cleanse the psyche.

Cherry Plum *Prunus cerasifera* (white) English Kit

Positive qualities: Spiritual surrender and trust, feeling guided and protected by a Higher Power; balance and equanimity despite extreme stress
Patterns of imbalance: Fear of losing control, or of mental and emotional breakdown; desperate, destructive impulses

Cross-references: Animals and Animal Care   Destructiveness   Eating Disorders Emergency   Faith   Fear   Hysteria   Inner Child   Mother and Mothering   Nervousness Overwhelm   Pregnancy   Release   Stress   Surrender   Trust

There are times when the soul has difficulty bearing the weight of its incarnation. The circumstances of life oppress and condense the soul, so that it literally feels that it cannot take any more pressure or stress. There is the fear that one will lose control and become erratic, destructive, or even suicidal or insane. The soul tries to protect against this fear of losing control by tightening its grip, which only leads to more pressure and stress. At these extreme times, Cherry Plum is indicated. It helps the individual to re-connect with the Higher Self, to surrender ("Let go and let God"). Once the Self renews its trust in a Higher Power, the mind can then stabilize, and the individual feels the capacity to cope with life's challenges again. Cherry Plum flower essence brings strength and encouragement, helping the soul to overcome its extreme tension and fear.

Chestnut Bud *Aesculus hippocastanum* (green buds)   English Kit

Positive qualities: Learning the lessons of life experience, understanding the laws of karma; wisdom

Patterns of imbalance: Poor observation of life, failure to learn from experience; repeating mistakes

Cross-references: Addiction   Animals and Animal Care   Awakeness   Awareness
Children   Denial   Eating Disorders   Energetic Patterns   Escapism   Freedom
Habit Patterns   Healing Process   Inertia   Insight   Learning Difficulties   Manifestation
Morality   Release   Resistance   Study   Synthesis   Time Relationship   Wisdom

Three of the Chestnut remedies (Chestnut Bud, Red Chestnut, White Chestnut) address obsessive-compulsive behavior in the personality. Chestnut Bud is used to help break free of overly repetitive and habitual patterns which retard the soul's full development. It is indicated where there is a constant repetition of life experience without the ability of the soul to glean wisdom and insight. Chestnut Bud particularly stimulates the cognitive capacities so that the individual is able to grasp more completely and more rapidly the essential nature of the experience at hand, and learn the appropriate lessons. In this way, the individual is freed from the compulsive need to repeat mistakes and re-create regressive patterns. This remedy is obviously helpful in many learning situations, and is also useful in a broader way when the soul needs to break through deeply resistant karmic patterns.

Chicory *Cichorium intybus* (blue)   English Kit

Positive qualities: Selfless love given freely, respecting the freedom and individuality of others

Patterns of imbalance: Expressing love by being possessive, demanding, and needy; getting attention through negative behavior; self-centeredness

Cross-references: Abandonment   Aging   Altruism   Animals and Animal Care
Attachment   Attention   Children   Co-Dependence   Egotism   Inner Child   Irritability
Love   Manifestation   Martyrdom   Mother and Mothering   Personal Relationships
Possessiveness   Power   Rejection   Release   Responsibility   Self-Concern   Selfishness
Sharing

Chicory is a very important remedy for emotional congestion and misdirected love forces. Those in need of this essence must learn to distinguish between personal emotions and desires, and genuine impersonal love and caring for another.

Otherwise, the individual becomes selfish rather than selfless, manipulating the emotions of others for his or her own needs and desires. The energy which would ordinarily flow out from one's heart is thwarted, so that emotions of self-pity, neediness and even martyrdom are experienced. A guise of seemingly loving behavior is very often used as an inappropriate way of soliciting and manipulating the psychic energy and attention of others. Particularly with children, the Chicory pattern manifests as negative attention-getting, fussiness and tantrums which pull on the other members of the family. Chicory flower essence nourishes the inner neediness of such souls and helps to re-balance and re-direct psychic currents of energy, especially as they flow through the heart and solar plexus.

Chrysanthemum *Chrysanthemum morifolium* (red-brown)
Research Kit

Positive qualities: Shifting the ego identification from one's personality to a higher spiritual identity; feeling oneself as transpersonal and transcendent
Patterns of imbalance: Fear of aging and mortality, identification with youth and lower personality; mid-life crisis

Cross-references: Acceptance Addiction Aging Alienation Anxiety Attachment Avoidance Courage Death and Dying Denial Depression and Despair Egotism Escapism False Persona Father and Fathering Fear Greed Individuality Life Direction Lower Self Materialism and Money Mid-Life Crisis Non-Attachment Nostalgia Power Release Resistance Self-Actualization Selfishness True to Self

The soul-spiritual part of ourselves is immortal; it chooses to continuously grow and evolve by incarnating in a particular body and expression of personality. If the soul loses connection with its true immortality, or if it overinflates the importance of a particular life, there will be great fear and avoidance of physical death. Such a soul has a psychological need to firmly establish its personality in the world as a defense against death and mortality. He or she seeks fame and fortune and falls too deeply into the forces of materialism. The spiritual part of the soul is often obliterated or blocked, although it will attempt to make its presence known through a strong awareness crisis (for instance, at mid-life), through a life-threatening illness, or through death itself. The Chrysanthemum flower gives such souls the ability to contact the true spiritual ego, and to contemplate the impermanent nature of earthly affairs in the light of the Higher Self.

Clematis *Clematis vitalba* (white)   English Kit

Positive qualities: Awake, focused presence; manifesting inspiration in practical life; embodiment
Patterns of imbalance: Avoidance of the present by daydreaming; other-worldly and impractical ideals

Cross-references: Addiction Aging Attention Avoidance Awakeness Body Children Concentration and Focus Daydreaming Disorientation Dreams and Sleep Earth Healing and Nature Awareness Escapism Groundedness Idealism Learning Difficulties Manifestation Procrastination Resistance Scatteredness Time Relationship

The soul in need of Clematis has a strong inner life; the ability to image and dream is particularly well-developed. But these capacities are so strong that they overwhelm and distort the soul's connection with the body and the concrete physical world. This results in a personality that is overly dreamy, lacking a vibrant emotional and physical presence in the here-and-now. Thus the great talents of the Clematis types are largely untapped, and physical illness easily takes hold of the body because the warm forces of the ego are lacking. In extreme states such souls will be attracted to drugs, particularly psychotropic drugs, in order to continue the soul's addiction to disincarnated psychic activity. Clematis helps such persons to realize that the great gifts within them can be constructively channeled into the physical world; in this way the soul forces grow warmer, richer, and more present for others.

Corn *Zea mays* (yellow-white)   Professional Kit

Positive qualities: Alignment with the Earth, especially through the body and feet; grounded presence
Patterns of imbalance: Inability to stay centered in the body; disorientation and stress, particularly in urban environments

Cross-references: Balance Body Centeredness City Life Disorientation Earth Healing and Nature Awareness Environment Feminine Consciousness Groundedness Mother and Mothering Overwhelm Pregnancy Spiritual Emergency or Opening

The Corn essence addresses the soul's need for spaciousness — its desire to live freely within the vast matrix of Nature and Cosmos. It is especially helpful for those ancient souls who find it extremely painful to "contract" into the modern conditions of living. They naturally prefer rural or uncrowded areas where they can feel in harmonious communion with the Earth. But these persons must also grow and evolve, learning how to make the body itself a microcosm of the Earth. The whole body, but especially the hands and feet, must learn to radiate this grounded spirituality. Without this shift in consciousness, the natural healing and teaching capacities which many of these souls harbor within them are never fully realized. Such individuals feel a great deal of pain and discomfort in the congestion and chaos of urban and technological environments or in any restricted living situations; and yet it is often necessary for them to experience just these conditions in order to promote the transition from a macrocosmic to microcosmic soul consciousness. Corn helps to balance and guide the soul in expressing its vast spiritual nature through the limitations of the physical world and physical body.

Cosmos *Cosmos bipinnatus* (red-purple/yellow) Research Kit

Positive qualities: Integration of ideas and speech; ability to express thoughts with coherence and clarity
Patterns of imbalance: Unfocused, disorganized communication; overexcited speech, overwhelmed by too many ideas

Cross-references: Animals and Animal Care   Awakeness   Awareness   Calm Communication   Concentration and Focus   Creativity   Disorientation   Dullness   Hysteria Impatience   Inspiration   Intellectualism   Learning Difficulties   Lightness   Mental Clarity Nervousness   Overwhelm   Self-Actualization   Self-Esteem   Self-Expression   Speaking Study   Synthesis   Thinking   True to Self   Wisdom

Cosmos helps those souls whose higher mental bodies are not properly integrated with the speaking and thinking functions of the nervous system. Such individuals often feel frustrated and overwhelmed as they attempt to convey the true inspiration of their Higher Self through their thoughts and especially through their speech. These persons can be flooded by too much information, rendering the speech patterns rapid and inarticulate; or the thoughts may be superficially glib but lacking in deeper concepts. In extreme cases the speech may actually become dulled and the soul forces introverted, as the personality no longer makes contact with the higher mental function. Cosmos harmonizes the thinking and speaking patterns with the higher soul functions, so that the true spirit can shine forth from the personality.

Crab Apple *Malus sylvestris* (white, tinged with pink)   English Kit

Positive qualities: Cleansing, bringing a sense of inner purity
Patterns of imbalance: Feeling unclean and impure, obsessed with imperfection

Cross-references: Acceptance Adolescence Body Cleansing Criticism Destructiveness Detail Dislike Earth Healing and Nature Awareness Eating Disorders Emergency Environment Hate Healing Process Home and Lifestyle Immune Disturbances Irritability Manifestation Massage Materialism and Money Menopause Morality Obsession Perfectionism Purification Rejection Self-Acceptance Self-Concern Sexuality Shame

The apple has strong mythological associations with Paradise, and of being cast out of Paradise. Indeed, the personality needing Crab Apple has difficulty accepting the imperfections of the physical plane. This manifests as rejection or disgust, and at its deepest level, a feeling of shame for the physical body and its imperfections. Such individuals are obsessively preoccupied with impurities, whether real or imagined. These feelings are also projected onto the environment, with an aversion to anything dirty or out of perfect order. It follows that such souls are prone to allergies and many forms of psychosomatic illness, because the body feels overwhelmed by the soul's impossibly high standards of perfection. While Crab Apple is indicated for those whose concern for cleanliness is inordinate, it can also be used in a general way for any activity of purification, such as fasting. This flower essence instills a balanced relationship of the soul to the body and to life on Earth, helping one to realize that it is only through suffering the pain of imperfection that the soul is afforded the possibility of true evolution, rather than static perfection.

Dandelion *Taraxacum officinale* (yellow)   Professional Kit

Positive qualities: Dynamic, effortless energy; lively activity balanced with inner ease
Patterns of imbalance: Overly tense, especially in the musculature of the body, overstriving and hard-driving

Cross-references: Body Grief Hardness Heart Masculine Consciousness Massage Mid-Life Crisis Perfectionism Relaxation Release Repression Resistance Study Tension Time Relationship Work and Career Goals

The soul needing Dandelion essence feels a natural intensity and love for life. Such individuals are compulsive "doers" who enter with great zeal and zest into many activities. Unfortunately, they can over-plan and over-form their lives beyond the natural capacity of the body to sustain such intensity. Furthermore, such persons may become unable to experience more contained moments of reflective activity. The unexpressed inner life of the soul and the harsh demands on the body collide to create extreme tension, especially in the musculature. The Dandelion flower teaches these individuals how to listen more closely to emotional messages and bodily needs. As tension is released the soul feels more inner ease and balance, allowing spiritual forces to flow *through* the body in a dynamic, effortless way.

Deerbrush *Ceanothus integerrimus* (white)   Professional Kit

Positive qualities: Gentle purity, clarity of purpose; sincerity of motive
Patterns of imbalance: Mixed or conflicting motives; subconscious feelings which propel outer actions

Cross-references: Clarity Cleansing Communication Denial Desire
Earth Healing and Nature Awareness Escapism Grace Guilt Healers Morality
Motivation Prejudice Purification Softness Soulfulness

It is essential that the soul acquire inner truthfulness, acting with clear intention and nobility of purpose. Deception and illusion are great stumbling blocks along the path of soul initiation. Self-observation demands constant inner scrutiny by the personality, in order to align inner motive with outer deed. As much as we may be wary of others who deceive us, it is far more often that we deceive ourselves by lack of honesty in our relationships with others and in the countless affairs of daily life. Deerbrush helps the soul to attain purity; not the purity which is associated with a set of moral dictates, but consonance of mind and heart with motive and deed. As the soul grows in its ability to realize inner virtue, the outer actions become more resonant with the inner being. Such persons radiate truth and harmony, and heal others by their very presence.

Dill *Anethum graveolens* (yellow) Professional Kit

Positive qualities: Experiencing and absorbing the fullness of life, especially its sensory aspects
Patterns of imbalance: Overwhelm due to overstimulation, hypersensitivity to environment or to outer activity, sensory congestion

Cross-references: Animals and Animal Care   Awakeness   City Life   Clarity
Earth Healing and Nature Awareness   Eating Disorders   Emergency   Insomnia   Irritability
Moderation   Overwhelm   Relaxation   Restlessness   Stress

The cacophony of modern living conditions can stun, and even stifle, the sensory capacities of most persons. With the advent of the technological age, the soul is literally bombarded with countless sense impressions — what one sees, hears, tastes, smells and touches in the course of a day can be quite staggering. Soul hygiene requires that these sensorial impressions be assimilated; otherwise psychic indigestion and nervous overwhelm result. In prior times, those who wished to develop spiritually sought remote environments and ascetic living conditions which diminished sensorial stimulation and freed the soul for higher spiritual work. Dill flower essence helps to harmonize the psychic life within the context of daily work and modern living. Through the Dill flower, the soul learns not only to discriminate and regulate sense experience, but even more importantly to allow *the sense life itself to become a vehicle for enlightenment*. Rather than being dulled and subdued, the senses can be refined and clarified, becoming ever more luminous and transparent. By consciously encountering sensory experience, a new kind of clairvoyance and clairsentience arises in the modern soul. Dill flower essence assists the soul in transforming sensory overwhelm into an ability to perceive the sense world as a manifestation of spiritual archetypes.

Dogwood *Cornus nuttallii* (yellow/white bracts) Professional Kit

Positive qualities: Grace-filled movement, physical and etheric harmony
Patterns of imbalance: Awkward and painful awareness of the body; emotional trauma stored deep within the body

Cross-references: Abuse   Awkwardness   Body   Children   Communication   Creativity
Destructiveness   Erratic Behavior   Flexibility   Grace   Hardness   Inner Child   Massage
Rejection   Release   Sexuality   Softness

When we say that a soul is full of grace, we are referring to a particular fullness and flexibility of the etheric body, the most immediate sheath which surrounds the physical body. If there is repeated violation to the body — either through physical or sexual abuse, or by very harsh physical and materialistic living circumstances — the etheric body shrivels, and consequently the physical body hardens. The soul suffers greatly from an inability to live properly within the physical-etheric body. The emotions can become hardened, and the body is felt as awkward and ungainly. Quite often such a person unconsciously repeats earlier patterns of degradation by choosing abusive relationships or exhibiting self-destructive or accident-prone tendencies. The beautiful Dogwood flower essence helps to expand the etheric body and soften the physical body. The individual is able to feel more gentleness and inner sanctity, as the soul regains its state of grace through harmonious communion with the life or etheric body.

Easter Lily *Lilium longiflorum* (white)   Seven Herbs Kit

Positive qualities: Inner purity of soul, especially the ability to integrate sexuality and spirituality
Patterns of imbalance: Feeling that sexuality is impure, unclean; inner conflicts about sexuality

Cross-references: Ambivalence Cleansing Conflict Desire Feminine Consciousness Instinctual Self Lower Self Menopause Morality Pregnancy Purification Sexuality Shame

The white lily has long been a symbol of purity, as well as sexuality and child-bearing. It is extremely challenging for the soul to integrate the sexual life with the spiritual life. For good reason, many spiritual paths require celibacy as a condition of spiritual development. It is possible, however, for modern souls to reconcile these seeming polarities; in fact, new and important soul capacities will emerge as a result. Easter Lily is an important remedy to help those individuals who feel a great inner tension between their sexuality and spirituality. These conflicts can be in either direction — towards promiscuity which degrades and damages the astral body, or towards prudishness which severs the soul from the life forces of the lower body. It is an especially important remedy for women, and can help when there are impurities and disturbances in the sexual and reproductive organs. The most fundamental gift of the Easter Lily is to enable the soul to fully utilize the psychic energy currents which are associated with the sexual and reproductive organs.

Echinacea *Echinacea purpurea* (pink/purple) Research Kit

Positive qualities: Core integrity, contacting and maintaining an integrated sense of Self, especially when severely challenged

Patterns of imbalance: Feeling shattered by severe trauma or abuse which has destroyed one's sense of Self; threatened by physical or emotional disintegration

Cross-references: Abuse Children Earth Healing and Nature Awareness Emergency Exhaustion and Fatigue Healing Process Immune Disturbances Individuality Inner Child Loneliness Menopause Rejection Self-Acceptance Self-Actualization Self-Esteem Shock Strength Transcendence True to Self

One of the most important initiations in the contemporary life of the soul is that of coming in right relationship to the Self, or spiritual ego. While inflation of the ego can be a formidable problem, there are equally devastating assaults to the positive spiritual identity of the human being. Until recent times, family, community, and Nature have provided the context for a certain kind of self-identity. But the increasing anonymity of modern civilization, along with countless other mechanizing and alienating forces, leaves many souls bereft of earthly or human nourishment. More importantly, acts of crime, violence, and sexual or emotional degradation, often beginning even in early childhood, shatter the dignity of the Self. Many souls live a phantom-like existence, seeming to have a functioning persona when in fact only a meager connection to the true spiritual Self exists. This is one of the underlying reasons, at the level of soul reality, for the vast outbreak of immune-related diseases. Echinacea flower essence stimulates and awakens the true inner Self. This is a fundamental remedy for many soul and physical illnesses, especially when the individual has experienced shattering and destructive forces. Echinacea restores the soul's true self-identity and essential dignity, in relationship to the Earth and to the human family.

Elm *Ulmus procera* (reddish brown) English Kit

Positive qualities: Joyous service, faith and confidence to complete one's task
Patterns of imbalance: Overwhelmed by duties and responsibilities, feeling unequal to the task required

Cross-references: Altruism Ambition Anxiety Challenge Children Co-Dependence Community Life and Group Experience Confidence Depression and Despair Dutifulness Exhaustion and Fatigue Failure Father and Fathering Guilt Inadequacy Inner Child Leadership Loneliness Martyrdom Masculine Consciousness Mid-Life Crisis Mother and Mothering Overwhelm Perfectionism Relaxation Responsibility Stress Time Relationship Work and Career Goals

The healthy soul expresses itself by wanting to care for and serve others, but at times this positive altruistic impulse can be stymied. Becoming responsible requires that one rightly assesses one's "ability to respond." Over-perfectionist or unrealistic goals can result in fatigue and overwhelm at a later point when the individual is simply unable to measure up to the tasks assumed. Feelings of self-doubt, despondency, and deep feelings of loneliness can set in when the soul feels it must face an overwhelming task relying solely on its own ego forces. It is necessary at these times to shift the identity from that of hero or rescuer to an alignment with the true energy and inspiration of the Higher Self. In this way the individual is able to receive help from others and from the spiritual world. Elm balances the natural leadership capacities within the soul, especially by integrating these with the true directives of the Higher Self.

Evening Primrose *Onenothera hookeri* (yellow)   Research Kit

Positive qualities: Awareness and healing of painful early emotions absorbed from the mother; ability to open emotionally and form deep, committed relationships

Patterns of imbalance: Feeling rejected, unwanted; avoidance of commitment in relationships, fear of parenthood; sexual and emotional repression

Cross-references: Abandonment Abuse Alienation Ambivalence Avoidance Barriers Catharsis Children Cleansing Courage Dreams and Sleep Eating Disorders Escapism Feminine Consciousness Grief Inadequacy Inner Child Insecurity Intimacy Involvement Loneliness Mother and Mothering Personal Relationships Pregnancy Purification Rejection Release Repression Self-Esteem Sexuality

The soul is most open, and receives its first impressions of life on Earth, while in utero or in very early infancy. At this time it is more of a moon-like being than a sun-being, receiving and reflecting the soul light of the parents, especially the mother. These early experiences of light and love are as formative for emotional development as proper nutrition is for the physical fetus. If the soul is neglected or abused while in utero or in very early infancy, a profound and deeply unconscious feeling of pain and rejection resides in the individual. Such persons feel unwanted and often cope by avoiding deep emotional contact or bonding; they retain a moon-like coldness in their souls and are unable to radiate warmth and love from their own center. There can also be a deeply repressed aversion to sexuality, particularly if the reproductive act which brought in the incarnating child was filled with turmoil, violence, or debased lust. Evening Primrose helps to catalyze the emotional awareness of such souls, especially regarding the original, core incarnation experiences which were so devastating. Evening Primrose literally rebirths the soul, providing a matrix of emotional nutrients that were lacking in the soul's earliest feelings about incarnation.

Fairy Lantern *Calochortus albus* (white)   Research Kit

Positive qualities: Healthy maturation; acceptance of adult responsibilities
Patterns of imbalance: Immaturity, helplessness, neediness, childish dependency; unable to take responsibility

Cross-references: Acceptance Addiction Adolescence Alienation Ambivalence
Authority Avoidance Body Children Co-Dependence Confidence Eating Disorders
Escapism False Persona Father and Fathering Fear Feminine Consciousness Freedom
Healing Process Hesitation Home and Lifestyle Inadequacy Individuality Inner Child
Insecurity Life Direction Masculine Consciousness Menopause Mid-Life Crisis
Mother and Mothering Nostalgia Personal Relationships Power Resistance
Responsibility Self-Effacement Self-Esteem Seriousness Sexuality Strength
True to Self Work and Career Goals

The early developmental process of childhood is critical for the human soul. When this is disturbed, many problems will manifest which inhibit full adult maturation. The soul who needs Fairy Lantern still clings to a childlike personality. In some instances, the true identity of the child was suppressed during its development and not allowed its rightful expression. More frequently, the parents or other family members excessively reinforce or restrict the personality in its identity as an immature child. Such a person learns that she or he will receive love only by remaining in an arrested, over-dependent childlike state. These souls become delicate and needy, lacking in inner strength to face the world or shoulder responsibility. They play the role of the *puer eterna* (eternal child) who needs to unconsciously repeat childhood throughout adult life, hoping to somehow transform this arrested stage of development. Fairy Lantern can also be used during childhood and adolescence for retarded phases of physical or emotional development. Fairy Lantern helps souls to move through these emotional blocks in the maturation process by maintaining a healthy relationship to the inner child, but as a fully functioning, mature adult.

Fawn Lily *Erythronium purpurascens* (yellow with purple)   Research Kit

Positive qualities: Accepting and becoming involved with the world; sharing one's spiritual gifts with others

Patterns of imbalance: Withdrawal, isolation, self-protection; overly delicate, lacking the inner strength to face the world

Cross-references: Acceptance Alienation Aloofness Ambivalence Avoidance Balance Barriers Body Children City Life Community Life and Group Experience Compassion Conflict Courage Daydreaming Devitalization Eating Disorders Escapism Father and Fathering Fear Feminine Consciousness Groundedness Heart Home and Lifestyle Idealism Intimacy Involvement Love Meditation Mother and Mothering Perfectionism Psychosomatic Illness Self-Concern Selfishness Service Sharing Spiritual Emergency or Opening Vitality Warmth Work and Career Goals

Souls in need of Fawn Lily have very highly developed forces of spirituality, so much so that it is difficult for them to cope with the stresses and strains of modern society. Such persons are naturally inclined to states of contemplation, meditation, and prayer. It is easier for them to stay in these modes of spirituality, rather than to be involved with the world. However, the soul can become overripe and overdeveloped in its spirituality. Such persons need to disseminate the great gifts which have accumulated in their beings in order to evolve and progress; otherwise they become too introverted and spiritually cold, lacking the ability to draw strength and vitality from the physical world. Fawn Lily stimulates the natural healing and teaching capacities of such individuals, so that the soul evolves from its archetype of cosmic virgin to world mother, or world-server.

Filaree *Erodium cicutarium* (violet)   Professional Kit

Positive qualities: Star-like vision, a cosmic overview which holds the events of ordinary life in perspective

Patterns of imbalance: Disproportionate and obsessive worry; unable to gain a wider perspective on daily events

Cross-references: Anxiety Calm Community Life and Group Experience Concentration and Focus Criticism Detail Escapism Fear Home and Lifestyle Manifestation Materialism and Money Non-Attachment Obsession Overview Perfectionism Perspective Release Self-Concern

There are times when the soul loses its proper perspective, becoming entirely too enmeshed and overly concerned with the mundane affairs of daily life. Such persons spend a great deal of time and psychic energy absorbed in small problems and compulsive concerns. It is essential for the soul's development that these "energy leaks" be recognized. Such persons must marshal their psychic and physical energy for truly productive tasks; otherwise, the larger destiny goes unfulfilled or only partially addressed. They have tremendous inner strength and reserve, which can be of great value when it is properly channeled. Filaree helps such individuals to make a fundamental shift in their perspective by instilling a more cosmic overview, thus helping to put the affairs of the daily world in proper perspective. Filaree especially liberates overly suppressed psychic energy, allowing greater receptivity to spiritual inspiration and vision.

Five-Flower Formula   English Kit

a combination of Cherry Plum, Clematis, Impatiens, Rock Rose, and Star of Bethlehem

Positive qualities: Calmness and stability in any emergency or time of high stress
Patterns of imbalance: Panic, disorientation, loss of consciousness

Cross-references: Addiction   Animals and Animal Care   Body   Breakthrough   Calm   Centeredness   Challenge   Children   Death and Dying   Disorientation   Emergency   Energetic Patterns   Fear   Hysteria   Pregnancy   Relaxation   Scatteredness   Shock   Stress

The Five-Flower Formula can be regarded as a single composite remedy for formulas, or used alone. It is most effective during any profound trauma or emergency, helping the person to cope with extreme pain and shock. This formula literally helps the soul-spiritual part of the Self to stay incarnated or connected with the physical body, even under extreme stress. It brings immediate balance and harmony in acute situations. It is less often indicated in the long-term therapeutic work of soul development; however, it can be employed in early stages when it seems difficult to make contact with the Higher Self, or when the Self needs to be stabilized before inner work can begin.

Forget-Me-Not *Myosotis sylvatica* (blue) Research Kit

Positive qualities: Awareness of karmic connections in one's personal relationships and with those in the spiritual world; deep mindfulness of subtle realms; soul-based relationships

Patterns of imbalance: Loneliness, isolation; lack of awareness of spiritual connection with others

Cross-references: Acceptance Awareness Brokenheartedness Certainty Clarity Communication Death and Dying Denial Dreams and Sleep Dullness Escapism Faith Listening Loneliness Love Meditation Mother and Mothering Nostalgia Personal Relationships Perspective Pregnancy Receptivity Soulfulness Spiritual Emergency or Opening Transition Trust

If we are to heal the wounds imposed on human culture by its overly materialistic viewpoint, it is necessary to lift our consciousness of the human family to include those souls who live outside the earthly dimension. Our hearts can naturally feel grief and concern for a living child who is abandoned and lacks the loving care and attention of a family; however, our materialistic bias makes us totally oblivious to the needs of souls who have departed from the physical realm. This blindness prevents us from providing sustenance and support to such souls, and also from receiving guidance and counsel from them for our earthly affairs. Yet establishing healthy contact with souls beyond the physical dimension is not easy. Many attempt unlawful contact through lower astral currents using drugs, sexuality, mediumism, or dangerous occult techniques. Rather than using these methods, we must be able to make contact with such souls in a heartfelt, conscious manner. The path of soul communion beyond the earthly threshold is a path of love — it depends on our ability to believe in the continued existence of the soul who has departed from physical form; remaining faithful to, and continuing to nurture the bonds of love which began on Earth. Forget-Me-Not helps awaken the soul to this higher level of heart exchange. It is an important essence to consider following the initial stage of grief after the death of a loved one, and can be very helpful for those who have never fully resolved their feelings of isolation and abandonment following the loss of an important family member or friend during childhood. Forget-Me-Not can also be used by expectant parents who wish to establish a conscious link with the soul seeking to be incarnated through them, or it can be beneficial when one wishes to understand the deeper, karmic soul connection which inspires or challenges any current relationship. In all these instances, Forget-Me-Not guides us toward greater love for the human family, and greater awareness of the incredible depth, beauty, and possibility of soul-based relationships.

Fuchsia *Fuchsia hybrida* (red/purple)   Professional Kit

Positive qualities: Genuine emotional vitality, ability to express deep feelings
Patterns of imbalance: False states of emotionality which cover more deeply-seated pain and trauma; psychosomatic symptoms

Cross-references: Acceptance Anger Avoidance Awareness Body Breakthrough Catharsis Energetic Patterns Escapism Grief Harmony Healing Process Honesty Hysteria Inner Child Insight Lower Self Menopause Psychosomatic Illness Release Repression Resistance Sexuality

The soul can be trapped and hindered in its progress through suppression and denial of core emotions. The individual needing Fuchsia tends to mask true feelings with various states of hyper-emotionality or psychosomatic symptoms. Such persons may cry easily or have myriad physical complaints such as headaches or stomachaches. This false emotionality or suffering acts as a foil or cover for the deeper emotions which appear too powerful and overwhelming for the psyche to integrate. The soul longs to express feelings, but hopes it can do so without taking the "plunge" into more awesome and painful emotions. Fuchsia helps such an individual towards emotional catharsis, so that the feeling life becomes more genuine, and conveys greater depth and presence. Emotions such as grief, deep-seated anger, or rejection can be encountered and effectively transformed through Fuchsia. The individual learns how to recognize pain and other strong feelings more immediately, thus freeing the soul life to become emotionally authentic and vital.

Garlic *Allium sativum* (violet)   Professional Kit

Positive qualities: Unitive consciousness, sense of wholeness which imparts strength and active resistance
Patterns of imbalance: Fearful, weak or easily influenced, prone to low vitality

Cross-references: Anxiety Body Calm Confidence Courage Devitalization Fear Immune Disturbances Influence Insecurity Nervousness Protection Speaking Spiritual Emergency or Opening Tension

Garlic flower essence is a very important healing agent for those souls who become too diffuse in their astrality, and therefore subject to entities of many kinds. These souls have enormous psychic forces which are scattered or splintered, leaving them host to many other entities who prey off their life forces and gain unlawful entry into the auric field. A wide spectrum of disturbances can be treated by Garlic essence, from poor immune response with a tendency to parasitic or viral infection, to low-grade psychism, mediumism, or possession. Garlic addresses many forms of nervous fear which arise from the overly intense activity of various elemental beings in the astral body. In all of these cases there is a characteristic vacancy in the eyes and paleness of features, with the impression that soul-color and vitality is being drained or siphoned from the individuality. Garlic flower restores wholeness for such souls, helping them to consolidate and unify the astral body, and to bring it into greater harmony with the physical and etheric bodies and the spiritual ego.

Gentian *Gentiana amarella* (purple)   English Kit

Positive qualities: Perseverance, confidence; faith to continue despite apparent setbacks
Patterns of imbalance: Discouragement after a setback; doubt

Cross-references: Adolescence Aging Challenge Depression and Despair Discouragement Escapism Failure Frustration Healing Process Learning Difficulties Life Direction Manifestation Perfectionism Perseverance Pessimism Rejection

The soul can become strong and vibrant only by becoming resilient. Obstacles and problems test the soul's ability to respond, and to trust in the unfoldment of life. Those in need of Gentian become too easily discouraged and disheartened when problems and setbacks occur. Such souls view impediments as insurmountable problems, and are unable to discover solutions. The individual needs to learn that such vexing situations occur because they are exactly those lessons which are needed for growth and strength. Gentian gives encouragement, especially helping the soul to shift its mental perspective and see the long view. The doubting and skeptical qualities which the soul harbors are gradually transformed into deeper faith. Gentian flower essence helps the soul to acquire great inner fortitude and unwavering trust in the outcome of life events.

Golden Ear Drops *Dicentra chrysantha* (yellow) Professional Kit

Positive qualities: Contacting one's childhood experience as a source of emotional well-being; releasing painful memories from the past
Patterns of imbalance: Suppressed toxic memories of childhood; feelings of pain and trauma about past events which affect present emotional balance

Cross-references: Abuse Alienation Awareness Catharsis Cleansing Dryness
Forgiveness Grief Guilt Healing Process Inner Child Masculine Consciousness
Purification Release Repression Resistance Shame

Emotional amnesia is a survival mechanism for the soul, especially during childhood, or any period of life when the individual is vulnerable to exploitation or abuse. This unconscious residue of traumatic memories must eventually be encountered with more awareness, or else it works like a toxic poison which corrodes the present emotional life. Golden Ear Drops helps the soul to remember and feel unpleasant or painful episodes. This essence is an especially powerful cleanser of the heart, and may stimulate tears as a form of emotional discharge. Once the individual experiences this cleansing process, there is also the ability to contact the positive aspects of the past. This is especially true regarding the events of one's childhood — when the personality suppresses painful aspects of the childhood experience, connection with the archetypal child as a source of positive spirituality is also severed. Golden Ear Drops helps the soul to remember and reclaim this past, so that it becomes a source of strength, wisdom, and insight.

Golden Yarrow *Achillea filipendulina* (yellow)   Research Kit

Positive qualities: Remaining open to others while still feeling inner protection; active social involvement which preserves the integrity of the Self

Patterns of imbalance: For outgoing people who are overly influenced by their environment and by other people; protecting oneself from vulnerability to others by withdrawal and social isolation

Cross-references: Action Addiction Adolescence Ambivalence Anxiety Body Centeredness Children City Life Community Life and Group Experience Competitiveness Confidence Courage Creativity Eating Disorders Emergency Fear Groundedness Healers Immobility Inadequacy Insecurity Intimacy Involvement Manifestation Nervousness Protection Self-Actualization Sensitivity Softness Speaking Strength Tension True to Self Vulnerability

One of the greatest challenges in the life of the soul is that of learning to stay open and balanced, without compromising one's basic integrity and health. Golden Yarrow assists with this balance, and is indicated for those whose natural inclination is to avoid public limelight or performance because of acute sensitivity. In such situations the soul becomes imprisoned in its introversion, unable to learn how to open itself within proper limits. This situation is especially pronounced for artists whose very involvement in the arts requires profound soul refinement. Such persons often find it difficult to cope with their sensitivity, and can turn to drugs or other activities which blunt and harden the soul. Unfortunately, this choice is self-defeating, for it also severs the individual from true artistic capacity and sensitivity. Golden Yarrow helps such a person to build a sheath which shields and protects, while still providing access to its innate sensitivity. In this way the soul comes to anchor inviolable light and strength within itself, which protects and encourages the delicate and gentle expression of the Self.

Goldenrod *Solidago californica* (yellow)   Professional Kit

Positive qualities: Well-developed individuality, inner sense of Self balanced with group or social consciousness
Patterns of imbalance: Easily influenced by group or family ties; inability to be true to oneself, subject to peer pressure or social expectations

Cross-references: Adolescence Anxiety Balance Barriers Centeredness Certainty Co-Dependence Community Life and Group Experience Eating Disorders Egotism Envy False Persona Greed Honesty Inadequacy Individuality Inner Child Insecurity Non-Attachment Personal Relationships Prejudice Rejection Seeking Self-Esteem True to Self

Our earliest sense of Self unfolds within the context of others — parents, extended family, and community. Gradually, through a healthy maturation process, the soul acquires a clear sense of its individuality. Some souls do not successfully complete this individuation process, remaining too subject to group morés and family ties. These souls need to establish their own inner values and beliefs, otherwise their inherent weakness is easily exploited. They tend to be adversely influenced by social pressures and conventions, conforming their behavior to social norms in order to win approval and acceptance. In some situations such souls will also display antisocial or obnoxious behavior as an extreme measure to acquire a self-image — this is especially true during adolescence. Goldenrod essence helps such persons to find a true relationship to the Higher Self. It encourages a vertical or individuated axis to counterbalance the overly broad, horizontal social axis, which influences the personality too strongly. In this way the soul acquires greater strength and inner conviction, learning to successfully balance the polarities of Self and Other.

Gorse *Ulex europaeus* (golden yellow)   English Kit

Positive qualities: Deep and abiding faith and hope; equanimity and light-filled optimism
Patterns of imbalance: Discouragement, darkness, hopelessness, resignation

Cross-references: Apathy Darkness Depression and Despair Discouragement Doubt Gloom Healing Process Manifestation Motivation Pessimism Pregnancy Time Relationship

The soul must learn to live in equilibrium between the polarities of light and dark. Those needing Gorse have internalized darkness or pessimism in their outlook on life. This pessimism gives too much weight and depression to the soul, and erodes the soul's natural buoyancy. Gorse restores hope to such souls, so that they are able to look with a brighter, more expectant, and joyful outlook on life situations. This quality of hope deeply affects physical as well as emotional healing, because the life force is nourished by light. Such persons need to counter the darkness they feel within themselves with strong forces of inner light and luminous insight. Through Gorse, the soul learns to use light as an alchemical agent for change and healing, directing a powerful, illuminating beacon even in the most trying moments and bleakest situations.

Heather *Calluna vulgaris* (pink, purple)   English Kit

Positive qualities: Inner tranquillity; emotional self-sufficiency
Patterns of imbalance: Over-talkative, self-absorbed; over-concerned with one's own problems

Cross-references: Adolescence Aging Attention Community Life and Group Experience Compassion Healing Process Listening Loneliness Martyrdom Obsession Personal Relationships Self-Concern Self-Esteem Self-Expression Selfishness Speaking

Heather flower essence helps those who become too absorbed in their own problems and worries. Such persons are deeply lonely and in great pain, but they seek contact with others in a dysfunctional manner. Feeling empty inside, the Heather type hopes to assuage its hunger by "feeding" off the psychic attention and sympathy of others. In most cases this excessive self-concern repels others from forming a truly empathetic bond. Thus the Heather type becomes increasingly lonely and dysfunctional. In extreme states, such a person may learn to manipulate psychic energy so that others are compelled to listen to and attend to their problems. Heather nourishes the soul's feeling of profound emptiness so that it can become stronger within itself, and realize compassion. This is the key to experiencing love, for one is healed from one's own suffering by learning to care for and perceive the suffering of others. Heather heals the soul by reversing psychic currents of energy which are directed too strongly toward the Self. By learning to find itself in caring for others, the Heather soul becomes *self-fulfilled* rather than *self-absorbed*.

Hibiscus *Hibiscus rosa-sinensis* (red)   Research Kit

Positive qualities: Warmth and responsiveness in female sexuality; integration of soul warmth and bodily passion
Patterns of imbalance: Inability to connect with one's female sexuality; lack of warmth and vitality, often due to prior exploitation or abuse

Cross-references: Abuse Aging Body Desire Devitalization Dryness Feminine Consciousness Groundedness Instinctual Self Intimacy Lower Self Menopause Rejuvenation Repression Sexuality Vitality Warmth

One of the most tragic assaults to the soul dignity of women is the exploitation and commercialization of female sexuality. This deeply wounds the souls of many women so that they no longer feel a warm connection to their sexuality. Often the sexuality is divorced from deeper feelings of love and warmth which come from the heart. In many cases sexual expression becomes cold and unresponsive, because the Soul can no longer contact this part of the Self and infuse it with love and caring. Hibiscus essence helps women to reclaim their sexuality, and to restore these soul forces with vitality and authenticity. It can aid many women who have been sexually traumatized, and is also generally beneficial for all modern women who have unconsciously absorbed media images and other stereotypes of dehumanized sexuality. This remedy is sometimes also indicated for men who need to develop a stronger relationship to feminine warmth and positive sexuality. Hibiscus creates flowing warmth throughout the body and soul, especially healing the sexuality.

Holly *Ilex aquifolium* (white, tinged with pink)   English Kit

Positive qualities: Feeling love and extending love to others; universal compassion, open heart

Patterns of imbalance: Feeling cut off from love; jealousy, envy, suspicion, anger

Cross-references: Abandonment Acceptance Adolescence Aging Anger Animals and Animal Care Appreciation Brokenheartedness Catharsis Children Cleansing Community Life and Group Experience Compassion Competitiveness Conflict Cooperation Cynicism Death and Dying Destructiveness Dislike Egotism Envy Fear Forgiveness Grace Hate Heart Hostility Inner Child Joy Love Morality Negativity Paranoia Personal Relationships Prejudice Rejection Resentment Selfishness Sharing Soulfulness

Above all else, the soul seeks in its evolution to experience real love. This is the most fundamental lesson for the soul, and at the same time the most challenging. Holly is therefore a foundational remedy with many broad-based applications, for it restores the soul's ability to feel unity and wholeness. When we feel separate from others we can take no joy or compassionate interest in their affairs; instead our isolation is compounded into negative states of jealousy, envy, suspicion or anger. The soul grasps for its share of love as though it were a limited commodity, rather than realizing that love is an infinite resource which is divinely available to all. Holly essence nourishes the heart, helping the individual to make and sustain the shift from a limited and narrow conception of the Self, to one which is expansive and inclusive of others. In this way, the soul experiences wholeness or "holiness," for it feels permeated with divine love. This sense of sacred unity is the very special gift and teaching of Holly flower essence.

Honeysuckle *Lonicera caprifolium* (red/white)   English Kit

Positive qualities: Being fully in the present; learning from the past while releasing it

Patterns of imbalance: Nostalgia; emotional attachment to the past, longing for what was

Cross-references: Aging Avoidance Brokenheartedness Concentration and Focus Daydreaming Envy Escapism Grief Home and Lifestyle Loneliness Mid-Life Crisis Nostalgia Prejudice Rejection Release Resistance Time Relationship

Time is the life current of the incarnated soul. If it does not navigate the stream of time, it drowns in the past or parches its future possibilities. The soul needing Honeysuckle stifles life force and denies its true evolution by living too much in past events, places and relationships. Such a soul needs more inner flexibility and adaptability. Rather than face the challenge of change, it clings emotionally to a past which seems to have been more appealing. This perception is usually an illusion; for example, a past relationship or an earlier phase of one's life can be glossed over with dreamy reverie, ignoring the actual pain and trauma that was part of the experience. The essential lesson of Honeysuckle has to do with the soul's perceptive faculties; being able to learn from previous life experiences by seeing clearly their meaning and message. When this occurs it frees the soul to grow and change, to experience life with intention and purpose, as an ever-unfolding present and ever-possible future.

Hornbeam *Carpinus betulus* (yellow/green)   English Kit

Positive qualities: Energy, enthusiasm, involvement in life's tasks
Patterns of imbalance: Fatigue, weariness; daily tasks seen as an overwhelming burden

Cross-references: Action Challenge Cheerfulness Depression and Despair Devitalization Dreams and Sleep Dullness Dutifulness Energetic Patterns Exhaustion and Fatigue Involvement Joy Manifestation Overwhelm Procrastination Resistance Seriousness Sluggishness Time Relationship Work and Career Goals

The soul makes unlimited reserves of energy available to the body; unfortunately, these are seldom tapped to their full potential. At the soul level, energy is produced not by calories or fuel, but by full attention and positive connection to one's work or life tasks. Those individuals who experience monotonous routine, or lack genuine interest or involvement in their work, can feel extreme tiredness and exhaustion completely out of proportion to the real capacity of the physical body. The Hornbeam essence re-orients the soul so that it can freshly perceive work or habits which may have become overly dull or routine. Hornbeam sometimes brings an inner realization that a new approach or new lifestyle is necessary to completely recapture one's full energy. Above all, Hornbeam nourishes the soul with renewed strength and vitality so that it may live more effectively and more joyfully in the world.

Hound's Tongue *Cynoglossum grande* (blue/white)   Professional Kit

Positive qualities: Holistic thinking; perceiving the physical world and physical life with spiritually clear thoughts

Patterns of imbalance: Seeing the world in materialistic terms, weighed down or dulled by a mundane or overly scientific viewpoint

Cross-references: Creativity   Denial   Earth Healing and Nature Awareness   Body Cynicism   Dullness   Eating Disorders   Insight   Inspiration   Intellectualism   Lightness Masculine Consciousness   Materialism and Money   Meditation   Mental Clarity   Perspective Study   Thinking   Transcendence   Wisdom

The modern soul is evolving in its ability to think; this is a true spiritual gift which carries enormous creative potential. However, this thinking force is threatened in its development by overly intellectual and materialistic attitudes. For example, we may exactly analyze a tree for its fuel or timber capacity without ever seeing its spiritual identity. We may think of the sun as simply an explosion of hydrogen atoms, or the stars as a result of the "big bang," without realizing that real spiritual forces and beings live and breathe in the movements of the sun and stars. This is tantamount to seeing the human being as only a physical body composed of highly defined parts like bones, cartilage, cellular tissue, and DNA, without ever apprehending the wholeness and spiritual complexity of the *being* which stands before us. Sensitive persons rebel against this materialistic consciousness, but often do so in a way that denies the real thinking capacities. Hound's Tongue stimulates and enlivens the thinking activity. It restores a sense of wonder and reverence for life, while also helping the soul to think in clear and specific ways about the spiritual dimensions of the physical world.

Impatiens *Impatiens gladulifera* (pink/mauve) English Kit

Positive qualities: Patience, acceptance; flowing with the pace of life and others
Patterns of imbalance: Impatience, irritation, tension, intolerance

Cross-references: Abuse   Acceptance   Aggressiveness   Anger
Animals and Animal Care   Children   Community Life and Group Experience
Competitiveness   Destructiveness   Earth Healing and Nature Awareness   Eating Disorders
Erratic Behavior   Exhaustion and Fatigue   Frustration   Healers   Healing Process   Heart
Home and Lifestyle   Impatience   Irritability   Joy   Learning Difficulties   Listening
Manifestation   Masculine Consciousness   Meditation   Moderation   Mother and Mothering
Perfectionism   Resistance   Restlessness   Stress   Tension   Thinking   Time Relationship
Tolerance   Work and Career Goals

The souls who need Impatiens find it difficult to be within the flow of time; their tendency is to rush ahead of experience. In doing so, they deny themselves full immersion in life, even though they may appear very busy and engaged. In particular, these individuals miss the more gentle and subtle exchanges which can occur with others, or with the world around them. Their overabundance of fiery force flares up easily into irritation, impatience, intolerance, and anger. Although quite mentally agile and extremely capable, the great inner tension and excitability of such souls leads to various physical disease states or premature aging due to "burnout." The Impatiens type needs to experience not only the powerful flaming of life, but also its gentle flowering. Through the Impatiens essence, the soul learns to still the attention and deepen the breathing so that the inner Self becomes more receptive to the unfolding moment. The precious flower of life is then experienced in all of its fleeting fragility and delicate beauty.

Indian Paintbrush *Castilleja miniata* (red)   Professional Kit

Positive qualities: Lively, energetic creativity, exuberant artistic activity
Patterns of imbalance: Low vitality and exhaustion, difficulty rousing physical forces to sustain the intensity of creative work; inability to bring creative forces into physical expression

Cross-references: Body Breakthrough Catalyst Creativity Devitalization Dryness Energetic Patterns Exhaustion and Fatigue Frustration Groundedness Inspiration Manifestation Rejuvenation Spiritual Emergency or Opening Vitality Will

When the soul is engaged in highly creative work, it must integrate itself with its physical vehicle in the right way. If the body does not stay grounded and energized during creative work, it will suffer from low vitality, exhaustion and other forms of physical illness. Many souls do not fulfill their true artistic and creative potential because they are unable to harness spiritual energy in the right way. This phenomenon is similar to an electrical current of energy which needs to be properly polarized and grounded. Indian Paintbrush is very specific for this level of imbalance. It shows the soul how to use the will or lower metabolic forces to polarize spiritual energy, so that the physical body reflects a healthy alignment between Earth and Heaven. Indian Paintbrush also helps artists with the qualitative expression of their art, especially if such work lacks substance or connection with the physical world and natural processes. All in all, this essence helps the soul to learn how to use creative potential in a manner which is richly resonant with the physical world.

Indian Pink *Silene californica* (red)   Professional Kit

Positive qualities: Remaining centered and focused, even under stress; managing and coordinating diverse forms of activity

Patterns of imbalance: Psychic forces which are easily torn or shattered by too much activity; inability to stay centered during intense activity

Cross-references: Action   Calm   Centeredness   City Life   Concentration and Focus Disorientation   Emergency   Environment   Erratic Behavior   Home and Lifestyle Irritability   Mother and Mothering   Nervousness   Overwhelm   Quiet   Scatteredness Strength   Stress   Time Relationship

It is easy for the soul to experience equanimity when removed from daily stress and activity; but it is a far greater challenge to maintain one's inner center despite chaos or pressure. Indian Pink helps those who are particularly vulnerable in this way, finding it difficult to anchor and center themselves. This remedy is quite specific to movement and activity. Those in need of Indian Pink are attracted to doing many things at once and live with much intensity. However, the astral body spins out of control, no longer stabilized by the ego, or spiritual Self. These individuals identify too much with the periphery of the circle and its agitated movement, rather than the point which remains fixed and inviolable. They are very tense and emotionally volatile, and can appear haggard and depleted because the etheric body is ravaged by too much astrality. Indian Pink assists such persons to identify with their spiritual center. By remaining more self-contained, they learn to orchestrate activity from the conscious Self, and therefore experience more health and harmony.

Iris *Iris douglasiana* (blue-violet)

Professional Kit

Iris (Blue Flag) *Iris versicolor* (blue-violet)

Seven Herbs Kit

Positive qualities: Inspired artistry, deep soulfulness which is in touch with higher realms; radiant, iridescent vision and perspective

Patterns of imbalance: Lacking inspiration or creativity; feeling weighed down by the ordinariness of the world; dullness

Cross-references: Action Body Breakthrough Children Creativity Dryness Dullness Earth Healing and Nature Awareness Eating Disorders Environment Feminine Consciousness Freedom Frustration Home and Lifestyle Immobility Inadequacy Inner Child Inspiration Learning Difficulties Lightness Manifestation Materialism and Money Menopause Mid-Life Crisis Mother and Mothering Rejuvenation Self-Actualization Self-Expression Soulfulness Spiritual Emergency or Opening Spontaneity Study Tension Transcendence Work and Career Goals

It is the soul's mission to build a rainbow bridge between spirit and matter. The pure light of the spirit needs to be ensouled, or colored with feeling. The rich darkness of matter needs to become luminous and filled with inner meaning. This is the path of the artist, and it is really true that every soul should express itself as an artist. As the physical body needs air to breathe, so does the soul need inspiration in order to live. As the physical body circulates blood in order to nourish itself, so does the soul live through the streaming and weaving of radiant color. Many modern individuals lack soul vitality; a gray pallor stifles them, they suffocate in the mundane and mechanical. Iris is a fundamental remedy for restoring and revitalizing the soul. It is indicated not only for those who are on a specific artistic path, but also for many individuals who need to bring passionate creativity to their life work. Iris essence impels the soul to create and cultivate beauty, within itself and within the world. It is an excellent, universally applicable remedy for initiating and sustaining development through flower essence therapy and other allied healing arts; *for the flowers are the soul colors of Nature.* Thus Iris helps the inner life of the human soul harmonize with the Soul of Nature, and in this way to become alive, vibrant, and truly "iridescent."

Lady's Slipper
Seven Herbs Kit

Yellow Lady's Slipper *Cypripedium parviflorum* (yellow)
Showy Lady's Slipper *Cypripedium reginae* (pink and white)

Positive qualities: Integration of spiritual purpose with daily work, bringing spiritual power into the root chakra; spiritualized sexuality and grounded spirituality
Patterns of imbalance: Estranged from one's inner authority, inability to integrate higher spiritual purpose with real life and work; nervous exhaustion, sexual depletion

Cross-references: Alienation   Authority   Community Life and Group Experience   Conflict   Desire   Energetic Patterns   Exhaustion and Fatigue   Feminine Consciousness   Groundedness   Leadership   Life Direction   Manifestation   Nervousness   Power   Restlessness   Self-Actualization   Sexuality   Spiritual Emergency or Opening   Vitality   Work and Career Goals

Lady's Slipper helps the soul to incorporate its spirituality more completely into the body. It especially balances the relationship between the crown chakra and the lower energy centers. Those in need of this remedy are often unable to realize their inherent power and ability, so that their daily work or career is only a dim reflection of what is possible. A congestion of spiritual forces in the upper chakras results in psychic energy which is not properly circulated throughout the body. Such persons often suffer from weariness and exhaustion, especially depletion of their sexual forces. Lady's Slipper is a tonic for the nervous system; it frees those spiritual capacities which reside in the upper energy centers to radiate more fully through the body. This redistribution of psychic energy is particularly pronounced in the feet; indeed, the ability to follow one's destiny or "walk" one's path has very much to do with intuitive powers which reside in the limbs. Lady's Slipper calms and re-stabilizes the nervous system, helping the individual to regain inner composure and spiritual strength.

Larch *Larix decidua* (red f./yellow m.)   English Kit

Positive qualities: Self-confidence, creative expression, spontaneity
Patterns of imbalance: Lack of confidence, expectation of failure, self-censorship

Cross-references: Adolescence Anxiety Blame Calm Children Communication
Confidence Courage Creativity Discouragement Doubt Failure Father and Fathering
Fear Hesitation Immobility Inadequacy Indecision Inner Child Life Direction
Manifestation Masculine Consciousness Motivation Perfectionism Perseverance
Pessimism Pride Procrastination Rejection Repression Self-Acceptance
Self-Effacement Self-Esteem Self-Expression Sexuality Shame Shyness Speaking
Spontaneity   Work and Career Goals

Larch helps those individuals who suffer from great self-doubt and poor
self-esteem. The soul is lacking in confidence and thus projects failure, poor
performance, or harsh judgment by others, far beyond the objective situation. In this
way, the soul capacities stagnate, for such individuals severely censor and constrict
their creative expression, and stifle their spontaneity. They are afraid to try anything
new or risky, and therefore do little to grow and evolve. The Larch essence
particularly heals the throat, or communication and creativity chakra. Many of those
who need Larch are very closed down in this center, and may even have a physical
affliction of the throat or other speaking impediments. Larch flower essence frees
creative potential, giving the individual renewed confidence and expressiveness.
Larch impels the soul from a self-limiting to a self-transcending mode of behavior.

Larkspur *Delphinium nuttallianum* (blue-violet)   Professional Kit

Positive qualities: Charismatic leadership, contagious enthusiasm, joyful service
Patterns of imbalance: Leadership distorted by self-aggrandizement or
burdensome dutifulness

Cross-references: Aggressiveness Altruism Ambition Cheerfulness Community Life
and Group Experience Dutifulness Egotism Enthusiasm Idealism Influence Joy
Leadership Lightness Martyrdom Masculine Consciousness Materialism and Money
Power Responsibility Self-Aggrandizement Service Work and Career Goals

At many stages of its evolution, the soul assumes leadership responsibilities, in
both large and small circles of influence. Unfortunately, leadership tasks are often
assumed for the wrong reasons, and the soul either becomes weighted with
burdensome duty, or inflated with self-importance. True spiritual leadership requires

the radiance of charisma and contagious enthusiasm. When the soul is fired from within by positive identification with its inner ideals, its altruism can nourish and inspire others. Such leadership is not a matter of a forceful will which manipulates others, or dutiful execution of one's responsibilities; rather, it is an inner joyfulness which energizes others. Larkspur helps those who are in positions of leadership to align their feeling life with their spiritual ideals. From this place, the soul learns to radiate inspired charismatic energy which motivates and encourages others.

Lavender *Lavandula officinalis* (violet) Professional Kit

Positive qualities: Spiritual sensitivity, highly refined awareness
Patterns of imbalance: Nervousness, overstimulation of spiritual forces which depletes the physical body

Cross-references: Addiction Aging Calm Dreams and Sleep Emergency Energetic Patterns Exhaustion and Fatigue Harmony Healing Process Immune Disturbances Insomnia Irritability Massage Meditation Menopause Moderation Nervousness Overwhelm Perfectionism Pregnancy Protection Psychosomatic Illness Relaxation Restlessness Sensitivity Shock Soothing Spiritual Emergency or Opening Stress Study Tension Time Relationship

The Lavender flower helps those souls who are highly absorbent of spiritual influences. They tend to be very awake and quite mentally active, with a strong attraction to spiritual practices and various forms of meditation. However, they often absorb far more energy than can actually be processed through the body. "High-strung" and "wound-up" are words typically used to describe such personalities. They especially suffer from afflictions to the head, such as headaches or vision problems, and neck and shoulder tension. They are quite often plagued by insomnia or other nervous maladies. Lavender first works to sedate and soothe such persons; at a deeper level, it teaches one how to moderate and regulate one's spiritual-psychic energy. In this way the soul learns to use its highly sensitive capacities in balance with the physical needs of the body.

Lotus *Nelumbo nucifera* (pink)   Professional Kit

Positive qualities: Open and expansive spirituality, meditative insight and synthesis
Patterns of imbalance: Spiritual pride, inflated spirituality

Cross-references: Balance Egotism False Persona Grace Harmony Lower Self
Meditation Perfectionism Pride Receptivity Self-Aggrandizement Self-Esteem
Spiritual Emergency or Opening Synthesis Toner Wisdom

   The soul is meant to wear a crown of light, and quite literally bears a subtle energy center called the crown chakra. This chakra gives the soul its sense of dignity, and awareness of its own regal or divine nature. Although the crown of light is a regal attribute, it can only be rightly worn by the soul which has acquired inner humility. Lotus is particularly indicated for imbalances in the crown chakra. It acts as a spiritual elixir or harmonizer, helping the soul to open itself to its inner divinity. However, an individual can also become overly developed in its spirituality. If the crown is overactive in relation to the other energy centers — especially the heart — the Lotus flower will re-direct and balance the spiritual forces. It particularly heals the tendency toward spiritual pride, or the illusion that one is "spiritually correct or superior." Lotus is an excellent, all-purpose remedy for enhancing and harmonizing the higher consciousness, and especially for integrating spirituality in a balanced way with the other energy centers.

Love-Lies-Bleeding *Amaranthus caudatus* (red) Research essence
(Amaranthus)

Positive qualities: Transcendent consciousness, the ability to move beyond personal pain, suffering or mental anguish by finding larger, transpersonal meaning in such suffering; compassionate awareness of and attention to the meaning of pain or suffering

Patterns of imbalance: Intensification of pain and suffering due to isolation; profound melancholia due to the over-personalization of one's pain

Cross-references: Acceptance Animals and Animal Care Attachment Awareness Body Brokenheartedness Catharsis Challenge Community Life and Group Experience Compassion Death and Dying Depression and Despair Emergency Escapism Feminine Consciousness Grief Healing Process Heart Immune Disturbances Loneliness Love Martyrdom Non-Attachment Release Self-Concern Sensitivity Spiritual Emergency or Opening Surrender Transcendence Vulnerability

The Love-Lies-Bleeding (Amaranthus) flower enables the soul to encounter and to transmute pain and suffering. Such pain is felt in an intense manner, either as mental anguish, deep-seated bodily torment, or disease. While such suffering usually has a physical component, the experience of agony is also deep within the soul itself. The effect of such torment is to push the consciousness deeply *inward*; such a person is truly *deep-pressed*, or in the throes of depression. Love-Lies-Bleeding does not play the role of an analgesic; it does not provide direct relief from such distress. It helps by moving the soul consciousness *outward* from over-personal identification and isolation, to transpersonal awareness of the meaning and purpose of such an experience. This energetic shift can often be experienced directly in the physical body, in the cessation of symptoms of pain or as a general stimulus to the immune system. However, more typically the individual is able to experience physical and mental suffering differently, within the context of a larger, shared human experience. For example, one suffering from a personal illness, a particular handicap, or addiction may be impelled to reach out to others who suffer similarly. The deepest teaching of Love-Lies-Bleeding is centered around the meaning of compassion and sacrifice. This realization within the soul is often called "Christ consciousness" — the capacity to suffer or to "bleed" not for ourselves but for all of humanity and for the redemption of the Earth itself. The ability to understand that one's own pain is part of a larger, deeper experience of the human condition is the key to being able to truly experience love and compassion for all living beings.

Madia *Madia elegans* (yellow/red spots) Professional Kit

Positive qualities: Precise thinking, disciplined focus and concentration
Patterns of imbalance: Becoming easily distracted, inability to concentrate, dull or listless

Cross-references: Aging Attention Awareness Clarity Concentration and Focus Daydreaming Decisiveness Detail Disorientation Environment Home and Lifestyle Learning Difficulties Manifestation Mental Clarity Quiet Scatteredness Speaking Study Time Relationship

The healthy soul needs to learn to contract as well as expand — it must be able to narrow the consciousness, and limit the experience. One who can do this is able to focus and direct energy in a very clear and productive manner. Lacking this ability, the soul becomes easily distracted, or "spacey." This latter word is a good description of the person in need of Madia. Such an individual literally lives too much in *space* and not enough in present *time*; therefore its psychic forces are easily scattered. Madia is indicated for this basic imbalance in the soul life, but can also be helpful for seasonal distress, especially during the summer when hot weather makes one listless and distracted, or for a similar unfocused feeling which can occur in mid-afternoon. Madia pulls the soul into its center, so that the field of consciousness is pinpointed and focused. Its helps the soul to incarnate and direct its vast spiritual potential.

Mallow *Sidalcea glauscens* (pink-violet) Professional Kit

Positive qualities: Warm and personable, open-hearted sharing and friendliness
Patterns of imbalance: Socially insecure, fear of reaching out to others; creating barriers

Cross-references: Abandonment Adolescence Aloofness Awkwardness Barriers Children Community Life and Group Experience Compassion Healers Insecurity Intimacy Involvement Loneliness Personal Relationships Receptivity Rejection Self-Esteem Sharing Shyness Trust Warmth

The soul flourishes through friendship and social exchange. Physical warmth is the basis of life, and likewise social warmth sustains the life of the human soul. Many individuals suffer from an inability to reach out to others. Often this stems from early childhood, but can also be due to other cultural or karmic factors. Such a personality has not learned to trust others, nor to trust his/her own capacity to radiate warmth to others. There is a profound inability to feel or to receive the warm flow of exchange which occurs when two souls touch energetically. Instead, the heart feels frozen, and those places which should be like portals are more like walls or barriers. The Mallow flower gently opens these obstructions to the feeling life, so that the soul can begin to experience the rich glow of social warmth that comes from loving exchange with others. Mallow helps the soul learn to trust the feelings buried in the heart, encouraging the individual towards greater social involvement.

Manzanita *Arctostaphylos viscida* (white-pink) Professional Kit

Positive qualities: Embodiment, integration of spiritual Self with the physical world

Patterns of imbalance: Estranged from the earthly world; aversion, disgust or revulsion toward the bodily Self and physical world

Cross-references: Adolescence Alienation Ambivalence Appreciation Awareness Awkwardness Body Children Desire Destructiveness Dislike Earth Healing and Nature Awareness Eating Disorders Groundedness Healing Process Instinctual Self Massage Mid-Life Crisis Perfectionism Pregnancy Resistance Sexuality

The soul is a bridge between body and spirit; its task is a physical one every bit as much as a spiritual one. In some persons there is a particular aversion to the physical world and physical body. This can be the result of a current religious philosophy or spiritual program, or it can stem from deeply unconscious beliefs about the physical world which the soul has acquired in previous incarnations. This inner illness manifests as a feeling that the body is ugly and corrupted, or that it has little intrinsic worth compared to the spirit. The body is often highly objectified, exploited, or deprived through strict spiritual or ascetic regimens. Such an individual may have especially strong restrictions or rituals relating to food, with tendencies toward bulimia or anorexia. This harsh view of physical life and physical matter often hardens the body prematurely and can result in many illnesses, despite "perfect" health programs. Manzanita helps the individual to soften its relationship to the physical world, and re-direct its spiritual focus toward the body. Thus the soul comes to understand the body as a sacred shrine or temple of the spirit. Manzanita encourages the soul's involvement with the physical world, especially the body; and imparts the teaching that matter is dead or inferior only to the degree that it remains unembraced by the soul's consciousness.

Mariposa Lily *Calochortus leichtlinii* (white/yellow center/purple spots)
Professional Kit

Positive qualities: Maternal consciousness, warm, feminine and nurturing; mother-child bonding, healing of the inner child

Patterns of imbalance: Alienated from mother or from mothering, feelings of childhood abandonment or abuse

Cross-references: Abandonment Abuse Adolescence Alienation
Animals and Animal Care Children Co-Dependence Compassion Death and Dying
Eating Disorders Feminine Consciousness Forgiveness Healers Healing Process Heart
Home and Lifestyle Inner Child Intimacy Involvement Love Menopause
Mother and Mothering Personal Relationships Pregnancy Protection Receptivity
Rejection Self-Acceptance Service Sexuality Softness Soothing Trust Warmth

The ability of the human soul to show nurturing and caring attention for others depends very much on whether it has received such nurturing itself. Each person should be able, as a divine birthright, to receive maternal love and unconditional support as a young infant and child. Many souls are deprived of a positive relationship to the mother. Especially in the modern world, cultural conditions de-humanize the relationship of the infant to the mother through birthing and child-rearing practices. Further deprivation may result from family trauma, divorce, economic hardship, or extreme situations of abuse, abandonment, and neglect. If the soul is crippled in its early relationship to the feminine, it feels cold and empty inside, and at its core, experiences itself as unloved and unwanted. The maturation process into adulthood is usually distorted — for males a rejection of or hostility to the feminine, and for females an alienation from their own mothering instincts. Mariposa Lily helps such souls heal this trauma by coming to terms with the painful past. It is an extremely important remedy, not only for infants and children, but also for many phases of adult therapy and positive parenting. Despite the wounding which may have occurred through an imperfect human mother, the soul can learn to forgive and heal, by experiencing the presence of the divine or archetypal mother who embraces the entire human family with gentle mercy and nurturing. This ability of the soul to feel and embrace the warm, loving presence of the maternal is the very important gift of the Mariposa Lily.

Milkweed *Asclepias cordifolia* (red-purple)   Research Kit

Positive qualities: Healthy ego strength; independence and self-reliance
Patterns of imbalance: Extreme dependency and emotional regression, dulling the consciousness through drugs, alcohol, overeating; desire to escape from self-awareness

Cross-references: Addiction Alienation Awakeness Co-Dependence Community Life and Group Experience Denial Depression and Despair Desire Disorientation
Dreams and Sleep Eating Disorders Escapism Healing Process Inadequacy
Individuality Inner Child Learning Difficulties Meditation Mental Clarity
Mother and Mothering Self-Actualization Spiritual Emergency or Opening Strength
True to Self

Milkweed is indicated for extreme states of soul dependency and regression, characterized by lack of an independent ego identity. Such a condition can develop for many reasons — an accident or other life trauma which has made the individual overly dependent on family or institutionalized care; or gradual addiction to drugs, especially narcotics such as sedatives, opiates, and tranquilizers. Milkweed can sometimes be indicated for those on spiritual paths who deny the awake conscious ego function, or who believe that initiation can proceed only if the ego is annihilated. These regressive tendencies may also be the result of a disturbed maturation process in childhood which creates an unconscious desire for the ego to return to an infantile state. At its deepest karmic level, some souls may incarnate with impairments which disturb the natural maturation of the ego function. Because the core identity is poorly defined, there is difficulty coping with the normal demands and responsibilities of the adult ego. The soul seeks to blot out consciousness through drugs, overeating, excessive sleep, accidents, illness, or extreme spiritual practices. Milkweed nourishes the soul at a very deep level, leading to the ability to rebirth that part of the core self which has regressed. As the soul learns to experience the healthy function of its ego, it grows in strength and independence.

Mimulus *Mimulus guttatus* (yellow, red spots)   English Kit

Positive qualities: Courage and confidence to face life's challenges
Patterns of imbalance: Known fears of everyday life; shyness

Cross-references: Aging   Animals and Animal Care   Anxiety   Calm   Children
Confidence   Courage   Escapism   Faith   Fear   Hesitation   Home and Lifestyle   Insecurity
Nervousness   Self-Concern   Self-Effacement   Shyness   Speaking   Time Relationship

Mimulus is one of the most basic remedies for fear. Those needing this essence are hypersensitive and live with a great many small fears of ordinary and everyday events. They are especially afflicted in the solar plexus, which churns with great anxiety and unease. Eventually, if these fears are not met and transformed, the soul becomes quite darkened and introverted as it withdraws more and more from the stresses of daily living. Mimulus brings the light of courage back to such souls. It helps the individual shift its fixation from myriad lesser fears to awareness of a more basic, usually unconscious fear. This is a fear of the physical body, or of physical life itself, which can sometimes be traced to actual hesitation at the moment of incarnation. A pattern is thus set deep within the substrata of the soul which must be healed. Mimulus helps the soul to contact the strength and purpose of its Higher Self, and thus sets it free to experience life with greater curiosity, exuberance, and joy.

Morning Glory *Ipomoea purpurea* (blue)   Professional Kit

Positive qualities: Sparkling vital force, feeling awake and refreshed, in touch with Life
Patterns of imbalance: Dull, toxic, or "hung over," inability to fully enter the body, especially in the morning; addictive habits

Cross-references: Addiction   Attachment   Awakeness   Balance   Breakthrough
Destructiveness   Devitalization   Dreams and Sleep   Dullness   Earth Healing and Nature
Awareness   Eating Disorders   Energetic Patterns   Erratic Behavior   Escapism   Exhaustion
and Fatigue   Freedom   Habit Patterns   Hardness   Home and Lifestyle   Immobility
Immune Disturbances   Inertia   Moderation   Nervousness   Rejuvenation   Relaxation
Resistance   Restlessness   Sluggishness   Time Relationship   Toner   Transition   Vitality

The soul must constantly be on guard to align its astral body with its physical/etheric components. The astral (or star) body is naturally akin to the forces of night, and, if left unregulated, will not hesitate to devour the etheric (or life) body. Individuals with this imbalance typically crave late-night activity and have erratic eating and sleeping rhythms. The etheric body is more akin to the forces of day-time, especially early morning, and is greatly abused by such astrality. If such abuse continues over a long period of time, the individual will experience increasing difficulty incarnating in the body, not only in the morning, but throughout the day. Unable to use the natural energy of the etheric body, the person will crave stimulants such as caffeine, and in extreme cases, cocaine or amphetamines. As this astrality continues to predominate, the individual will display increasingly erratic patterns, possibly deteriorating into destructive and violent tendencies. Many levels of physical illness may occur, especially compromised immune response, nerve depletion, and disturbances in vital organs such as the liver. Morning Glory helps the soul come to greater awareness and respect for life and the life processes of the body. The individual learns to adjust its rhythm so that it is more in tune with the cycles of Nature. Through Morning Glory, the soul learns to experience more natural states of energy, and thus the gift of life itself.

Mountain Pennyroyal *Monardella odoratissima* (violet)

Professional Kit

Positive qualities: Strength and clarity of thought, mental integrity and positivity
Patterns of imbalance: Absorbing negative thoughts of others, psychic contamination or possession

Cross-references: Addiction Clarity Cleansing Healing Process Home and Lifestyle Influence Mental Clarity Negativity Protection Purification Release Sensitivity Spiritual Emergency or Opening Strength Thinking Vitality

Hygiene is as important to the life of the soul as it is for the physical body. Mountain Pennyroyal particularly addresses an individual's mental field which may be devitalized due to psychic congestion from too many negative or chaotic thought forms. There can also be mediumistic tendencies in such persons, so that they unconsciously absorb the negative thoughts of other persons or entities. When developed to an extreme state, the individual may no longer be able to think clearly for him/herself, or make rational decisions. There may be a tendency to possession, especially if the person is prone to using alcohol or other drugs. In these cases, seemingly conscious actions are actually carried out at the behest of others' intentions rather than those of the true Self. Mountain Pennyroyal works as a purgative; it has the powerful ability to cleanse and expel negative thoughts, or the unhealthy intrusion of entities in the astral body. This essence clarifies the mental body and leads to greater vitality of the mental life, especially positive, clear thinking.

Mountain Pride *Penstemon newberryi* (magenta)   Professional Kit

Positive qualities: Forthright masculine energy; warrior-like spirituality which confronts and transforms
Patterns of imbalance: Vacillation and withdrawal in the face of challenge; lack of assertiveness, inability to take a stand for one's convictions

Cross-references: Action Aggressiveness Breakthrough Challenge Community Life and Group Experience Competitiveness Confidence Courage Cynicism
Death and Dying Decisiveness Dutifulness Earth Healing and Nature Awareness
Escapism Fear Idealism Leadership Manifestation Masculine Consciousness Morality
Motivation Perseverance Power Prejudice Responsibility Self-Expression Service
Strength Will

In learning to distinguish good from evil, or truth from untruth, the soul is compelled to take a stand in the world. The ability to act on what one knows to be true is of enormous importance. Especially in our modern world, it is of utmost urgency that the individual learn to transform feelings of dissatisfaction or disillusionment with the world into positive energy for change. Mountain Pride imparts to the soul the archetype of the spiritual warrior — the radiation of the positive masculine for both male and female souls. It is an especially important remedy for those persons who confuse peace with passivity. Such individuals must learn that positive activity is an important healing agent, not only for personal strength and soul development, but also for real peace in the world. Through Mountain Pride the soul learns to take a stand *in* the world and *for* the world, by aligning its own personal identity with forces of goodness and truth.

Mugwort *Artemisia douglasiana* (yellow)   Professional Kit

Positive qualities: Integrating psychic and dream experiences with daily life; multi-dimensional consciousness
Patterns of imbalance: Inability to harmonize psychic forces, tendency to hysteria or emotionality, overactive psychic life out of touch with the physical world

Cross-references: Awareness Balance Daydreaming Dreams and Sleep
Feminine Consciousness Hysteria Insight Insomnia Inspiration Massage Meditation
Pregnancy Receptivity Sensitivity Spiritual Emergency or Opening Toner

The soul is only half alive if it does not experience itself when asleep. The body may vegetate during sleep, but the soul has the capacity to awaken to another dimension of life. Mugwort enhances the receptive quality of the psyche, allowing greater awareness of dreams, so that the Self can gain insight about the affairs of daily life and can access guidance and direction from the spiritual world. This essence particularly helps the soul to navigate within the flow of psychic life, so that it is neither lost nor overwhelmed. It helps to balance transitions between day and night consciousness, assisting the individual to remain connected in a healthy way with the practical and physical world. This balance is very important, for when the moon forces become too predominant or inappropriately expressed, the soul becomes irrational, hysterical, or overly emotional. Mugwort helps to direct the psychic life into its proper sphere, gradually opening the soul to expanded consciousness.

Mullein *Verbascum thapsus* (yellow)   Professional Kit

Positive qualities: Strong sense of inner conscience, truthfulness, uprightness
Patterns of imbalance: Inability to hear one's inner voice; weakness and confusion, indecisiveness; lying or deceiving oneself or others

Cross-references: Certainty Choice Decisiveness Denial Escapism Guilt Honesty Indecision Individuality Judgment Listening Morality Pregnancy Prejudice Receptivity Self-Actualization True to Self

Consciousness must also include conscience; as the soul gains greater awareness of itself it also acquires an inner voice or moral life. This morality must be generated from within; as long as laws or dictates are stamped on the personality from the outside, the Self will not develop real strength of character. Mullein essence helps the individual at those times when it must wrestle with its own conscience. It can be extremely beneficial for those who lack moral fortitude, and who may resort to dishonesty or deceit in conducting the affairs of daily life. Through Mullein the soul awakens to its inner voice and develops the capacity to listen and respond to its true Self. This remedy can be especially helpful when one must take a stand for personal authenticity, despite social pressure or confusing social mores. The Mullein flower assists the soul in achieving greater moral uprightness, infused with qualities of Light and Truth.

Mustard *Sinapis arvensis* (yellow)   English Kit

Positive qualities: Emotional equanimity, finding joy in life
Patterns of imbalance: Melancholy, gloom, despair; generalized depression without obvious cause

Cross-references: Acceptance Adolescence Anxiety Cheerfulness Courage
Darkness Depression and Despair Destructiveness Discouragement Gloom
Healing Process Joy Lightness Loneliness Martyrdom

Mustard is one of the important remedies for the soul's experience of darkness. The soul in need of this essence feels suddenly overwhelmed with feelings of gloom and despair. This mood does not appear connected with obvious episodes or situations surrounding the person's life. Instead, the feelings are much deeper and more overpowering, especially because the consciousness finds it difficult to penetrate to the cause or meaning of such depression. The reason for this experience lies deep within the subconscious memory, and often points to karmic circumstances beyond the present life. If the events preceding the depression are carefully reviewed the individual can usually identify an image, a word, a person, or a place which served as a trigger point for the unconscious to activate this darker material of the psyche. Mustard assists this healing response, helping one to come to terms with deep, unreconciled parts of the past. This essence is very helpful for complex states of depression, such as manic-depressive mood swings. It brings equilibrium and equanimity by helping the Self to balance extreme polarities of light and dark. Rather than experiencing light as *separate* from darkness, the soul is able to experience darkness as a *transformative process*. In this way, Mustard flower essence helps the soul to anchor and stabilize its light, leading to a sustained experience of gentle joyfulness and quiet radiance.

Nasturtium *Tropaeolum majus* (orange-red) Professional Kit

Positive qualities: Glowing vitality, flaming, radiant energy and warmth
Patterns of imbalance: Feeling overly "dry" or intellectual; depletion of life-force and emotional verve

Cross-references: Balance Body Creativity Devitalization Dryness
Earth Healing and Nature Awareness Energetic Patterns Exhaustion and Fatigue
Immune Disturbances Intellectualism Massage Rejuvenation Seriousness Study
Thinking Vitality Warmth

Nasturtium is indicated for those times when the soul overuses or overextends the thinking forces, so that they are no longer in alignment with the lower, metabolic forces of life and warmth. This remedy is very helpful for students, those whose career demands strong intellectual activity, or for any phase of life where the intellect predominates. If these head forces are allowed to prevail, the soul life will become cold and disconnected from its physical body and from the larger physical body of the Earth. This imbalance predisposes the individual to many forms of physical illness, from colds and congestion in the head, to immune dysfunction and general hardening of the body. Nasturtium flower essence teaches the Self that the polarity of Light, or consciousness, must always be balanced with the opposite pole of Life, or experience. This essence brings warmth and vitality to the thinking process and, furthermore, helps the individual to direct its light into the practical experiences of daily life and physical reality.

Nicotiana *Nicotiana alata* (white)   Research essence
(Flowering Tobacco)

Positive qualities: Peace which is deeply centered in the heart; integration of physical and emotional well-being through harmonious connection with the Earth
Patterns of imbalance: Numbing of the emotions accompanied by mechanization or hardening of the body; inability to cope with deep feelings and finer sensibilities

Cross-references: Addiction Aggressiveness Aloofness Anxiety Avoidance Balance Body Calm City Life Cynicism Denial Devitalization Earth Healing and Nature Awareness Eating Disorders Energetic Patterns Escapism False Persona Hardness Heart Loneliness Lower Self Masculine Consciousness Nervousness Power Repression Sensitivity Strength Tension Vulnerability

In the struggle to achieve balance, the soul needs to receive strength and stability from the Earth. However, if the heart is not sufficiently engaged in this process, the finer etheric sensibilities and feelings may be stymied. This soul disposition can be healed by Nicotiana, or Flowering Tobacco. The worldwide physical addiction to nicotine as a smoking substance is a remarkably rapid and pervasive phenomenon, occurring only since the European discovery of the Americas. During this same period of time, the soul's relationship to the Earth has changed dramatically. The Earth is now seen largely as a source for exploitation rather than nurturing, with its resources used to promote an increasingly technological and machine-based culture. A hardening has occurred in the physical bodies of most modern people, accompanied by a blunting of the emotions and reduced appreciation for that which is subtle and soulful. Those who are addicted to nicotine seek a way to stay grounded and to cope with the harsh forces they feel around them. Tobacco smoking is usually experienced as a sensation of relaxation and greater bodily ease, although more accurately this practice produces a numbing of the feelings. This reduction in the feeling life of the heart, accompanied by greater stimulation to the physical heart, enables the individual to adapt and even thrive in the harder, denser world of modern technology. While the flower essence of Nicotiana is strongly indicated for those who are healing their addiction to tobacco, it also has a much wider application, representing a soul condition which pervades the whole of modern culture. Nicotiana is a very important remedy for the heart, helping it to find true energy and sustenance which is not divorced from the life of feelings. It is very helpful for those who cope by numbing their feelings, hiding behind a tough or "cool" persona, or for those who seek stimulants of any kind that harden or falsify the body's experience of the Earth. The flower essence of Nicotiana re-instills the true spiritual teaching of the Tobacco plant, which is used reverently and judiciously in peace pipe ceremonies by Native Americans. This teaching is that real peace arises from being able to feel deeply with the heart, and that these deep feelings give us our true connection to the Earth and all living beings.

Oak *Quercus robur* (red) English Kit

Positive qualities: Balanced strength, accepting limits, knowing when to surrender
Patterns of imbalance: Iron-willed, inflexible; overstriving beyond one's limits

Cross-references: Acceptance Ambition Attachment Competitiveness Egotism
Exhaustion and Fatigue Failure Flexibility Hardness Healers Leadership Martyrdom
Masculine Consciousness Mid-Life Crisis Overwhelm Perseverance Release
Responsibility Strength Surrender Will Work and Career Goals

Oak addresses many positive masculine soul traits of endurance, strength, and
perseverance. These are the admirable qualities of the Mars-like hero, but they
become a source of illness and dysfunction when they are not balanced with
Venusian grace and gentle surrender. The Oak personality presses the limits of
endurance; such persons are capable of enormous achievement. They are able to
truly serve and help others because of their tremendous wellspring of willpower.
However, this very strength can also become too rigid; the unrelenting demands
and expectations which they have for themselves eventually take a toll on the
physical health and inner happiness of the soul, until finally the individual is forced
by circumstances to acknowledge that he/she is not all-powerful. Oak flower
essence teaches such persons the positive attributes of surrender and acceptance of
limitation. Through Oak the naturally strong capacities of the soul are balanced with
the inner feminine Self, which learns to yield and to receive help from others when
necessary.

Olive *Olea europaea* (white)   English Kit

Positive qualities: Revitalization through connection with one's inner source of energy
Patterns of imbalance: Complete exhaustion after a long struggle

Cross-references: Addiction   Body   Depression and Despair   Devitalization
Energetic Patterns   Exhaustion and Fatigue   Healing Process   Immune Disturbances
Massage   Menopause   Pregnancy   Rejuvenation

Olive essence relieves extreme physical symptoms of exhaustion and weariness. Despite the seemingly physical character of this remedy, it is nevertheless connected to a definite state of soul consciousness. Those needing this essence are usually over-identified with the physical body or the physical dimension. The healing crisis which they experience is actually a spiritual opening, which prompts them to look beyond the purely physical for health and sustenance. For many people, Olive can be their first spiritual opening, bringing the realization that the physical body is sustained by metaphysical forces. They learn that despite the fact that their physical forces are entirely spent, they can tap into another dimension of consciousness which gives renewal and restoration. Olive is helpful for many related, but lesser states of transformation — any time the physical body experiences utter fatigue and breakdown and the individual needs to reach to a higher place for its revitalization. Olive helps bring the awareness that the physical self is profoundly connected with higher states of soul-spiritual consciousness.

Oregon Grape *Berberis aquifolium* (yellow)   Professional Kit

Positive qualities: Loving inclusion of others, positive expectation of good will from others, ability to trust
Patterns of imbalance: Feeling paranoid or self-protective; unfair projection or expectation of hostility from others

Cross-references: Abandonment   Aggressiveness   Appreciation   Blame   City Life
Community Life and Group Experience   Cynicism   Dislike   Faith   Fear   Hate   Hostility
Inner Child   Loneliness   Masculine Consciousness   Negativity   Paranoia
Personal Relationships   Pessimism   Prejudice   Rejection   Resentment   Trust

To trust in the goodness of others is to be nourished by the milk of human kindness. Regrettably, many souls are malnourished; they are unable to receive the sustaining love of others. Oregon Grape is indicated for those persons who are filled with paranoia; they see the world and those around them as hostile and unfair. These patterns were learned in childhood from the family or culture, and have not been healed; instead they fester in the soul and go on to infect all human relationships and social situations. Unfortunately, the soul who is gripped by this paranoid state creates the very reality he/she projects, for those who are treated in a hostile or mistrustful manner usually respond with an equal measure in return. Oregon Grape is widely applicable, but is especially indicated for the tension and ill-will which predominates in many urban environments. Through Oregon Grape the soul learns to break the basic pattern of mistrust. It realizes that it can look instead for the positive intentions of others, and create situations which generate good will and loving inclusion.

Penstemon *Penstemon davidsonii* (violet-blue)   Professional Kit

Positive qualities: Great inner fortitude despite outer hardships; perseverance

Patterns of imbalance: Feeling persecuted or sorry for oneself; inability to bear life's difficult circumstances

Cross-references: Acceptance Adolescence Aging Animals and Animal Care Barriers Body Challenge Children Competitiveness Confidence Courage Death and Dying Discouragement Doubt Failure Frustration Healing Process Learning Difficulties Manifestation Martyrdom Masculine Consciousness Perseverance Personal Relationships Pessimism Pregnancy Prejudice Self-Acceptance Strength Will

The soul lesson of Penstemon is reminiscent of the biblical story of Job, where unusually harsh or severe life circumstances test the soul's uttermost faith and tenacity. Those who need Penstemon seem to have been dealt an unfair blow in life; they may be born handicapped or become physically impaired through an accident. They may have lost a loved one, home, or possessions through a criminal act of violence or a natural catastrophe. Such souls have good reason to feel victimized; yet, in these moments of sorrow and pain, the soul must have the courage to rebuild itself and the faith to trust in a higher power. Penstemon has enormous strengthening powers, enabling the soul to tap into reservoirs of courage and resilience which are normally inaccessible to human consciousness. At its deepest level of transformation, Penstemon essence shows the soul that it has freely chosen even the harshest circumstances for its growth and evolution.

Peppermint *Mentha piperita* (violet)   Professional Kit

Positive qualities: Mindfulness, wakeful clarity, mental alertness
Patterns of imbalance: Dull or sluggish, especially mental lethargy; unbalanced metabolism which depletes mental forces

Cross-references: Addiction Aging Apathy Awakeness Body Clarity
Concentration and Focus Dullness Eating Disorders Energetic Patterns
Exhaustion and Fatigue Learning Difficulties Lightness Mental Clarity Sluggishness
Study Thinking Vitality

Peppermint imparts alert clarity and mental vibrancy. Those who need this remedy have a soul struggle between the lower and upper parts of their being, especially between the metabolic/digestive forces and the thinking/creative forces. In these cases, the life or metabolic forces overwhelm the consciousness with too much warmth, making the mental capacity dull and lethargic. Peppermint is at once cooling and warming. It cools down the lower organs, especially the liver, so that the consciousness can be freed for higher activity. It also stimulates the thinking forces so that they have a "digestive capacity" of a higher nature, making the thinking more lively, vital, and penetrating. Many people who need Peppermint have profound issues around eating and consciousness. They may crave the stimulation of food, only to find themselves sluggish and mentally incapacitated afterwards. It is as though two parts of the Self are warring for attention. Peppermint brings great healing and balancing energy, freeing the mind for higher thought, and helping the digestive, life forces work in their proper sphere.

Pine *Pinus sylvestris* (red f./yellow m.)   English Kit

Positive qualities: Self-acceptance, self-forgiveness; freedom from inappropriate guilt and blame

Patterns of imbalance: Guilt, self-blame, self-criticism, inability to accept oneself

Cross-references: Abuse Acceptance Blame Co-Dependence Criticism
Depression and Despair Destructiveness Father and Fathering Forgiveness Grace Guilt
Hardness Hate Healing Process Inadequacy Inner Child Judgment Lower Self
Manifestation Morality Perfectionism Prejudice Rejection Self-Acceptance
Self-Effacement Shame Softness Time Relationship

Objective acknowledgment of one's faults is an important soul virtue; when taken to an extreme, however, one can be wracked with undue guilt and misery. Those who need Pine get stuck in self-blame. At times a real circumstance from the past may result in deep feelings of regret and remorse; however, the Pine type often feels guilt which is entirely disproportionate to the actual events. These feelings may arise from childhood, when the person learned to internalize blame for dysfunction in the family system, or they may stem from a religious background which emphasizes sin and error more than salvation and grace. Pine helps the Self to learn true forgiveness by quite literally being *for giving:* learning to give oneself nourishment rather than withholding love from oneself; learning to release rather than retain energy. The individual is encouraged to move forward rather than stay entangled in self-deprecation and emotional paralysis. At its highest level, Pine teaches self-acceptance and inner esteem as a pathway to the soul's realization of its own sacredness and divinity.

Pink Monkeyflower *Mimulus lewisii* (pink)   Research Kit

Positive qualities: Emotional openness and honesty; courage to take emotional risks with others

Patterns of imbalance: Feelings of shame, guilt, unworthiness; fear of exposure and rejection, hiding essential Self from others, masking one's feelings

Cross-references: Abandonment Abuse Acceptance Addiction Adolescence Aloofness Anxiety Attention Avoidance Awkwardness Barriers Body Brokenheartedness Children Co-Dependence Communication Community Life and Group Experience Courage Cynicism Eating Disorders Escapism False Persona Father and Fathering Fear Feminine Consciousness Freedom Guilt Hardness Healers Healing Process Heart Honesty Inadequacy Inner Child Insecurity Intimacy Loneliness Love Masculine Consciousness Massage Obsession Personal Relationships Psychosomatic Illness Rejection Release Repression Resistance Self-Effacement Sensitivity Sexuality Shame Sharing Shock Softness Toner Vulnerability

Pink Monkeyflower treats a type of fear which resides in the deepest recesses of the soul: the fear of being *exposed*, of others seeing one's pain and vulnerability. Such persons experience a profound sense of shame, and thus have a need to hide or mask themselves as a form of protection. The Pink Monkeyflower type withdraws in a way that is more pronounced than ordinary shyness, for the soul is attempting to cover deeply internalized wounds from the past. Most frequently, early childhood trauma or abuse — or exploitative and debasing experiences at any phase in life — are the hidden factors in such behavior. These souls are highly sensitive and bear deep pain within themselves. They very much want to reach out and be loved by others, but often fail at making real contact. Such individuals are highly sensitive to being seen, both literally and metaphorically. They are also very vulnerable to being touched and making physical contact with others. Pink Monkeyflower gently opens such souls by helping them to take emotional risks again. In this way, they begin to experience the love and the contact which they so desperately need and want. Pink Monkeyflower is a remedy which is especially effective for the heart, teaching that it is only by remaining open and risking vulnerability that one can experience the warmth of human love and affection.

Pink Yarrow *Achillea millefolium* var. *rubra* (pink-purple)

Professional Kit

Positive qualities: Loving awareness of others from a self-contained consciousness; appropriate emotional boundaries

Patterns of imbalance: Unbalanced sympathetic forces, overly absorbent auric field, lack of emotional clarity, dysfunctional merging with others

Cross-references: Abuse   Animals and Animal Care   Blame   Calm   Children   City Life   Co-Dependence   Community Life and Group Experience   Compassion   Concentration and Focus   Death and Dying   Devitalization   Eating Disorders   Energetic Patterns   Environment   Feminine Consciousness   Guilt   Healers   Healing Process   Heart   Home and Lifestyle   Hysteria   Influence   Inner Child   Intimacy   Irritability   Love   Massage   Menopause   Negativity   Nervousness   Overwhelm   Paranoia   Personal Relationships   Power   Pregnancy   Protection   Sensitivity   Strength   Stress   True to Self   Vulnerability

Every human soul seeks at its deepest level to be compassionate, to open its feeling life to others. The Pink Yarrow type needs to distinguish authentic compassion from overly sympathetic identification with others. For such persons, the boundaries between the Self and others are quite loose and ill-defined. This extreme openness predisposes the soul to easily "bleed," or merge with its environment, particularly the emotional aura of others. As a consequence, such individuals experience emotional confusion and oversensitivity, unable to identify which feelings originate from the Self and which from others. Sometimes this emotional merging is unconscious; at other times, the individual willingly sponges up emotional debris. Such a soul is extremely "allergic" to emotional confusion and disharmony, and hopes to dissipate such discord by internalizing it. Pink Yarrow flower essence imparts greater objectivity and containment. It teaches that true compassion comes from the heart which is in touch with its own spiritual strength. Such a person learns to give love that does not absorb, but radiates; that heals not by sympathetic merging, but by compassionate presence.

Poison Oak *Rhus diversiloba* (greenish-white)   Research Kit

Positive qualities: Emotional openness and vulnerability, ability to be close and make contact with others

Patterns of imbalance: Fear of intimate contact, protective of personal boundaries; fear of being violated; hostile or distant

Cross-references: Aggressiveness Alienation Anger Avoidance Barriers Compassion   Earth Healing and Nature Awareness Environment Escapism Fear Feminine Consciousness Hardness Hostility Impatience Intimacy Irritability Masculine Consciousness Materialism and Money Negativity Personal Relationships Protection Resistance Sensitivity Softness Vulnerability

Many souls have difficulty coping with their softer, more vulnerable feelings. This can be especially true for men, who are culturally influenced to display little intimacy or emotion. Those who need Poison Oak actually have within themselves very deep sensitivity, and can feel quite insecure about their personal boundaries. They fear that if they are too open or too intimate with others, their personal defenses will be violated. Such persons, however, rarely show their vulnerability and sensitivity, for they learn to cope by projecting an overly tough, Mars-like exterior. They erect negative barriers between themselves and others by showing hostility, anger, and irritability, thus keeping a "safe" emotional distance. At the deepest level, such persons are afraid of the inner feminine or of being engulfed by feminine values. This attitude can sometimes extend to feelings about Nature, so that the individual develops a relationship with Nature only through sports or activities that conquer the elements. Poison Oak teaches such souls to open gently by learning to identify and accept the softer side of themselves. In doing so, the soul creates boundaries that are inclusive rather than exclusive, learning that the essential strength of the Self also includes the most sensitive and gentle aspects.

Pomegranate *Punica granatum* (red)   Professional Kit

Positive qualities: Warm-hearted feminine creativity, actively productive and nurturing at home or in the world

Patterns of imbalance: Ambivalent or confused about the focus of feminine creativity, especially between values of career and home, creative and procreative, personal and global

Cross-references: Adolescence Ambivalence Balance Body Choice Conflict Creativity Decisiveness Feminine Consciousness Instinctual Self Life Direction Menopause Mother and Mothering Pregnancy Psychosomatic Illness Sexuality Work and Career Goals

The individual who seeks to evolve through her feminine incarnation is given great possibility and choice in our modern era. Within the feminine soul are strong creative forces which can be used for biological mothering and family nurturing. But these same womb forces can also be used in the larger sphere of "world mother." Many women feel torn in their allegiance to traditional values of family and home, or service in the larger world. Those who attempt to balance both possibilities may feel that their energies are drained and compromised, so that neither role provides full, creative satisfaction. This crisis in the feminine soul may come at a particular stage in the life cycle, such as mid-life or menopause. The psychological tension may be so profound that physical illness is created, especially in the sexual organs. Without conscious awareness of this struggle, the soul does not have the power to choose and act freely. In the end many women short-change their ability to fully realize their feminine creative forces because of the inner confusion and turmoil which they feel. Pomegranate promotes conscious alignment with the feminine creative Self, so that a woman can see more clearly her right destiny and choices. Pomegranate helps the soul to stay connected to the Mother-Spirit-of-Love in all that it gives to the world.

Pretty Face *Triteleia ixioides* (yellow, brown stripes)   Research Kit

Positive qualities: Beauty that radiates from within; self-acceptance in relation to personal appearance

Patterns of imbalance: Feeling ugly or rejected because of personal appearance; over-identified with physical appearance

Cross-references: Abuse Adolescence Aging Alienation Anxiety Awkwardness Body Communication Confidence Darkness Eating Disorders Envy False Persona Feminine Consciousness Healing Process Home and Lifestyle Inadequacy Inner Child Insecurity Lightness Menopause Mid-Life Crisis Perfectionism Prejudice Pride Rejection Self-Acceptance Self-Effacement Self-Esteem Shame

Perhaps at no other time in history have human beings sought so desperately to insure their self-worth by exterior standards of beauty. True beauty is a genuine attribute of the soul which every human being is capable of attaining. But great spiritual illness is created in those who seek to identify themselves only with cultural, cosmetic standards of beauty. Tremendous energy is drained from the soul when one tries to wear a cosmetic "mask" which can never be part of the true, living Self. Pretty Face is indicated for many different situations — for those born with physical deformities or ungainly features, and are especially karmically challenged to find their own inner worth and goodness; for those who, despite normal features, feel the need to excessively groom and alter their appearance; or for those who fear the aging process. In all these cases Pretty Face shifts the soul's awareness from looking outside itself, to finding beauty within. This flower essence encourages the soul to contact its true inner luminosity, for it is this soul radiance which is the real component of beauty.

Purple Monkeyflower *Mimulus kelloggii* (purple)

Research essence

Positive qualities: Inner calm and clarity when experiencing any spiritual or psychic phenomenon; the courage to trust in one's own spiritual experience or guidance; love-based rather than fear-based spirituality

Patterns of imbalance: Fear of the occult, or of any spiritual experience; fear of retribution or censure if one departs from religious conventions of family or community

Cross-references: Abuse Aging Authority Body Calm Children Community Life and Group Experience Confidence Death and Dying Emergency False Persona Freedom Hysteria Individuality Inner Child Meditation Morality Nervousness Obsession Paranoia Protection Repression Self-Esteem Sensitivity Sexuality Shame Spiritual Emergency or Opening Tension Trust

Like the other Mimulus (Monkeyflower) species, Purple Monkeyflower addresses a state of fear within the soul. This flower particularly addresses fear related to experiences of a spiritual or psychic nature. Most typically, the Purple Monkeyflower is beneficial for those individuals whose great need for security and safety causes them to cling to conventional social-religious structures, even though these may not meet the real evolutionary needs of the soul. This prompts an inner conflict between the spiritual impulses received as inner guidance versus outer conventions or expectations. The fear of "going astray" and following one's own authentic path can further be accentuated by harsh or judgmental religious dogma which includes threats of retribution or condemnation. This remedy is a powerful cleanser and stabilizer for projections based on cultural-religious superstition. Purple Monkeyflower is also indicated for intense fear, hallucinations, or paranoia that may result from abrupt or unexpected psychic opening, such as through drugs, cultic ritual abuse, or psychic manipulation. In such cases the soul develops profound fear of the spiritual world as being demonic or horrific. The path of healing for such souls is that of *courage* — to gain one's own authentic experience by encountering spiritual phenomena in a calm and conscious manner. Through this courage, the soul is able to find true spiritual guidance, sustenance and support for life on Earth.

Quaking Grass *Briza maxima* (green)   Professional Kit

Positive qualities: Harmonious social consciousness, finding higher identity in group work, flexibility

Patterns of imbalance: Dysfunctional in group settings, inability to balance individual sense of Self and higher needs of group

Cross-references: Animals and Animal Care   Appreciation   Communication Community Life and Group Experience   Conflict   Cooperation   Desire   Egotism Flexibility   Harmony   Listening   Overview   Personal Relationships   Prejudice   Resistance Tolerance   Work and Career Goals

The soul must constantly balance its individuality with its social identity. A weak sense of Self can give nothing to the world; but too strong an ego can receive nothing from others. Quaking Grass is indicated for those who need to learn how to balance their sense of Self within a group context. This essence is not only very important for individuals, but also for entire groups or family systems to take together. It helps to create a group awareness which is greater than any single person, yet remains conscious of each individual identity. Most importantly, Quaking Grass helps the individual to see her/himself within a larger social matrix. Just as all parts of the physical body form one wholeness, so each individual can learn to see her/his role within a larger social body. This harmonious social consciousness is the special gift of the Quaking Grass flower.

Queen Anne's Lace *Daucus carota* (white)　　　Research Kit

Positive qualities: Spiritual insight and vision; integration of psychic faculties with sexual and emotional aspects of Self
Patterns of imbalance: Projection and lack of objectivity in psychic awareness; distortion of psychic perception or physical eyesight due to sexual or emotional imbalances

Cross-references: Balance　Clarity　Aging　Attention　Awareness　Body Concentration and Focus　Creativity　Denial　Disorientation　Emergency　Groundedness Insight　Instinctual Self　Judgment　Lightness　Lower Self　Meditation　Perspective Psychosomatic Illness　Sensitivity　Sexuality　Spiritual Emergency or Opening　True to Self

Clairvoyance is often thought of in pseudo-mystical terms, but in fact, all human beings are clairvoyant to some extent. Whenever one is able to see not only the physical thing itself, but also the inherent qualities which emanate from the physical, one is seeing clairvoyantly. True clairvoyance is refined to ever more subtle levels in a gradual way, through inner purification of the emotional and instinctual life. Old forms of clairvoyance usually required that the individual sever conscious connection with the physical body and ordinary reality; however, modern clairvoyance depends very much on the ability to form a warm and grounded connection with the physical world. Queen Anne's Lace is an important remedy for this transition of consciousness. It helps to remove debris in the emotional lens of the soul which distorts "clear-seeing." These imbalances in the "third eye" chakra, the center of clairvoyant faculties, often arise from disturbances in the lower chakras, when emotional and instinctual energies such as sexuality are not properly integrated by the individual. Queen Anne's Lace harmonizes both "higher" and "lower" energies, so that one can stay connected with the Earth, yet also be emotionally clear and objective in one's spiritual insight and vision. This essence is helpful for many who are seeking balanced psychic opening, or who may experience vision problems connected with emergent clairvoyance. The Queen Anne's Lace flower helps to ground and stabilize, as well as to refine and sensitize the soul's "clear-seeing."

Quince *Chaenomeles speciosa* (red)   Professional Kit

Positive qualities: Loving strength, balance of masculine initiating power and feminine nurturing power

Patterns of imbalance: Inability to catalyze or reconcile feelings of strength and power with essential qualities of the feminine; distorted connection with the masculine Self or animus

Cross-references: Balance   Co-Dependence   Conflict   Father and Fathering Feminine Consciousness   Hardness   Mother and Mothering   Power   Pregnancy Self-Actualization   Softness   Strength

Love is a force which emanates from the heart, or feeling life, while power radiates primarily from the will sphere of the human being. Yet both these parts of the soul must eventually be integrated. Quince helps those who have difficulty reconciling these seeming opposites. It is especially indicated for women who need to come to terms with the "animus," or inner masculine part of their souls. Until it is consciously integrated, this masculine part may overwhelm the soul, creating a hard or calculating persona which is not consonant with the true feelings of the heart. At other times, Quince may be indicated for men or women who need to use their loving nature in a way that does not compromise their essential dignity and strength. Quince flower essence can be especially important for parents who must demonstrate nurturing and gentle qualities, as well as firm discipline and objectivity. The soul learns through the Quince essence that real power can be loving, and that true love also empowers.

Rabbitbrush *Chrysothamnus nauseosus* (yellow)   Professional Kit

Positive qualities: Active and lively consciousness; alert, flexible and mobile state of mind

Patterns of imbalance: Easily overwhelmed by details; unable to cope with simultaneous events or demanding situations

Cross-references: Attention Awakeness Awareness Concentration and Focus Detail Flexibility Mental Clarity Overview Overwhelm Perspective Scatteredness Study Synthesis Thinking Work and Career Goals

Rabbitbrush is one of the essences which stimulates and vitalizes the awareness faculties of the soul. Its special gift is the ability to combine two seemingly opposite polarities: focused attention to detail, and a wide-ranging perspective which can encompass the "big picture." Most souls are able to master, at best, one of these modalities of awareness. If they develop focus and concentration, it is only by shutting out from their field of vision all that would distract. If they learn to see the full landscape of a situation, then the details blur, leaving only the broad outlines visible. The lesson of the person needing Rabbitbrush is to maintain a clear, precise awareness of a range of individual details, while simultaneously extending the field of awareness to include the larger, organizing principles which interrelate the various individual parts. Rabbitbrush essence is indicated for people who feel overwhelmed by the amount of detail, or by the jumble of simultaneous events which need attention. Many of the jobs in our modern society present such challenges — for example, managing a busy office. By developing the capacity to integrate many simultaneous details while maintaining awareness of the total situation, the soul acquires great agility and flexibility. The person who unconsciously draws the soul's energy out of the body, and resists becoming fully engaged and fully focused in the physical world, will not be able to develop this potential, and will shrink from the seemingly overwhelming challenges of modern life. Rabbitbrush can help such souls to take greater interest in the world around them, thereby strengthening one's ability to learn from physical existence.

Red Chestnut *Aesculus carnea* (red)   English Kit

Positive qualities: Caring for others with calm, inner peace, trust in the unfolding of life events

Patterns of imbalance: Obsessive fear and worry for well-being of others, fearful anticipation of problems for others

Cross-references: Attachment Calm Co-Dependence Doubt Fear Healers
Insomnia Mother and Mothering Obsession Perfectionism Pregnancy Relaxation
Responsibility Sensitivity

To genuinely care for another is a great virtue of the human soul. But this caring can cross the boundary of healthy compassion and turn instead into negative worry and anxiety for another. This is particularly true in a family system or other close relationship, when a parent or spouse is too closely identified with its role as caretaker, and thus becomes unconsciously enmeshed in the psychic space of another. Red Chestnut particularly addresses the mental imbalance which this condition produces. It shows the soul how worry and concern drain the individual of positive vital energy, and does little to help heal the actual situation. When the soul pulls back into its own sphere of consciousness it can effectively anchor itself and become an agent for real healing. The greatest of healing gifts which one can bestow upon another is the ability to radiate calm, loving thoughts. This unconditional regard for another's welfare is the great gift of Red Chestnut.

Red Clover *Trifolium pratense* (pink-red) Professional Kit

Positive qualities: Self-aware behavior, calm and steady presence, especially in emergency situations

Patterns of imbalance: Susceptible to mass hysteria and anxiety, easily influenced by panic or other forms of group thought

Cross-references: Animals and Animal Care Calm Centeredness Challenge Co-Dependence Death and Dying Disorientation Emergency Gloom Hysteria Inner Child Leadership Overwhelm Prejudice Protection Speaking Vulnerability

The ability to maintain one's own sense of individuality can be severely challenged in adverse situations, particularly where conditions of strong "mass consciousness" prevail. It is well known that many people lose their capacity to think and respond when caught in highly-charged "webs" of emotional energy, such as the group panic or hysteria which can arise during natural disasters, war, economic crisis, or when public emotions are inflamed by political or religious demagoguery. Conditions such as these can be seen from another level as a severe form of psychic infectious disease, which rapidly inflames a crowd of people, feeding on currents of fear and confusion. The individual loses his or her own identity and is used as a vehicle to serve the needs of an unleashed force of negativity. This situation can also arise in a family, especially during emergencies or crises, when the blood ties of the family become stronger than the self-awareness of the single individual, who is then propelled by hysterical or destructive energy. Red Clover flower essence is a powerful cleanser and balancer; it is especially related to the psychic properties of the blood, where the spiritual ego of each individual resides. Red Clover infuses strong forces of self-awareness so that the individual can think in a calm and steady way, and act from his/her own center of truth.

Rock Rose *Helianthemum nummularium* (yellow)   English Kit

Positive qualities: Self-transcending courage, inner peace and tranquillity when facing great challenges
Patterns of imbalance: Deep fear, terror, panic; fear of death or annihilation

Cross-references: Challenge Children Courage Death and Dying Emergency Fear Hysteria Immobility Non-Attachment Spiritual Emergency or Opening Surrender Transcendence

Rock Rose flower essence addresses the soul's need for courage, especially in very extreme circumstances. This remedy is indicated for moments when the soul has stepped almost completely outside the body and is in a survival mode of consciousness. The Self is forced to address a severe emergency, usually of life-threatening proportions such as violent attack or a traumatic accident. This remedy can also be indicated for the process of dying, when the ego is gripped by the fear that it will be utterly annihilated or destroyed. Rock Rose restores sun-like forces of courage to the human soul so it can meet these tremendous challenges with self-transcending strength. Although Rock Rose can be used alone, it is most commonly used in the composite "Five Flower Formula" (Star of Bethlehem, Impatiens, Cherry Plum and Clematis) for maximum benefit.

Rock Water solarized spring water English Kit

Positive qualities: Flexibility, spontaneity, and flowing receptivity; following the spirit rather than the letter of the law
Patterns of imbalance: Rigid standards for oneself, asceticism, self-denial

Cross-references: Barriers Criticism Desire Dutifulness Eating Disorders Flexibility Habit Patterns Hardness Idealism Martyrdom Masculine Consciousness Morality Obsession Perfectionism Repression Resistance Seriousness Spiritual Emergency or Opening Spontaneity Tolerance

Rock Water, one of the original English remedies, is not made from a plant, but from the essence of a sacred, underground spring, where the Earth forces are concentrated and consecrated. Rock Water treats a condition of soul which is more mineral than plant-like; it is for those who have extremely rigid attitudes toward life. Although such souls have high philosophical ideals, they suffer from an inability to enjoy life, and their thoughts quickly crystallize into hardened dogma. They adopt schedules for work, or life patterns for eating and sleeping, which are overly restrictive and mechanical. If they are following a spiritual path, such individuals tend towards harsh asceticism, attempting to fit their lives into strict and narrow concepts of spiritual behavior. The essence of Rock Water helps such souls to develop more inner flexibility, and especially to feel the living, pulsing currents of their emotional life. In this way, such persons come more in touch with their feelings, which stream and flow from the inner being much as water courses from the Earth. This essence is sometimes indicated for those beginning flower essence therapy, or for those who cannot feel the results of flower essences. Rock Water opens the soul to the plant realm of consciousness, by helping it to experience the flowering, flowing qualities of the feeling life.

Rosemary *Rosmarinus officinalis* (violet-blue)   Research Kit

Positive qualities: Warm physical presence; embodiment; vibrantly incarnated

Patterns of imbalance: Forgetfulness, poorly incarnated in body, lacking physical/etheric warmth; higher ego forces which are not integrated with the physical body

Cross-references: Abuse Addiction Aging Awakeness Body Centeredness Concentration and Focus Devitalization Disorientation Dreams and Sleep Eating Disorders Energetic Patterns Groundedness Healing Process Inner Child Insecurity Massage Menopause Mental Clarity Nervousness Spiritual Emergency or Opening Stress Warmth

Rosemary flower essence is a strong awakening and incarnating remedy. It is indicated for those souls whose incarnation is weak or disturbed, especially when the higher spiritual or thought faculties cannot work properly through the physical vehicle. This results in a reduced state of consciousness in the body, with a tendency toward absent-mindedness, forgetfulness, or hypoglycemic tendencies. In particular, the soul forces are lacking in warmth and full-bodied presence. Quite literally, this means that the physical extremities of the body are often cold and devitalized. At a deeper level, this lack of warmth stems from with the soul's feeling of insecurity in the physical body. This can sometimes be traced to a karmic disposition of the soul which feels ambivalent about its incarnation and has learned to use its spiritual forces outside the world of physical matter. Very often this soul illness is caused by early childhood trauma, where extreme physical abuse or stress has forced the soul out of the body, so that it no longer trusts its connection with the physical world. Rosemary gives such persons the ability to feel warm and secure in their physical bodies. Through these renewed forces, the spirit's flame burns more brightly in the body and gives its light and consciousness to the physical world.

Sage *Salvia officinalis* (violet)   Research Kit

Positive qualities: Drawing wisdom from life experience; reviewing and surveying one's life process from a higher perspective

Patterns of imbalance: Seeing life as ill-fated or undeserved; inability to perceive higher purpose and meaning in life events

Cross-references: Acceptance Aging Appreciation Attachment Authority Awareness Blame Community Life and Group Experience Cynicism Death and Dying Faith Father and Fathering Forgiveness Insight Leadership Life Direction Masculine Consciousness Materialism and Money Menopause Mid-Life Crisis Non-Attachment Overview Perspective Quiet Self-Esteem Time Relationship Wisdom

Sage flower essence enables the Self to learn and reflect about life experience, particularly enhancing the capacity to experience deep inner peace and wisdom. This remedy addresses a natural distillation process which occurs as the healthy person ages. Throughout the course of life, trials and tribulations are placed in the soul's path so that it can distill impurities and volatile emotions, reaching an ever more clarified and refined state. Through the aging process, the soul should be able to attain increasing inner stability and peaceful acceptance of its condition. If one is unable to experience this graceful maturation process, life events seem ill-fated and undeserved, without higher purpose or meaning. The Sage remedy can be helpful during various life phases and transitions, when one needs to step back and consider the unfolding events of life. However, it is particularly indicated for advanced stages of the life biography, when the Self must learn to survey life experience, and to glean wisdom and insight. Through Sage, the soul comes more in touch with its own spiritual meaning and purpose, and thus acquires profound wisdom to heal and counsel others.

Sagebrush *Artemisia tridentata* (yellow)

Professional Kit
Seven Herbs Kit

Positive qualities: Essential or "empty" consciousness, deep awareness of the inner Self, capable of transformation and change

Patterns of imbalance: Over-identification with the illusory parts of oneself; purifying and cleansing the Self to release dysfunctional aspects of one's personality or surroundings

Cross-references: Addiction Adolescence Attachment Breakthrough Cleansing Creativity Death and Dying Depression and Despair Desire Egotism False Persona Freedom Greed Grief Habit Patterns Healing Process Home and Lifestyle Honesty Individuality Life Direction Materialism and Money Menopause Mid-Life Crisis Non-Attachment Purification Quiet Receptivity Release Self-Esteem Soulfulness Time Relationship Transcendence Transition True to Self

If the soul is not prepared to go through the psychological experience of "the abyss," or emptiness, it robs itself of the essential precondition for rebirth, or transformation. Especially in our modern culture which emphasizes materialism and ego-inflation, it is difficult for the personality to voluntarily practice emptiness and detachment. Many people cling too tightly to exterior props of existence through over-identification with possessions, lifestyle or social recognition, and thereby deny themselves the opportunity for true soul evolution. Often, the Higher Self intervenes by setting up a condition to cleanse the false persona through illness or misfortune. Sagebrush helps one to come in touch with the naked, essential Self, for it is here that truly free and spacious spiritual forces reign. As the soul recognizes what is absolutely essential to its identity and releases what no longer serves its evolution, it moves forward in its destiny with far greater forces of discrimination and inner freedom.

Saguaro *Cereus giganteus* (white, yellow center)   Professional Kit

Positive qualities: Awareness of what is ancient and sacred, a sense of tradition or lineage; ability to learn from elders
Patterns of imbalance: Conflict with images of authority, sense of separateness or alienation from the past

Cross-references: Acceptance Adolescence Alienation Ambivalence Authority
Blame Conflict Criticism Destructiveness Father and Fathering
Feminine Consciousness Prejudice Resistance Will Wisdom

In the soul's struggle for freedom and self-determination, it can sometimes react negatively to all which has come from the past. In these instances, the individual lacks the insight to acknowledge that it has freely chosen its incarnation in a particular subculture, race, folk-soul, or family constellation. When these deep connections are not understood, the very influences from which the personality seeks liberation are often unconsciously internalized and negatively re-enacted in a subsequent phase of life. Saguaro addresses rebellious tendencies of the emotional life, refining these into positive qualities of awareness and insight. This remedy is particularly indicated for the adolescent and young adult phases of life. Saguaro can also be helpful when the individual requires a deeper understanding of his or her tradition, lineage, or culture, or needs to establish a more conscious relationship to elder authority and guidance. By actively embracing and understanding its past, the soul is free to grow and change in a more conscious and clear way.

Saint John's Wort *Hypericum perforatum* (yellow)   Professional Kit

Positive qualities: Illumined consciousness, light-filled awareness and strength
Patterns of imbalance: Overly expanded state leading to psychic and physical vulnerability; deep fears, disturbed dreams

Cross-references: Shock Aging Awakeness Certainty Children Confidence Darkness Daydreaming Death and Dying Devitalization Dreams and Sleep Emergency Fear Groundedness Insecurity Insomnia Lightness Massage Protection Sensitivity Spiritual Emergency or Opening   Trust   Vulnerability

As flowers need sunlight in order to grow, so also the soul needs light — both physical and spiritual — to flourish. However, some souls lose themselves in light because they have not developed proper rooting. Saint John's Wort is indicated for those persons who are quite sensitive or over-receptive to the effects of light; they may be fair-skinned, easily sunburned, or find themselves adversely affected by intense heat or light. They are prone to many forms of environmental stress, including allergies. These individuals have a very active psychic life — the astral body expands greatly during sleep, often distorting its connection with the physical and etheric bodies, or with the ego. This weak association to the other bodies results in a propensity for invasion or attack from negative elemental forces or other entities, especially during sleep; dream disturbances, bed-wetting, or night sweats can be common symptoms. Saint John's Wort flower essence has marvelous restorative powers; it provides protection and strength when the soul is in an overly expanded state. While it is generally indicated for those who are oversensitive to light, it can also be helpful for those deprived of light, such as Seasonal Affective Disorder. At its deepest level of transformation, Saint John's Wort helps the soul to circulate light through the body and into the Earth. Rather than experiencing light as an external and merely physical reality, light works within the Self as a spiritual force which can illumine and anchor the consciousness.

Scarlet Monkeyflower *Mimulus cardinalis* (red)   Professional Kit

Positive qualities: Emotional honesty, direct and clear communication of deep feelings, integration of the emotional "shadow"
Patterns of imbalance: Fear of intense feelings, repression of strong emotions; inability to resolve issues of anger and powerlessness

Cross-references: Addiction Anger Avoidance Awareness Breakthrough Catharsis Communication Courage Death and Dying Denial Destructiveness Escapism Father and Fathering Fear Freedom Hate Honesty Inner Child Instinctual Self Lower Self Masculine Consciousness Menopause Mother and Mothering Negativity Perfectionism Personal Relationships Power Rejection Repression Resistance Shadow Consciousness Shame

The Scarlet Monkeyflower treats a particular state of fear within the human soul: the soul's fear of its own "shadow self" or lower emotions. Those who need this remedy often keep a "lid" on unpleasant emotions. These feelings remain bottled up in the psyche, subject to increasing levels of tension and pressure, until the individual explodes in blind rage or other raw emotions. Unfortunately, these episodes seem to confirm the worst fears — that there is an explosive, demonic force lurking inside — and so the soul is often caught in a vicious cycle of repressing emotional material, only to have it ooze out or explode full force when the ego's "lid" can no longer hold it in. Scarlet Monkeyflower gives the soul courage to actively acknowledge and confront such feelings. These emotions of anger or other intense feelings often have a legitimate basis, but because they are not dealt with in a timely fashion, they loom out of proportion in the psyche. As these experiences are more quickly and honestly acknowledged, the soul learns that it is healthier to integrate such material than to repress it. Scarlet Monkeyflower imparts emotional depth, honesty, and vitality to the soul in its journey toward true wholeness.

Scleranthus *Scleranthus annuus* (green)   English Kit

Positive qualities: Decisiveness, inner resolve, acting from the certainty of inner knowing

Patterns of imbalance: Hesitation, indecision, confusion, wavering between two choices

Cross-references: Ambivalence Balance Breakthrough Certainty Choice Confidence Conflict Decisiveness Desire Doubt Erratic Behavior Escapism Hesitation Immobility Indecision Judgment Life Direction Manifestation Morality Pregnancy Psychosomatic Illness Restlessness Scatteredness

The experience of living on Earth is one of duality; the soul must constantly learn to establish its own inner balance through the tension of polarity. The individual who needs Scleranthus finds this level of inner activity to be very painful and challenging. Subconsciously, such a person longs for wholeness as a given external condition of life, not realizing that a far greater wholeness is achieved through the ability to choose and define who one is. Such individuals are by nature introverted and would prefer a quiet existence, but because of the need in their souls to evolve, they are often caught in one turmoil-creating incident or another. They tend to vacillate when making choices, and can postpone major, life-directing decisions for years. This extreme uncertainty drains the soul of much vitality and energy, and can permeate even into the physical body with numerous illnesses, especially characterized by a continual shifting of physical states and symptoms. Scleranthus flower essence helps such souls toward greater decisiveness and clarity of purpose. This enables the Self to make choices not only at the obvious, symptomatic level; at a deeper level the soul learns to choose greater involvement in its experience of earthly life.

Scotch Broom *Cytisus scoparius* (yellow)   Professional Kit

Positive qualities: Positive and optimistic feelings about the world and about future events; sun-like forces of caring, encouragement, and purpose

Patterns of imbalance: Feeling weighed down and depressed; overcome with pessimism and despair, especially regarding one's personal relationship to world events

Cross-references: Acceptance   Challenge   Darkness   Depression and Despair   Discouragement   Doubt   Earth Healing and Nature Awareness   Faith   Gloom   Manifestation   Motivation   Perseverance   Perspective   Pessimism   Service   Strength

We live in a time of great uncertainty, transformation, and upheaval. These powerful conditions can predispose many souls to feel very anxious and depressed about their lives and the future of the Earth. Such persons may be morbidly attracted to apocalyptic scenarios of the future, or exposure to mass media portrayal of world events may arouse intense feelings of pessimism and despair. These feelings burden the soul with extreme emotional weight so that the soul becomes heavy and "deep-pressed." At the core of such illness is the feeling of "What's the use?" or "Why try?" The depression such persons experience is characterized not only by feelings about their personal lives, but about the world as a whole and their relationship to world events. Thus the soul is paralyzed in the positive use of its forces, unconsciously adding to the darkness of the "world-psyche." Scotch Broom gives tenacity and strength, enabling the individual to move from personal despair to impersonal service and concern for the welfare of the world. This essence helps the soul to meet the challenges of our times as opportunities for self-growth and for helping others. In making this transition, the soul shifts from its unconscious identification with world darkness to the vision of a more hopeful, positive world future.

Self-Heal *Prunella vulgaris* (violet)   Professional Kit

Positive qualities: Healthy, vital sense of Self; healing and beneficent forces arising from within oneself, deep sense of wellness and wholeness

Patterns of imbalance: Inability to take inner responsibility for one's healing, lacking in spiritual motivation for wellness, overly dependent on external help

Cross-references: Addiction Aging Ambivalence Animals and Animal Care Body Children Cleansing Confidence Conflict Denial Doubt Eating Disorders Emergency Energetic Patterns Escapism Exhaustion and Fatigue Faith Healers Healing Process Immune Disturbances Individuality Inner Child Learning Difficulties Massage Menopause Mid-Life Crisis Psychosomatic Illness Rejuvenation Resistance Seeking Self-Acceptance Self-Actualization Shock Toner Trust Vitality

Self-Heal flower essence is one of the most fundamental and broadly applicable remedies for true soul healing and balance. Its very name is exquisitely evocative of its profound qualities; this essence addresses the capacity of the Self to become involved with and take responsibility for its own healing journey. No variety of outer measures and techniques can bring about genuine healing at any level unless the individual is quickened from within and motivated to seek and affirm the wholeness of life. Self-Heal flower essence addresses a very special relationship between the etheric, or life body, and the Spiritual Self. On the physical level, the etheric body restores wholeness to wounds and other afflictions by quite literally *"re-covering"* the body with its life sheath. The Higher Self can also draw upon this etheric life force and the possibility for *recovery.* Self-Heal flower essence is especially indicated for those who have lost belief in their own capacity to be well, or who have abdicated this inherent responsibility to healers or others. It is a very beneficial remedy for those who face great healing challenges, whether physical, mental, or spiritual. The great lesson and the powerful gift of Self-Heal is to enable the Self to affirm and to draw from the deep wellspring of etheric life, toward true recovery and restoration.

Shasta Daisy *Chrysanthemum maximum* (white/yellow center)
Professional Kit

Positive qualities: Mandalic or holistic consciousness, synthesizing ideas into a living wholeness

Patterns of imbalance: Over-intellectualization of reality, especially seeing information as bits and pieces rather than parts of a whole

Cross-references: Awareness   Children   Community Life and Group Experience Concentration and Focus   Creativity   Detail   Harmony   Healers   Healing Process Home and Lifestyle   Insight   Inspiration   Intellectualism   Manifestation   Mental Clarity Overview   Perspective   Scatteredness   Study   Synthesis   Thinking   Toner   Wisdom

The thinking part of the soul functions by dividing phenomena into smaller, more easily understood components. However, if the analytical aspect of the mind holds too great a sway, the consciousness can no longer experience greater wholeness and meaning in its understanding of life. This is an especially powerful tendency in our modern culture, where the thinking and intellectual life is given great prominence and emphasis. Shasta Daisy imparts insight into the broader meanings and larger patterns of mental and emotional experience. This remedy can be very helpful for those involved in writing, teaching, research, or other intellectual professions. It is also beneficial in any therapeutic process where the essential emotional experience is broken into smaller parts. Shasta Daisy enables the Self to re-integrate and re-pattern the emotional life into new wholeness and self-identity. Shasta Daisy helps the soul become more capable of archetypal or wholistic consciousness, stimulating great forces of intelligence and insight into life experience.

Shooting Star *Dodecatheon hendersonii* (violet/pink) Professional Kit

Positive qualities: Humanized spirituality, cosmic consciousness warmed with caring for all that is human and earthly

Patterns of imbalance: Profound feeling of alienation, especially not feeling at home on Earth, nor a part of the human family

Cross-references: Alienation Ambivalence Awkwardness Body Children Choice Earth Healing and Nature Awareness Environment Escapism Groundedness Inner Child Intimacy Involvement Life Direction Personal Relationships Pregnancy Rejection

Shooting Star is a very special remedy for those souls who hold back from full participation in earthly life. They may have waited for a long period of time before seeking earthly incarnation, and may have sojourned in other cosmic dimensions which feel more familiar. These souls suffer in a profound way — an affliction which often receives little understanding from family or friends, or even from therapists. Such persons have often been preoccupied, even from childhood, with stories of extra-terrestrial existence, and they may feel that they are actively in touch with such forms of life. It is common for these individuals to have birth trauma or complications, since the soul often hesitates or pulls back at the moment of contraction into matter. Shooting Star helps such persons to find their right connection to earthly life. Rather than feeling merely imprisoned in matter, the soul comes to experience its body as a vehicle for true self-containment and awareness. In this way such individuals come to understand the meaning of love, for love is experienced in a uniquely human way through that which streams freely from the self-aware human heart. At its deepest level, Shooting Star teaches such souls that the Earth is the right place to humanize one's cosmic consciousness, for it is the place to learn about heart-impelled love.

Snapdragon *Antirrhinum majus* (yellow)   Research Kit

Positive qualities: Lively, dynamic energy; healthy libido; verbal communication which is emotionally balanced

Patterns of imbalance: Verbal aggression and hostility; repressed or misdirected libido; tension around jaw

Cross-references: Abuse   Aggressiveness   Anger   Animals and Animal Care   Authority   Blame   Body   Communication   Community Life and Group Experience   Creativity   Criticism   Destructiveness   Eating Disorders   Feminine Consciousness   Hate   Honesty   Hostility   Instinctual Self   Irritability   Lower Self   Negativity   Personal Relationships   Power   Repression   Self-Aggrandizement   Self-Expression   Sexuality   Shadow Consciousness   Speaking   Strength   Tension   Will

The positive Snapdragon type possesses strong physical presence. Such persons are highly energetic, with powerful wills and libidos. In some cases, these energies are so pronounced that they override the other chakras of the body. In other instances, these forces may have been culturally repressed, causing the energy to be improperly released elsewhere in the body. With both these patterns of imbalance, the individual will misdirect digestive and sexual forces which rightly belong in the lower energy centers, distorting them through expression in the communication center. The spoken word is misused in a harsh or destructive way, with the tendency toward biting sarcasm or lashing criticism. There can be extreme tension in the jaw and mouth, grinding of the teeth, or the need to eat foods which provide continuous biting, crunching, and chewing activity. Snapdragon helps such persons re-direct their powerful metabolic and sexual energy into its rightful channels. At its deepest level, the Snapdragon helps the soul to distinguish its use of creative forces — especially those which radiate from the lower energy centers, and those which are used for the spoken word. By harmonizing the relationship between these energy centers, the soul evolves in its use of creative power.

Star of Bethlehem *Ornithogalum umbellatum* (white)   English Kit

Positive qualities: Bringing soothing, healing qualities, a sense of inner divinity

Patterns of imbalance: Shock or trauma, either recent or from a past experience; need for comfort and reassurance from the spiritual world

Cross-references: Abuse Addiction Animals and Animal Care Body Calm Children Death and Dying Emergency Grief Psychosomatic Illness Sensitivity Shock Soothing Stress

Star of Bethlehem is a deeply restorative remedy, with calm, soothing properties for people who have experienced shock or trauma. It is particularly helpful for individuals who have never adequately addressed a disturbance from the past. Such persons often seek to anesthetize this trauma in inappropriate ways, such as through drugs, occult ritual, or a numbing of awareness. There is a longing and seeking for a part of the Spiritual Self which seems inaccessible. The nervous system often becomes deadened, and the mental faculties are lacking in vibrancy and coherency. In some essential way, the personality is out of alignment with its higher components, and is stymied from full and vibrant functioning. Star of Bethlehem helps bring about this much-needed psychic and spiritual adjustment, although other therapeutic and counseling measures are often necessary to help the individual fully access the trauma and its causes. Star of Bethlehem is also one of the ingredients in the Five-Flower Formula indicated by Dr. Bach for broad-based emergency and first aid use.

Star Thistle *Centaurea solstitialis* (yellow)   Professional Kit

Positive qualities: Generous and inclusive, a giving and sharing nature, feeling an inner sense of abundance
Patterns of imbalance: Basing actions on a fear of lack, inability to give freely and openly, or to trust a higher providence

Cross-references: Community Life and Group Experience   Cynicism   Fear   Greed
Insecurity   Materialism and Money   Morality   Mother and Mothering
Personal Relationships   Possessiveness   Resistance   Selfishness   Sharing

Star Thistle addresses the capacity for generosity and sharing in the human soul. It is particularly indicated for "fear of lack," or the feeling that there is not enough. Such persons are malnourished at a deep level. There is often a disturbance in the bond with the mother, which is transferred as an unhealthy bond to matter (the Latin word *mater* means *mother*). Such persons seek to establish a matrix of security for the essential Self by gaining firm hold of the material world, with a tendency to hoard and carefully guard their material possessions. This state of consciousness can be present whether the individual is outwardly wealthy or poor. The Star Thistle type is often socially reclusive or antipathetic, having a difficult time learning to trust, or to share his/her Self or resources in an open, generous way. They are susceptible to premature physical aging, especially hardening or sclerotic diseases or disturbances in the liver. Despite possible wealth or status, such persons are often lonely at their deepest core, and feel profoundly unnourished and unfulfilled. Star Thistle helps such souls to feel more secure within themselves and therefore less dependent on external things. As the soul feels fuller, it learns to open itself, and to share and give more freely. The Star Thistle teaches that it is through giving that one finds inner nourishment, and through the sharing of the Self that one becomes richer and more abundantly "full"-filled.

Star Tulip *Calochortus tolmiei* (white/purple)

also known as Cat's Ears

Professional Kit

Seven Herbs Kit

Positive qualities: Sensitive and receptive attunement; serene, inner listening to others and to higher worlds, especially in dreams and meditation

Patterns of imbalance: Feelings of being hardened or cut-off, inability to feel quiet inner presence or attunement, unable to meditate or pray

Cross-references: Addiction Aging Awareness Barriers Clarity Creativity Death and Dying Denial Dreams and Sleep Dullness Environment Feminine Consciousness Grace Hardness Harmony Home and Lifestyle Insight Inspiration Intimacy Listening Masculine Consciousness Massage Meditation Mother and Mothering Pregnancy Purification Quiet Receptivity Resistance Sensitivity Softness Soulfulness Spiritual Emergency or Opening Toner Wisdom

Star Tulip is an exquisite remedy for gently opening and expanding the life of the soul. It can be characterized as a "listening" remedy, helping the soul to become more aware of subtle influences, or of guidance from higher realms. This remedy is very beneficial for those who feel unable to contact their Higher Self, or who feel they cannot meditate or pray effectively. Star Tulip has a strong relationship to the "anima," or inner feminine. It is an excellent remedy for men who have denied their softer, more receptive side, or for women who may have built a shell of protection around themselves. Star Tulip opens and sensitizes the soul, making it more aware of its connection to higher worlds. It enhances dreaming, prayer, meditation, and all intuitive capacities. It is an important essence for the beginning stages of the therapeutic process, helping to open and "soften" the emotional life, enabling the individual to recognize and retrieve important information about the inner healing process. At its deepest expression, Star Tulip builds a chalice-like vessel in the human soul, creating the capacity to receive and contain higher thought and inspiration.

Sticky Monkeyflower *Mimulus aurantiacus* (orange)

Professional Kit

Positive qualities: Balanced integration of human warmth and sexual intimacy; ability to express deep feelings of love and connectedness, especially in sexual relationships

Patterns of imbalance: Repressed sexual feelings, or acting out inappropriate sexual behavior; inability to experience human warmth in sexual experiences; deep fear of sexuality and intimacy

Cross-references: Adolescence Awkwardness Desire Escapism Fear Inadequacy Instinctual Self Intimacy Loneliness Masculine Consciousness Menopause Obsession Personal Relationships Rejection Repression Sexuality Warmth

Through human sexuality one can come in deepest contact with another human being. The strongest soul ecstasy is afforded through such communion, but also the most painful soul illness. This distortion and suffering is especially pronounced in our modern society. That which is most profound is often the most profaned; indeed, human sexuality is publicized, commercialized, and exploited in every possible manner. Sticky Monkeyflower heals those who are challenged in their efforts to understand and affirm their true sexuality. Such persons have a deep fear of intimacy and human contact, sometimes avoiding relationships altogether. Often, they mask their fear by over-compensation, choosing numerous superficial sexual relationships which do not really engage full-hearted participation or emotional vulnerability. Such souls, at their very core, fear exposure of the Self to another human being. Thus, the expression of sexuality is often shallow or devoid of real presence. Sticky Monkeyflower helps such souls come in contact with the true feelings of the Self, and especially the relationship of sexual impulses and desires to the authentic emotions of the heart. When the soul honors this true Self, it is guided by the warmest impulses of love and compassion in its expression of human sexuality.

Sunflower *Helianthus annuus* (yellow)   Professional Kit

Positive qualities: Balanced sense of individuality, spiritualized ego forces, sun-radiant personality

Patterns of imbalance: Distorted sense of Self; inflation or self-effacement, low self-esteem or arrogance; poor relation to father or masculine aspect of Self

Cross-references: Action Addiction Adolescence Aggressiveness Alienation Authority Balance Children Co-Dependence Compassion Confidence Conflict Death and Dying Egotism False Persona Father and Fathering Feminine Consciousness Healers Healing Process Inadequacy Individuality Inner Child Leadership Masculine Consciousness Materialism and Money Personal Relationships Power Pride Self-Acceptance Self-Actualization Self-Aggrandizement Self-Effacement Self-Esteem Self-Expression Speaking Strength Transcendence

The healthy Self shines forth from the soul, not unlike the sun which shines in the sky. This benign and wondrous soul quality of radiance at once inspires with its light, and heals with its warmth. All human souls have within them this capacity to shine like the sun, but many are afflicted in their ability to emanate this solar power in a balanced way. Some people mask their true sun-nature with feelings of self-effacement and low self-esteem. This condition darkens the true luster of the Self; in these instances the Sunflower essence brings to the soul the quality of *light*. Others want their brilliance to shine too strongly, glaring others with pompous self-glory and ego-aggrandizement. For these people, Sunflower brings out the quality of *warmth*, or loving compassion. Just as the soul absorbs from the mother the moon-like qualities of receptivity and nurturing, so does the soul learn from the father the sun-like qualities of the shining, expressive Self. Sunflower heals disturbances or distortions in the soul's relationship to the masculine, often associated with a conflicted or deficient relationship with the father in childhood. This healing of the masculine Self is equally important for both men and women. The message of the Sunflower is so universal and foundational that it is beneficial at nearly every stage in the human life cycle. When the soul learns how to harness this great sun force within its Self, it is truly able to bless and heal other human beings and the Earth.

Sweet Chestnut *Castanea sativa* (green f./yellow m.)   English Kit

Positive qualities: Deep courage and faith which comes from knowing and trusting the spiritual world

Patterns of imbalance: Strong despair and anguish; experiencing the "dark night of the soul"

Cross-references: Abandonment Abuse Brokenheartedness Challenge Darkness Death and Dying Depression and Despair Faith Loneliness Martyrdom Mid-Life Crisis Rejection Spiritual Emergency or Opening Surrender Transcendence

Sweet Chestnut heals the deepest form of soul anguish and despair — that which is often referred to as the "dark night of the soul." The conditions which require Sweet Chestnut are extreme, and the individual is often in the most negative and acute form of suffering; however, this remedy is the harbinger of great spiritual transformation. The one who needs Sweet Chestnut is tested literally to the breaking point of endurance. Although the cause of such pain is based on a deeply personal situation, there is nevertheless a profound existential quality related to this state, for the soul feels utterly alone in its suffering. Sweet Chestnut is often indicated in drug addiction or suicide therapy, when the individual feels that he or she has hit "rock bottom." It can be indicated for many other extreme conditions, such as the death of a loved one or realization that one has a life-threatening illness. Through these forms of intense suffering, the Self surrenders to a Higher Power and is able to be reborn. It is precisely in this way that transformational healing is possible, for when the soul is stretched to its limits it also becomes transcendent. Sweet Chestnut helps the soul surrender and open to a new spiritual identity.

Sweet Pea *Lathyrus latifolus* (red-purple)   Professional Kit

Positive qualities: Commitment to community, social connectedness, a sense of one's place on Earth
Patterns of imbalance: Wandering, seeking, inability to form bonds with social community or to find one's place on Earth

Cross-references: Abandonment Adolescence Alienation Community Life
and Group Experience Conflict Earth Healing and Nature Awareness Environment
Escapism Father and Fathering Fear Groundedness Home and Lifestyle Involvement
Life Direction Loneliness Personal Relationships Rejection Scatteredness Seeking

Many souls are like pilgrims, searching and seeking for their place on Earth. When this condition is overemphasized, the individual is lost in wanderlust, unable to form true social bonds of caring and commitment. Such people move from one place to another, or from one community of friends to another, without becoming truly involved. They become hardened in their stance as "outsiders," and are deprived of true soul growth by being unable to establish roots in family or community life. At the heart of the suffering of one who needs Sweet Pea is a deep feeling of homelessness. Such persons do not have within themselves "a sense of place," or love for the Earth. This alienation can come from the experience of literal homelessness, or for those who were required to move a great deal during childhood. This imbalance is also related to urban and suburban living conditions — high-rise apartment complexes, urban ghettos, or anemic suburban developments — which rob the soul of its natural feeling of interest and connection to the Earth and the forces of Nature. The Sweet Pea helps such persons to come in contact with their feelings about "home." By acknowledging and experiencing this pain which has numbed the Self, the soul can begin to heal, and find its true connection to the Earth and to other human beings.

Tansy *Tanacetum vulgare* (yellow)   Professional Kit

Positive qualities: Decisive and goal-oriented, deliberate and purposeful in action, self-directed

Patterns of imbalance: Lethargy, procrastination, inability to take straightforward action; habits which undermine or subvert real intention of Self

Cross-references: Action Aloofness Apathy Body Breakthrough Catalyst Co-Dependence Decisiveness Desire Eating Disorders Energetic Patterns Hesitation Home and Lifestyle Immobility Indecision Inertia Manifestation Motivation Procrastination Repression Resistance Self-Actualization Sluggishness Time Relationship Will Work and Career Goals

Tansy flower essence addresses the consciousness of the Self in a very special way. Those who need this remedy exhibit a great deal of sluggish, lethargic energy; they are very often indecisive, tend to procrastinate when making decisions or commitments, and appear lazy, indifferent, or nonchalant. Although their will forces are indeed stymied, it is usually ineffective to treat the will, or physical energy level of such persons directly. Healing insight comes through understanding *why* such persons hold back the real expression of their Self. This soul type responds to intense overwhelm, excitement, or any feeling of pressure or tension by withdrawing and restricting physical energy. Sometimes this is a temporary response to current life situations, but generally speaking one will find this way of handling energy to be a deeply unconscious and ingrained pattern which is associated with family and early childhood trauma. Such persons have been exposed to a great deal of chaos, confusion, emotional instability, or even violence, and have learned to suppress their natural response to situations as a way of keeping peace, or avoiding further emotional overwhelm. They energetically "downshift" as an avoidance mechanism for emotional distancing and coping. Tansy stimulates the self-awareness of such persons, helping them to contact their true strength and purpose. In this way, such souls become more decisive and straightforward in their response to others and to life, and come to realize more fully their true Self.

Tiger Lily *Lilium humboldtii* (orange/brown spots)   Professional Kit

Positive qualities: Cooperative service with others, extending feminine forces into social situations; inner peace and harmony as a foundation for outer relationships
Patterns of imbalance: Overly aggressive, competitive, hostile attitude; excessive "yang" forces, separatist tendencies

Cross-references: Aggressiveness   Altruism   Ambition   Animals and Animal Care City Life   Community Life and Group Experience   Competitiveness   Cooperation Earth Healing and Nature Awareness   Feminine Consciousness   Hostility   Instinctual Self Leadership   Lower Self   Masculine Consciousness   Materialism and Money   Menopause Personal Relationships   Power   Service

The positive healing of ourselves and the larger world depends very much on the ability to shift from competitive, aggressive models of behavior to those which are cooperative and inclusive. This transition of consciousness involves the internalization of feminine values in the larger culture, especially in business and politics. Tiger Lily is an extremely beneficial remedy for helping the soul to transmute overly hostile or aggressive tendencies into positive social impulses. It helps the consciousness to move from a limited personal perspective toward values that include the greater whole. This essence especially benefits those who see themselves as separate from others, or as striving *against* others rather than working *for* the common good. In general, Tiger Lily balances overly *yang*, contracted energy, and is very helpful for many men who have not fully integrated the inner feminine *(anima)* part of themselves. Tiger Lily is also indicated for women who are addressing issues of the inner masculine *(animus)*, and is particularly valuable at the time of menopause when more masculine energy is available to the consciousness. While Tiger Lily is broadly associated with feminine energy, it is uniquely related to the *strength* of the feminine forces, or the ability of the feminine Self to work actively within yang or masculine structures or contexts. The Tiger Lily helps the human soul to harness its essential power and strength in the service of higher good and world evolution.

Trillium *Trillium chloropetalum* (purple)   Professional Kit

Positive qualities: Selfless service, altruistic sacrifice of personal desires for the common good, inner purity

Patterns of imbalance: Greed and lust for possessions and power; excessive ambition, overcome with personal needs and desires; materialism and congestion

Cross-references: Aggressiveness Altruism Ambition Attachment Competitiveness Cooperation Desire Envy Greed Instinctual Self Involvement Lower Self Masculine Consciousness Materialism and Money Mid-Life Crisis Morality Non-Attachment Overview Personal Relationships Possessiveness Power Self-Aggrandizement Selfishness Service Sharing Will Work and Career Goals

Trillium flower essence is a very effective cleanser and balancer for the lowest human energy center, referred to as the survival (base) chakra. A person needing Trillium has a disproportionate amount of energy directed toward issues of personal power or welfare. This excessive concern for personal well-being overrides other, more altruistic feelings within the soul. Such a person easily falls prey to the forces of materialism and greed, feeling a need for many possessions and other forms of material wealth and power. This remedy can also be indicated for one who is in poverty, but believes that acquisition of wealth and power would bring fulfillment. This soul imbalance can also be reflected in the body, especially when the body retains too much matter and does not effectively eliminate toxic waste. At the deepest level, such souls are disconnected from their spiritual strength; they seek to overcome an unconscious feeling of impotence by the exercise of social and material power. Because their awareness is limited to the physical plane, such souls can measure their self-worth only by material standards. Trillium encourages these individuals to shift their awareness to a transpersonal level, to derive a sense of personal well-being from a relationship to a *Higher Power*. Once the forces contained in the lowest chakra are purified and freed, such persons have great capacity to ground and harness spiritual forces in the service of others and of the Earth.

Trumpet Vine *Campsis tagliabuana* (red-orange)   Professional Kit

Positive qualities: Articulate and colorful in verbal expression; active, dynamic projection of oneself in social situations

Patterns of imbalance: Lack of vitality or soul force in expression; inability to be assertive or to speak clearly, impediments in speech

Cross-references: Aggressiveness Anxiety Children Communication Confidence Creativity Dryness Freedom Leadership Learning Difficulties Manifestation Self-Esteem Self-Expression Speaking Vitality

The capacity for human speech — to ensoul sound with thought and feeling — is one of the most extraordinary of human gifts. Yet for many souls, the ability to use the word as a creative force is stymied. Trumpet Vine flower essence is indicated for speech which tends to be mechanical, dull, or constricted, and can be very helpful for various speech impediments such as stuttering. It does not directly address fear or nervousness, but is nevertheless beneficial for many people who curtail their expression due to feelings of intimidation or shyness. With the help of Trumpet Vine, the soul is able to contact life energy residing in the lower chakras and to integrate these vital forces with the spoken word. Awareness and interest is brought to the expression itself, rather than focusing on the perception or judgment of others. Trumpet Vine awakens the warm and colorful feeling life of the soul, helping these qualities flow into the human speech. As the soul learns to project and express itself, it grows in its creative capacity to share its unique essence with others, and with the world.

Vervain *Verbena officinalis* (pink/mauve)   English Kit

Positive qualities: Ability to practice moderation, tolerance, and balance; "the middle way;" grounded idealism

Patterns of imbalance: Overbearing or intolerant behavior; overenthusiasm or extreme fanaticism; nervous exhaustion from overstriving

Cross-references: Animals and Animal Care   Balance   Body   Certainty   Enthusiasm   Exhaustion and Fatigue   Fanaticism   Grace   Groundedness   Idealism   Influence   Leadership   Moderation   Nervousness   Obsession   Perfectionism   Prejudice   Relaxation   Seriousness   Speaking   Stress   Tension   Tolerance   Will

Vervain soul types naturally possesses strong forces of passionate idealism. They give themselves fully and completely to the work or cause in which they believe. However, they can become so convinced of the rightness and urgency of their beliefs that their natural charismatic capacities degenerate into those of the zealot or fanatic. Their true leadership ability is afflicted, for the Vervain type's incredible intensity can overwhelm and prevent others from making their own energetic connection to the project or cause which is being promoted. Such an individual can be characterized as possessing not only great *intensity* but also great physical *tension*, which results in many nervous and digestive problems, and in extreme cases may lead to nervous breakdown. These persons are usually unaware of their true energy levels, and often push their bodies completely beyond their natural capacities. In fact, there is very little connection to the physical body or to the physical world, because this type lives so fervently in the world of ideas and ideals. Vervain is particularly an embodiment remedy, helping the soul to center and ground its tremendous enthusiasm. In this way, the body becomes a natural regulator and harmonizer for the abundant spiritual forces which pour out of such a person. When the fiery light of Vervain radiates through the medium of the body and the physical world, it becomes more luminous and contained. Such soul ardor is able to inspire, lead, and heal others.

Vine *Vitis vinifera* (green)

English Kit

Positive qualities: Selfless service, tolerance for the individuality of others
Patterns of imbalance: Domineering, tyrannical, forcing one's will on others

Cross-references: Abuse   Aggressiveness   Ambition   Animals and Animal Care
Authority   Children   Community Life and Group Experience   Earth Healing and
Nature Awareness   Egotism   Fanaticism   Father and Fathering   Greed   Influence
Leadership   Lower Self   Masculine Consciousness   Materialism and Money   Morality
Perfectionism   Power   Prejudice   Repression   Self-Aggrandizement   Service
Shadow Consciousness   Tolerance   Will   Work and Career Goals

The Vine personality possesses a strong will, with considerable power and force for leadership and organizational tasks. However, when these will forces are not aligned with the true Higher Self, they become *selfish* instead of *selfless*. The Vine soul type tends to impose its will on others, rather than leading them to their own power and self-awareness. The compulsive need to be in control creates a personality that is authoritative, domineering, tyrannical, and at its extreme, sadistic. The spiritual lesson for such an individual is contained in the words of Christ, "I am the Vine and ye are the branches." When the Vine soul type shifts identification from the lower willful self to the Higher Self, he or she learns that the essence of true leadership is not the ability to demand obedience from others, but rather inner obedience and devotion to a higher spiritual authority. The Vine essence helps such a soul to acquire true humility by realizing that spiritual service is the essence of authentic leadership. When such a soul shifts its archetypal consciousness from that of a king who rules to that of a shepherd who serves, the will forces become spiritualized and truly able to do good for others and for the Earth.

Violet *Viola odorata* (violet-blue) Professional Kit

Positive qualities: Delicate, highly perceptive sensitivity, elevated spiritual perspective; sharing with others while remaining true to oneself
Patterns of imbalance: Profound shyness, reserve, aloofness, fear of being submerged in groups

Cross-references: Alienation Aloofness Ambivalence Awkwardness Children Communication Community Life and Group Experience Escapism Fear Individuality Intimacy Involvement Loneliness Personal Relationships Receptivity Self-Effacement Self-Expression Sharing Shyness

The soul forces of the Violet type are highly refined, full of exquisite yet delicate sweetness. Such persons long to share themselves with others, but usually hold back due to a feeling of fragility in group situations, and fear that their sense of Self will be lost or submerged. Such a type often gravitates to a lifestyle or occupation where work is done silently and alone. The Violet personality inwardly feels a great deal of warmth, but he/she appears cool and aloof to others; even the body and especially the hands may be moist and cool. Although such persons may find a few others who are able to understand and accept their shyness, they suffer great feelings of loneliness, for they would like to share more of themselves than they actually do. The key to their unfoldment lies in being able to trust the warmth of others. Like the Violet flower, whose essential fragrance cannot be detected until the sun shines upon it and the air wafts it upward, so the Violet type must learn to let its essence flow into others. Violet flower essence helps such souls shift their awareness from fear of losing the Self, to trust that the Self will be warmed and revealed by others, so that their beautiful soul nature may be shared with the world.

Walnut *Juglans regia* (green) English Kit

Positive qualities: Freedom from limiting influences, making healthy transitions in life, courage to follow one's own path and destiny

Patterns of imbalance: Overly influenced by the beliefs and values of family or community, or by past experiences

Cross-references: Adolescence   Animals and Animal Care   Authority   Barriers Breakthrough   Co-Dependence   Concentration and Focus   Death and Dying   Desire Dutifulness   Eating Disorders   Escapism   Freedom   Habit Patterns   Healing Process Home and Lifestyle   Immune Disturbances   Influence   Life Direction   Manifestation Mid-Life Crisis   Pregnancy   Prejudice   Protection   Sensitivity   Strength   Transition True to Self

The human soul is akin to the plant in its patterns of growth. It grows slowly, almost imperceptibly from day to day, but there are moments when it makes radical, metamorphic changes, moving beyond its current form to something utterly new. Thus the plant transforms from root, to shoot, to leaf, to flower, to fruit, to seed. Walnut flower essence is an important remedy for times of great life transition; it assists the soul in making metamorphic change. It is indicated for those life passages when the Self must be completely and irrevocably transformed in order to continue its evolution. At these moments, the soul must be unwavering in its sense of inner purpose and conviction. If the mind experiences doubt or confusion, the progress of the Self is impeded, if not imperiled. Walnut is particularly helpful for those who may be easily influenced by family ties, community mores, social conventions, strong personalities, or past habits, and who are unable to muster the strength to make a break with the past and with the ideas of others. It is especially powerful in the mental field, helping to dispel any enchantment, illusion, or spell which may bind the soul to the past. This remedy can be broadly applied and is valuable for all life transitions including birth and death, moving, career changes, and ending or beginning relationships. Walnut helps the soul to perceive and follow its true Star of Destiny.

Water Violet *Hottonia palustris* (pale mauve, yellow center) English Kit

Positive qualities: Sharing one's gifts with others, appreciation of social relationships
Patterns of imbalance: Aloof, withdrawn, disdainful of social relationships

Cross-references: Alienation Aloofness Avoidance Barriers Communication Community Life and Group Experience Compassion Egotism Escapism Intimacy Involvement Perfectionism Personal Relationships Prejudice Pride Resistance Selfishness Service Sharing Shyness

The Water Violet personality is generally very quiet and self-contained, with soul qualities of gracefulness and equanimity. Their sedate, calm manner enables them to handle many different occupational and life situations in a very capable manner. However, it is difficult to know such persons well, or to feel a warm and personable connection with them. Such persons often appear distant or aloof; more extreme types seem proud, haughty, or arrogant. They may become involved in community affairs, but only in accordance with their professional standing. Many such souls have chosen to be born into families of wealth and social prominence, and they are well-cultured and educated. But even among Water Violet types without this obvious upper-class background, one feels a quality which sets such a person apart; the soul conducts itself with great dignity and refinement. It has no need to draw attention to itself, but neither does it seem to have much need to give of itself to others. Many such souls are in fact highly evolved, or they may be strongly influenced by the subconscious memory of a prominent past life. Such individuals are blocked in their further evolution until they realize that the Self can evolve only so far as a separate identity. The true spiritual Self must expand to include all of humanity. Water Violet helps such souls make a transition to a more inclusive state of consciousness, one that helps them experience a compassionate and joyful connection to the human family.

White Chestnut *Aesculus hippocastanum* (white with pink, red and yellow centers)   English Kit
also known as Horse Chestnut

Positive qualities: Inner quiet; calm, clear mind
Patterns of imbalance: Worrisome, repetitive thoughts, chattering mind

Cross-references: Aging Calm Children Clarity Concentration and Focus
Dreams and Sleep Exhaustion and Fatigue Inertia Insomnia Meditation Obsession
Quiet Relaxation Release Restlessness Speaking Thinking

White Chestnut flower essence is indicated for those who suffer from extreme mental agitation. Their thinking life is not free, but is highly compulsive and obsessive. The life energy is drained through excessive worry and anxiety, which is not directed outward toward others but is kept inside through a constant churning of the mind. Daily events, conversations, or other life episodes are continually replayed and analyzed, imprisoning the soul within the mental field. Such persons may suffer from insomnia, headaches, and other neurological disorders. They will often become addicted to sleeping pills, tranquilizers, aspirin, or other painkillers in an effort to subdue the mental pain and tension which they feel. White Chestnut helps such persons regain mental repose and inner peace. It redirects the extreme congestion of energy in the mental field, helping the individual to gain more awareness in the feeling life, especially in the solar plexus and in the heart. When these energy centers are re-balanced, the feelings are able to be processed before they become churning thoughts. White Chestnut frees the mental life for the calm, clear, and spacious activity of the Higher Mind.

Wild Oat *Bromus ramosus* (green)   English Kit

Positive qualities: Work as an expression of inner calling; outward life which expresses one's true goals and values; work experiences motivated by an inner sense of life purpose

Patterns of imbalance: Confusion and indecision about life direction; trying many activities but chronically dissatisfied, lack of commitment or focus

Cross-references: Adolescence   Certainty   Choice   Clarity   Concentration and Focus   Conflict   Decisiveness   Depression and Despair   Desire   Escapism   Freedom   Immobility   Indecision   Life Direction   Manifestation   Masculine Consciousness   Restlessness   Scatteredness   Seeking   Self-Actualization   Seriousness   Work and Career Goals

Soul health and happiness are very much dependent on the ability to realize one's true life purpose and vocation. If the soul does not have the opportunity to evolve and to serve through its basic life work, it will suffer great distress. By these standards, we can appreciate the depth of sickness in our modern, technological world. Many people are unknowingly enslaved to the forces of materialism, for their primary motivation to work is a monetary one (whether they make much or little money). This situation drastically drains the soul's true vitality; evenings, weekends, and holidays are spent simply recuperating or escaping from alienating or exploitative work situations. Dr. Bach recognized this fundamental soul ailment, and considered Wild Oat, along with Holly, to be one of the two basic remedies in his system. It is not improper to think of Wild Oat as relating to a particular type of person: one who is restless and seeking, who tries many jobs but is unable to commit to a true vocation. Indeed, many young people, or those experiencing mid-life crisis, have an acute need for this remedy. However, it is also important to regard Wild Oat as a broadly applicable polychrest, helping to transform the basic cultural illness of our age. Wild Oat helps the individual to recognize and respond to his/her true life calling, seeking forms of work that give the Self a sense of higher purpose and meaning, and the ability to truly serve and help others.

Wild Rose *Rosa canina* (pink or white) English Kit
also known as Dog Rose

Positive qualities: Will to live, joy in life
Patterns of imbalance: Resignation, lack of hope, giving up on life; lingering illness

Cross-references: Animals and Animal Care   Apathy   Challenge   Children
Depression and Despair   Exhaustion and Fatigue   Grief   Healing Process
Psychosomatic Illness   Surrender   Vitality   Will

The Wild Rose essence first developed by Dr. Bach addresses broad and important soul themes of motivation and interest in the world and in others. In this way, it is similar to the California Wild Rose. However, this English Rose specifically addresses the type of resignation in the soul which depletes one's vitality. Physical incarnation in a body is an experience fraught with difficulty and struggle, and for the Wild Rose personality the effort hardly seems worth making. Such apathy suppresses the soul's interest in life, and cuts off the individual from his or her inner sources of healing. This essence is very helpful for those who linger in long, drawn-out illness, and who seem to recover only fitfully and slowly. Wild Rose restores the vital forces of the soul, particularly its connection to the physical body and to the physical world, helping the individual regain an interest in earthly life. This essence teaches that life is a sacred and precious opportunity which the soul must make every effort to embrace, if it is to find the true meaning of love and physical incarnation.

Willow *Salix vitellina* (green) English Kit

Positive qualities: Acceptance, forgiveness, taking responsibility for one's life situation, flowing with life

Patterns of imbalance: Feeling resentful, inflexible or bitter; feeling that life is unfair or that one is a victim

Cross-references: Adolescence Aging Anger Blame Catharsis Co-Dependence Community Life and Group Experience Cynicism Death and Dying Denial Dislike Feminine Consciousness Flexibility Forgiveness Hate Inner Child Irritability Martyrdom Negativity Perfectionism Rejection Resentment Responsibility Tolerance

If the physical body does not keep flexible, it becomes stiff and contracted. The good health of the soul also depends on its ability to be yielding, flowing, and "for-giving." The Willow flower heals bitterness and resentment; it is for those who tend to "hold on" and become attached to negative emotions. Such persons often feel victimized by the circumstances of life — they feel that others are to blame for their misfortune; that life has been unfair to them; or they resent those who appear to have more status, prosperity, or felicity than themselves. The aging process is especially difficult for Willow types. At an energetic level, such persons are unable to flow with the streaming of their lives. Negative feelings are dammed up and then become magnified and internalized, congesting the inner being. The physical body also suffers from this stress, tending to manifest such problems as stiff joints, rheumatism, arthritis, and other aches and pains. *(It is interesting to note that Willow bark is the herbal precursor of aspirin, and is used particularly for such physical conditions.)* Willow restores a more "spring-like" disposition, helping the soul to respond with greater resilience and inward mobility to challenges and problems. In this way the Self takes more responsibility for its condition, and learns to flow more gently and graciously *with*, rather than *against*, the flow of life.

Yarrow *Achillea millefolium* (white) Professional Kit

Positive qualities: Inner radiance and strength of aura, compassionate awareness, inclusive sensitivity, beneficent healing forces

Patterns of imbalance: Extreme vulnerability to others and to the environment; easily depleted, overly absorbent of negative influences, psychic toxicity

Cross-references: Children City Life Devitalization Eating Disorders Emergency Energetic Patterns Environment Healers Immune Disturbances Irritability Learning Difficulties Lightness Massage Negativity Pregnancy Protection Sensitivity Spiritual Emergency or Opening Strength Stress Toner True to Self Vulnerability

As the soul becomes more spiritually open, it necessarily becomes more refined, sensitive, and absorbent. In the past, many of those on spiritual paths were removed and protected from the daily conditions of living, so that the soul could safely and harmoniously expand its boundaries. Modern conditions require that the path of spiritualization be connected to the physical world and to practical responsibilities. In this way, the light of the spirit is brought through the human soul right into the Earth as a healing force. Yarrow is a very important and highly beneficial remedy to harmonize this process. Those who typically need this remedy are easily affected by their surroundings, and can be prone to many forms of environmental illness, allergies, or psychosomatic diseases. Such persons have an extraordinary capacity for healing, counseling, or teaching, because they are readily able to receive psychic information and to understand the pain and suffering of others. At the same time they are easily depleted, and are quite vulnerable to the thoughts or negative intentions of others. Yarrow literally "knits together" the overly porous aura of such an individual so that it does not "bleed" so excessively into its environment. Furthermore, it helps such a person re-balance and stabilize the abundant light which radiates in the upper energy centers, directing it into the lower centers so that the Self has more vitality and solidity. Yarrow flower essence has nearly universal application, and should be considered in many formulas for the profound soul shifts of our age. Yarrow bestows a shining shield of Light which protects and unifies the essential Self, allowing compassionate healing qualities to flow freely from one's soul to others.

Yarrow Special Formula *Achillea millefolium* (white)
in a sea salt water base   Research essence

Positive qualities: Enhancing integrity of etheric body, of vital formative forces
Patterns of imbalance: Disturbance of life-force and vitality by noxious radiation, pollution, or other geopathic stress; residual effects of past exposure

Cross-references: City Life Devitalization Emergency Energetic Patterns Environment Immune Disturbances Negativity Pregnancy Protection Sensitivity Strength Stress Study Vulnerability

The very existence of our planet and the human species is threatened by the awesome and destructive force of nuclear weaponry and the extreme toxicity of nuclear waste. Nuclear energy is released through a process which directly attacks the "formative," or etheric qualities of matter, so that matter itself is literally "dis-integrated." This is distinguished from natural chemical processes, which transform matter but retain the essential quality of each element (e.g., forms of oxidation such as burning, rusting, or digestion). Nuclear reactions destroy the very integrity of the chemical elements involved, producing highly poisonous waste products which continue to disintegrate and destroy life. In essence, nuclear radiation is a death-oriented expression of light and fire, which assaults the very core of matter and the natural basis of life.

Yarrow Special Formula is indicated for exposure to nuclear radiation and other forms of noxious environmental or geopathic stress. It was originally developed in response to practitioner requests after the Chernobyl nuclear plant disaster in 1986. This remedy combines the remarkable light and fire processes of the Yarrow plant with the strong formative forces of potentized sea salt. By strengthening the etheric body with strong formative forces which can meet the harmful attack of radiation, Yarrow Special Formula directly counteracts the destructive effects of radiation on the human energy field. This remedy is indicated not only for obvious exposure to nuclear fallout, but also for the many ways in which nuclear radiation and other forms of aberrant and highly toxic energy infiltrate the modern world. Examples include video-display terminals, X-rays, radiation therapy, high-altitude radiation, detection devices at airport terminals, and invasive electromagnetic fields. Yarrow Special Formula is an immensely important remedy; it stands as a counter-shield to the destructive forces which threaten and plague human and planetary life, imparting powerful vitalizing and restorative properties.

Yellow Star Tulip *Calochortus monophyllus* (yellow)   Research Kit

Positive qualities: Empathy, receptivity to the feelings and experiences of others; acting from inner truth and guidance

Patterns of imbalance: Insensitivity to the sufferings of others; lack of awareness of the consequences of one's actions on others

Cross-references: Community Life and Group Experience Compassion Creativity Dullness Earth Healing and Nature Awareness Environment Feminine Consciousness Healers Insight Intimacy Listening Love Materialism and Money Morality Mother and Mothering Personal Relationships Pregnancy Receptivity Selfishness Sensitivity Service Softness Soulfulness Warmth

Yellow Star Tulip refines the soul life by developing one's capacity for receptive and insightful social presence. It does not work inwardly on the Self as much as it helps the soul direct all that has been developed within the inner life to go *outward* as a gift for helping and healing others, or working with the forces of Nature. Yellow Star Tulip develops the soul quality of *empathy*, so that one can intuit and act upon the deeper meaning and message of other beings. This remedy especially sensitizes one to the suffering of others, for without empathetic presence one cannot become truly compassionate. It can sometimes act as a "karmic truth serum," so that one feels more intensely the results of one's actions toward another. Yellow Star Tulip breaks down the dysfunctional and egotistical barriers of the Self, enabling one to make sensitive contact with others and truly learn from them. This remedy is particularly important for those involved in the healing and teaching professions, who need to expand and refine their empathetic qualities. Yellow Star Tulip can also be used more broadly for relationship healing, and for helping those who display more extreme soul states such as sociopathic tendencies. The essence of this delicately beautiful flower helps refine the sensitivity and awareness of the Self so that it becomes more actively responsible and truly compassionate and caring.

Yerba Santa *Eriodictyon californicum* (violet)

Professional Kit
Seven Herbs Kit

Positive qualities: Free-flowing emotion, ability to harmonize breathing with feeling; capacity to express a full range of human emotion, especially pain and sadness

Patterns of imbalance: Constricted feelings, particularly in the chest; internalized grief and melancholy, deeply repressed emotions

Cross-references: Awareness Body Brokenheartedness Children Cleansing Depression and Despair Exhaustion and Fatigue Grief Healing Process Heart Inner Child Massage Psychosomatic Illness Release Repression Soulfulness Strength Tension Toner

Yerba Santa (Spanish for "Holy Herb") addresses the inner sanctity of the human soul. There is within every human heart an inviolable space which must be kept open and free; the Self breathes its soul essence in and out from this center. This part of the human being is the most sensitive, the most deeply feeling, and the most psychic. It is especially vulnerable to emotions of sadness, grief, or other related soul pain. If such emotions are not actively addressed by the consciousness, they will be stored and buried away in this part of the heart. The individual becomes profoundly melancholic, bearing deep internalized sadness, which is not simply related to daily events, but which pervades and colors the entire emotional life. This soul illness grips the body. Most characteristically, the sacred part of the Self — the heart and chest area — becomes hollowed rather than hallowed. The breathing is congested and disturbed, resulting in the tendency toward degenerative diseases of the lungs such as chest congestion, pneumonia, asthma, tuberculosis, or addiction to tobacco. Such a person appears to be wasting away; quite literally the soul is being consumed by the intense forces of grief and sadness which work negatively *into* the Self. Yerba Santa reverses this soul consumption, promoting the release of trauma and emotional impurities. Often, the individual contacts profound unclaimed grief, such as the loss of a beloved friend or parent early in life. Yerba Santa gradually restores the temple space of the heart, making it more spacious and light-filled. Through this blessed flower, the soul re-establishes its sanctuary, freeing the human heart to experience the world with renewed emotional presence.

Zinnia *Zinnia elegans* (red)   Professional Kit

Positive qualities: Childlike humor and playfulness; experiencing the joyful inner child, lightheartedness, detached perspective on Self

Patterns of imbalance: Overseriousness, dullness, heaviness, lack of humor; overly somber sense of Self, repressed inner child

Cross-references: Cheerfulness Creativity Devitalization Dryness Dullness Dutifulness Earth Healing and Nature Awareness Enthusiasm Father and Fathering Healers Home and Lifestyle Inner Child Intellectualism Joy Lightness Masculine Consciousness Materialism and Money Menopause Mother and Mothering Seriousness Spontaneity Study Time Relationship Work and Career Goals

Humor is uniquely human. Other forms of life certainly experience joy and delight, but humor requires the ability to step outside oneself, and not take oneself so seriously. It is the human being, with its pronounced sense of Self, who has developed and very much needs the soul quality of humor. The capacity to laugh at one's self, or to be "light-hearted," is quite literally a necessary balance to the somber heaviness of self-consciousness. Zinnia is a most wonderful remedy for this state of soul, helping the Self to contact its inner child. Every child is born with the innate capacity to laugh and play, to enter into life with the full exuberance of the winged soul. The adult ego all too often stifles and suppresses this part of the Self. This remedy is clearly indicated for those who are overly grave and earnest, who take themselves and life too seriously, or who tend toward workaholism or other forms of unbalanced intensity. The message of the Zinnia is not that one's life should be frivolous or irresponsible, but rather that qualities of playfulness and laughter can be brought to one's work and daily responsibilities. Zinnia flower essence brings the soul quality of humor to one's humanness, teaching that the soul who is in "good spirits" is truly on a balanced spiritual path.

Contents of Flower Essence Kits

Professional Kit

Aloe Vera *Aloe vera*
Arnica *Arnica mollis*
Basil *Ocimum basilicum*
Black-Eyed Susan *Rudbeckia hirta*
Blackberry *Rubus ursinus*
Bleeding Heart *Dicentra formosa*
Borage *Borago officinalis*
Buttercup *Ranunculus occidentalis*
Calendula *Calendula officinalis*
California Pitcher Plant
  Darlingtonia californica
California Poppy
  Eschscholzia californica
California Wild Rose *Rosa californica*
Cayenne *Capsicum annuum*
Chamomile *Matricaria chamomilla*
  or *Anthemis cotula*
Chaparral *Larrea tridentata*
Corn *Zea mays*
Dandelion *Taraxacum officinale*
Deerbrush *Ceanothus integerrimus*
Dill *Anethum graveolens*
Dogwood *Cornus nuttallii*
Filaree *Erodium cicutarium*
Fuchsia *Fuchsia hybrida*
Garlic *Allium sativum*
Golden Ear Drops
  Dicentra chrysantha
Goldenrod *Solidago californica*
Hound's Tongue *Cynoglossum grande*
Indian Paintbrush *Castilleja miniata*
Indian Pink *Silene californica*
Iris *Iris douglasiana*
Larkspur *Delphinium nuttallianum*
Lavender *Lavandula officinalis*
Lotus *Nelumbo nucifera*
Madia *Madia elegans*
Mallow *Sidalcea glaucens*
Manzanita *Arctostaphylos viscida*
Mariposa Lily *Calochortus leichtlinii*
Morning Glory *Ipomoea purpurea*

Mountain Pennyroyal
  Monardella odoratissima
Mountain Pride *Penstemon newberryi*
Mugwort *Artemisia douglasiana*
Mullein *Verbascum thapsus*
Nasturtium *Tropaeolum majus*
Oregon Grape *Berberis aquifolium*
Penstemon *Penstemon davidsonii*
Peppermint *Mentha piperita*
Pink Yarrow
  Achillea millefolium var. *rubra*
Pomegranate *Punica granatum*
Quaking Grass *Briza maxima*
Quince *Chaenomeles speciosa*
Rabbitbrush
  Chrysothamnus nauseosus
Red Clover *Trifolium pratense*
Sagebrush *Artemisia tridentata*
Saguaro *Cereus giganteus*
Saint John's Wort
  Hypericum perforatum
Scarlet Monkeyflower
  Mimulus cardinalis
Scotch Broom *Cytisus scoparius*
Self-Heal *Prunella vulgaris*
Shasta Daisy
  Chrysanthemum maximum
Shooting Star
  Dodecatheon hendersonii
Star Thistle *Centaurea solstitialis*
Star Tulip *Calochortus tolmiei*
Sticky Monkeyflower
  Mimulus aurantiacus
Sunflower *Helianthus annuus*
Sweet Pea *Lathyrus latifolus*
Tansy *Tanacetum vulgare*
Tiger Lily *Lilium humboldtii*
Trillium *Trillium chloropetalum*
Trumpet Vine *Campsis tagliabuana*
Violet *Viola odorata*
Yarrow *Achillea millefolium*
Yerba Santa *Eriodictyon californicum*
Zinnia *Zinnia elegans*

Research Kit

Alpine Lily *Lilium parvum*
Angel's Trumpet *Datura candida*
Angelica *Angelica archangelica*
Baby Blue Eyes *Nemophila menziesii*
Calla Lily *Zantedeschia aethiopica*
Canyon Dudleya *Dudleya cymosa*
Chrysanthemum
    Chrysanthemum morifolium
Cosmos *Cosmos bipinnatus*
Echinacea *Echinacea purpurea*
Evening Primrose *Onenothera hookeri*
Fairy Lantern *Calochortus albus*
Fawn Lily *Erythronium purpurascens*
Forget-Me-Not *Myosotis sylvatica*
Golden Yarrow *Achillea filipendulina*
Hibiscus *Hibiscus rosa-sinensis*
Milkweed *Asclepias cordifolia*
Pink Monkeyflower *Mimulus lewisii*
Poison Oak *Rhus diversiloba*
Pretty Face *Triteleia ixioides*
Queen Anne's Lace *Daucus carota*
Rosemary *Rosmarinus officinalis*
Sage *Salvia officinalis*
Snapdragon *Antirrhinum majus*
Yellow Star Tulip
    Calochortus monophyllus

Seven Herbs Kit

Black Cohosh *Cimicifuga racemosa*
Easter Lily *Lilium longiflorum*
Iris (Blue Flag) *Iris versicolor*
Lady's Slipper (Yellow)
    Cypripedium parviflorum
    or **Showy Lady's Slipper**
    Cypripedium reginae
Sagebrush *Artemisia tridentata*
Star Tulip (Cat's Ears)
    Calochortus tolmiei
Yerba Santa *Eriodictyon californicum*

Other research essences

Love-Lies-Bleeding (Amaranthus)
    Amaranthus caudatus
Nicotiana (Flowering Tobacco)
    Nicotiana alata
Purple Monkeyflower *Mimulus kelloggii*
Yarrow Special Formula
    Achillea millefolium in sea salt

English Kit

Agrimony *Agrimonia eupatoria*
Aspen *Populus tremula*
Beech *Fagus sylvatica*
Centaury
    Centaurium erythaea / umbellatum
Cerato *Ceratostigma willmottiana*
Cherry Plum *Prunus cerasifera*
Chestnut Bud
    Aesculus hippocastanum
Chicory *Cichorium intybus*
Clematis *Clematis vitalba*
Crab Apple *Malus sylvestris*
Elm *Ulmus procera*
Gentian *Gentiana amarella*
Gorse *Ulex europaeus*
Heather *Calluna vulgaris*
Holly *Ilex aquifolium*
Honeysuckle *Lonicera caprifolium*
Hornbeam *Carpinus betulus*
Impatiens *Impatiens gladulifera*
Larch *Larix decidua*
Mimulus *Mimulus guttatus*
Mustard *Sinapis arvensis*
Oak *Quercus robur*
Olive *Olea europaea*
Pine *Pinus sylvestris*
Red Chestnut *Aesculus carnea*
Rock Rose
    Helianthemum nummularium
Rock Water *solarized spring water*
Scleranthus *Scleranthus annuus*
Star of Bethlehem
    Ornithogalum umbellatum
Sweet Chestnut *Castanea sativa*
Vervain *Verbena officinalis*
Vine *Vitis vinifera*
Walnut *Juglans regia*
Water Violet *Hottonia palustris*
White Chestnut
    Aesculus hippocastanum
Wild Oat *Bromus ramosus*
Wild Rose *Rosa canina*
Willow *Salix vitellina*
Five-Flower Formula *combination of*
    Cherry Plum, Clematis, Impatiens,
    Rock Rose, Star of Bethlehem